Patient Management Problems in Psychiatry

This book is dedicated to God Almighty, who made it possible for us to complete this work, and to our wives, Olukemi and Funmi, and our children, Omowonuola, Oluwatomisin, Olaotan and Semiloore, for their support and perseverance during the writing of this book.

Commissioning Editor: Michael Parkinson
Project Development Manager: Siân Jarman/Ailsa Laing
Project Manager: Frances Affleck
Designer: Erik Bigland

Patient Management Problems in Psychiatry

Olumuyiwa John Olumoroti
MBBS MSc MRCPsych

Specialist Registrar, Springfield University Hospital, London

Akim Abimbola Kassim
MBChB MRCPsych

Specialist Registrar in Old Age Psychiatry
South London & Maudsley NHS Trust,
Guy's Hospital, London

FOREWORD BY
Jim Bolton MRCPsych
Consultant Psychiatrist, St. Helier Hospital, Surrey,
Honorary Senior Lecturer,
St. George's Hospital Medical School, London

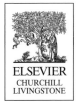

ELSEVIER
CHURCHILL
LIVINGSTONE

EDINBURGH LONDON NEW YORK OXFORD PHILADELPHIA
ST LOUIS SYDNEY TORONTO 2005

ELSEVIER
CHURCHILL
LIVINGSTONE

First published 2005

ISBN 0 443 10161 2

British Library Cataloguing in Publication Data
A catalogue record for this book is available from the British Library

Library of Congress Cataloging in Publication Data
A catalog record for this book is available from the Library of Congress

Note
Medical knowledge is constantly changing. Standard safety precautions
must be followed, but as new research and clinical experience broaden
our knowledge, changes in treatment and drug therapy may become
necessary or appropriate. Readers are advised to check the most current
product information provided by the manufacturer of each drug to be
administered to verify the recommended dose, the method and duration
of administration, and contraindications. It is the responsibility of the
practitioner, relying on experience and knowledge of the patient, to
determine dosages and the best treatment for each individual patient.
Neither the Publisher nor the authors assumes any liability for any injury
and/or damage to persons or property arising from this publication.

The Publisher

your source for books,
journals and multimedia
in the health sciences
www.elsevierhealth.com

The
Publisher's
policy is to use
paper manufactured
from sustainable forests

Printed in China

Foreword

In psychiatric practice, each patient we meet poses a different problem. The PMP examination tests a candidate's ability to approach a new clinical scenario in a structured way. This is something we do every working day. So why is the exam so anxiety-provoking?

None of us likes being put on the spot, especially when we feel that our ignorance might be exposed to our senior colleagues. For this reason viva voce examinations are particularly stressful. Candidates preparing for a PMP examination in psychiatry will be aware of the principles of behaviour therapy (if not, make sure that this is part of your revision) and will know that graduated exposure and habituation are important in overcoming fear. PMP questions are usually predictable because they are related to real clinical psychiatric practice. Sometimes candidates find it difficult to answer these questions because they think examiners are expecting something different from what they are used to. In reality, examiners are only expecting candidates to say what they would do in real life. Examiners are therefore quick to recognize candidates who are not approaching the task at hand from a real-life perspective.

This 'On the Spot' book is an excellent 'graduated exposure programme' to help candidates overcome exam nerves, particularly those preparing for the MRCPsych Part II examination and other postgraduate professional examinations such as the Irish and the South African Diplomas in Psychological Medicine (DPM), and the fellowship examination of the Australian and New Zealand Colleges of Psychiatrists (FRANZCP). The authors' suggestions for peer-group practice and detailed model answers also provide a unique revision aid, which will be welcomed by many anxious candidates.

In the ideal exam, candidates should be able to enter into a discussion with the examiners in much the same way that they discuss patients with colleagues at work. At the same time, candidates should demonstrate sufficient knowledge and clinical skill to pass the hurdle of the examination and reach the next stage in their training. Anything that helps to reduce anxiety and increase knowledge and skill should be mandatory for all those preparing for the exam. I certainly would have found this book helpful in overcoming my exam nerves!

Dr Jim Bolton
London, 2005

Acknowledgements

The authors gratefully acknowledge the assistance and advice received from the following colleagues and trainers who took time out of their busy schedules to comment on the earlier draft of this book. Our appreciation goes to Drs Jim Bolton, Joan Brunton, Wolfram Englehardt, Roger Farmer, Daniel Fekadu, Simon Fleminger, Nick Goddard, Quazi Haque, Chris Kenn, Tennyson Lee, Nicola Omu, Peter Pierzchniak, Gopinath Ranjith, Deji Sorinmade and Kim Stevens. We also thank several colleagues who supplied questions and volunteered to assist while testing the usefulness and suitability of many of the vignettes.

Our immense gratitude goes to Maggie Philpot, Deborah Yohanna-Washington and Chris Ford, who gave secretarial assistance, and Joanna Grant, who assisted with proofreading. This book would not have been completed on time, if not for the skill and dedication of the staff at Elsevier. We thank you all.

Contents

Abbreviations

ACTeRS	Abbreviated Connor's Teacher Rating Scale
ADH	Antidiuretic hormone
ADHD	Attention deficit hyperactivity disorder
ADIS	Autism Diagnostic Interview Schedule
ADL	Activities of daily living
ADOS	Autism Diagnostic Observation Schedule
AIDS	Acquired immunodeficiency syndrome
ASW	Approved social worker
BADS	Behavioural Assessment for Dysexecutive Syndrome
BDI	Beck's Depression Inventory
BMI	Body mass index
BNF	British National Formulary
BP	Blood pressure
BPRS	Brief Psychiatric Rating Scale
CAPE	Clifton Assessment Procedure for the Elderly
CAT	Cognitive analytical therapy
CBT	Cognitive behavioural therapy
CFS	Chronic fatigue syndrome
CJD	Creutzfeldt–Jakob disease
CMV	Cytomegalovirus
CPA	Care Programme Approach (in England and Wales)
CK	Creatine kinase
CPMS	Clozaril Patient Monitoring Service
CPN	Community psychiatric nurse
CPT	Continuous Performance Test
CSF	Cerebrospinal fluid
CSM	Committee on Safety of Medicines
CST	Card Sorting Test
CT	Computed tomography
CTO	Community Treatment Order
CTRS	Connor's Teacher Rating Scale
DBT	Dialectical behavioural therapy
DKA	Diabetic ketoacidosis
DMR	Dementia Scale for Mentally Retarded Persons

DSH	Deliberate self-harm
DSM–IV	Diagnostic and Statistical Manual of Mental Disorders (4th edition)
EBV	Epstein–Barr virus
ECG	Electrocardiograph(y)
ECT	Electroconvulsive therapy
EDNOS	Eating disorder not otherwise specified
EEG	Electroencephalography
EMI	Elderly mentally infirm
EPDS	Edinburgh Postnatal Depression Scale
EPSE	Extrapyramidal side-effects
ERP	Exposure and response prevention
ESR	Erythrocyte sedimentation rate
FBC	Full blood count
FME	Forensic medical examiner
FSH	Follicle-stimulating hormone
GCS	Glasgow Coma Scale
GHQ	General Health Questionnaire
GMC	General Medical Council
GMP	Guanosine monophosphate
GnRH	Gonadotrophin-releasing hormone
GP	General practitioner
HADS	Hospital Anxiety and Depression Scale
HAMD	Hamilton Rating Scale for Depression
HAS	Hamilton Anxiety Scale
HCR–20	Historical/Clinical/Risk Management 20-item Scale: violence risk assessment scheme
HDN	Haemorrhagic disease of the newborn
HIV	Human immunodeficiency virus
HRS	Hamilton Rating Scale
IADL	Instrumental Activity of Daily Living
ICD–10	International Classification of Diseases (10th edition)
ICP	Intracranial pressure
ICU	Intensive care unit
IMR	Inmate medical record
IPA	Individual patient assessment
IPT	Interpersonal therapy
IQ	Intelligence quotient
LFTs	Liver function tests
LH	Luteinizing hormone
MADRS	Montgomery–Asberg Depression Rating Scale
MAPP	Multi-Agency Public Protection team
MCI	Mild cognitive impairment

MCV	Mean corpuscular volume
MMSE	Mini Mental State Examination
MRI	Magnetic resonance image/imaging
MS	Multiple sclerosis
MSU	Medium secure unit
NART	National Adult Reading Test
NATs	Negative automatic thoughts
NICE	National Institute of Clinical Excellence
NMS	Neuroleptic malignant syndrome
NPH	Normal pressure hydrocephalus
NRT	Nicotine replacement therapy
NSAIDs	Non-steroidal anti-inflammatory drugs
NSF	National Service Framework for Older Adults
NTD	Neural tube defect
OCD	Obsessive-compulsive disorder
PALS	Patient Advisory Liaison Services
PCL-R	Hare's Psychopathic Checklist – Revised
PD	Panic disorder
PDD	Pervasive developmental disorders
PICU	Psychiatric intensive care unit
PMP	Patient management problems
prn	'as required' basis
PTA	Post-traumatic amnesia
PTSD	Post-traumatic stress disorder
RFTs	Renal function tests
RSU	Regional secure unit
SANS	Schedule of Affective and Negative Syndrome
SAPS	Schedule of Affective and Positive Syndrome
SDAT	Senile dementia of Alzheimer's type
SDQ	Strength and Difficulty Questionnaire
SIADH	Syndrome of inappropriate antidiuretic hormone secretion
SOTP	Sex Offenders Treatment Programme
SSRI	Selective serotonin re-uptake inhibitor
STD	Sexually transmitted disease
STR	Structured rehabilitation programme
TCA	Tricyclic antidepressant
TENS	Transcutaneous electric nerve stimulation
TFTs	Thyroid function tests
TIA	Transient ischaemic attack
TPHA	*Treponema pallidum* haemagglutination assay
TRS	Treatment-resistant schizophrenia
U and Es	Urea and electrolytes
UTI	Urinary tract infection

VDRL	Venereal Diseases Research Laboratory
WAIS–R	Wechsler Adult Intelligence Scale – Revised
WISC–R	Wechsler Intelligence Scale for Children – Revised
Y–BOCS	Yale–Brown Obsessive-Compulsive Scale

1

Introduction

The membership examinations of the major professional psychiatric bodies, such as the Royal Colleges of Psychiatrists of the United Kingdom (MRCPsych), the Australian and New Zealand Colleges of Psychiatrists (FRANZCP) and the Diplomas in Psychological Medicine (DPM) of other reputable colleges, have undergone considerable changes in the last decade. This has happened as the various professional and examination bodies look for better ways to improve the reliability and validity of their assessment procedures to make them reflect the acquisition of the expertise and knowledge required by trainees.

Changes to the patient management problems (PMPs) component of the Part II MRCPsych examinations became effective from Spring 2003. Examiners no longer supply their own scenarios, but use materials from a bank of structured vignettes established to assess candidates' core knowledge. The new structured PMP section continues to be 30 minutes in duration, and each candidate is given three vignettes to be discussed for 10 minutes each. In addition to the vignettes being read aloud, candidates are given written copies. For each of the vignettes, examiners have three probes, which may be used to promote further discussion. There are also five areas for discussion, which are relevant to the vignette but not necessarily all-inclusive. In essence, this means that examiners are looking for particular areas for discussion, sometimes using the probes available to them. The popular notion among candidates that there is no wrong or right answer for PMPs is no longer true. It is our opinion, however, that candidates are expected to give their answers and discuss them confidently within an acceptable and reasonable framework.

One effect of continual changes in examination format and procedures is that several revision aids and textbooks meant for examination preparation have become almost irrelevant. Increasing demands on consultants' and other seniors' time have also meant that trainees receive less supervision for examination purposes. The 'On the Spot' series is written with these realities in mind. The aim of this book is to help candidates who are preparing either alone or in groups to adopt a structured way of thinking and reasoning about a clinical scenario in order to arrive at a logical formulation and approach to management. This should not be far from what is achievable in day-to-day clinical practice.

HOW TO USE 'ON THE SPOT' PATIENT MANAGEMENT PROBLEMS

The layout of the book is such that it can be used among trainees who are preparing for the same examination. It is advised that pairs or small groups of candidates (maximum five) invite a senior with experience in examination preparation to put them 'on the spot' by using several different parts of the book. Candidates can also put each other on the spot, in an atmosphere similar to that of a real examination. We suggest that the questions be read out clearly by a member of the group to a trainee who must give a response within a period of not more than 8 minutes. The 2 remaining minutes should be used to probe the trainee further on relevant issues. As several of the questions and vignettes used in this book have been derived from a bank of material posed to candidates in previous years, it is likely that candidates may receive similar questions in their actual examination.

The format of this book, however, will not necessarily be suitable for every question. Candidates should be able to demonstrate flexibility and a strategy that shows good reasoning and thinking without deviating from the central theme of the question or vignette at hand. The layout of the book will also be useful in helping learners formulate management and treatment plans for specific scenarios met during the clinical and individual patient assessments (IPA) component of the different professional examinations.

This series of books is not in any way meant to replace the rigorous and structured academic and continuous professional development programmes to which all trainees should have access. They should be used to complement essential reading for the examinations, familiarization with the literature and current local practices, and supervision from trainers.

THE MAKING OF 'ON THE SPOT' PATIENT MANAGEMENT PROBLEMS

In an attempt to make the vignettes presented in this book similar to those used in actual examinations, candidates who have sat the examinations in the past (with variable outcomes) volunteered to discuss the questions they were asked by examiners. Some of these questions, which came up over a period of 3 years, formed a bank from which the scenarios in this book were derived. A selection of vignettes with similar themes was drawn up by the authors, who appointed a panel of four senior and eminent consultant psychiatrists with considerable experience in postgraduate psychiatry examinations to give advice about the vignettes' suitability. The four panellists have participated actively in the current changes to the Part II MRCPsych examinations, and were selected based on their extensive experience in general adult psychiatry and psychiatric subspecialties.

IMPORTANT NOTE

The authors are practising psychiatrists with considerable experience in general medicine, both in the UK and abroad. We have drawn on our clinical experience in posing and dealing with vignettes, which are meant to test the clinical management ability and styles of candidates in dealing with day-to-day encounters with psychiatric patients. We have not made reference to any real person, particularly our patients in the past or present.

Candidates are also reminded that local practices vary considerably, and references to the law, child protection procedures and legal rights mostly apply to the UK, where we currently practise. Answers to vignettes where the law and human rights are involved should be read in the knowledge that the authors and their advisers do not claim to be legally qualified. Appropriate expert clinical and legal advice should therefore be sought when difficult and complex situations arise.

HOW TO DO WELL IN PATIENT MANAGEMENT PROBLEMS EXAMINATIONS

A management problem usually begins with a discussion or meeting with a patient for interview or assessment. It has always been our advice that candidates should usually do no more in the examination than they would in a real-life situation. Most candidates sitting the Part II MRCPsych examination and the final part of other postgraduate professional examinations in psychiatry will have worked in general psychiatry and its subspecialties for anything up to 30 months. We always advise candidates to relax in the knowledge that they will have come across similar cases before. This is a psychological 'gimmick' and a well-tested anxiety management technique that works. It will also be reassuring to know that most candidates pass the oral examination and PMP. Candidates are advised to do what they would do in everyday practice, in a structured way that shows the examiner they have good judgment and the ability to put their answers into the perspective of what is being asked in individual test cases or vignettes. Throughout the book our approach is presented in a seven-stage format that encourages candidates to approach any viva voce, oral examination or patient management problem in a systematic manner to arrive at a solution. This solution should strike a reasonable balance between candidates' theoretical knowledge and the issues to be addressed in a particular setting. The seven-stage format (TICS-DAT) is described below.

1. TASK

Candidates should ask themselves 'What is the main task that I have been asked to carry out in this vignette?'. Such tasks, as in most PMPs, will include assessment and management; therefore assessment and management of the patient is the main task the candidate should perform. It is a common fault reported by examiners that candidates drift away from the case and proceed to answer questions from their textbooks or their well-rehearsed template. The new PMP format of the MRCPsych is such that candidates are given the vignettes on a card or paper; the vignettes are also read to the candidates. It is important to note that examiners no longer bring in their own questions and so there is little or no opportunity to clarify with the examiner what the vignette is all about.

2. ISSUES

Candidates are encouraged to raise, from the outset, the issues that they think are involved in a particular question, and then to give a more comprehensive assessment, with a view to expanding on the various points they need to cover. Some would argue that this is not compulsory and we quite agree. Apart from settling the candidates into the task and helping them to focus, listing issues gives the examiner the impression that the candidate has a good grasp of the question. We have heard candidates say things like 'I think there are three main issues in this question'. Unless they have been asked specifically how many issues are involved, we would encourage candidates to avoid this and say instead 'I think these are the issues' or 'These are the issues I want to focus on in answering this vignette'.

3. CLARIFY

Often in clinical practice, when we receive a referral or need to see a patient, we seek to clarify the patient's situation and also to make sure there are no urgent issues to be attended to. This will include ascertaining whether a patient is alone, has access to weapons, or needs immediate medical or surgical intervention. As far as possible, we have encouraged this approach in the full answers to vignettes detailed in this book.

4. SEEK MORE INFORMATION

In attending to most vignettes, a candidate would need to seek more information from a variety of sources, such as the patient, relatives, GP, current and old clinical notes, custodial records or inmate medical record, nurses' entry, and neuropsychological and other special assessments. Almost always you will need to carry out further investigations, and these should be organized into physical, psychological and social before you focus on the important ones for a particular scenario. Candidates should attempt to learn and master a few psychological investigations such as the Brief Psychiatric Rating Scale (BPRS), Hospital Anxiety Scale (HAS), Beck's Depression Inventory (BDI) and National Adult Reading Test (NART), and should understand the relevance of the components of the different Intelligent Quotient (IQ) tests. Candidates should say why they are asking for a particular investigation and what they expect to establish from it. This will prevent examiners from interjecting or taking control of the task meant for you. Some vignettes will state that several investigations have already been carried out and there is no point going over these again. You will only irritate the examiner.

5. DIFFERENTIAL DIAGNOSIS/DIFFICULTIES

What exactly is wrong with the patient and what may be contributing to the scenario at hand? Sometimes, direct questions are asked about differential diagnosis and it is important to answer these first before moving on to other parts of the answer, irrespective of the structure you may have had in mind. It might be useful to organize your thoughts into whether differential diagnoses are organic or functional, mentioning things that are common before detailing other less likely possibilities.

6. APPROACH TO MANAGEMENT

What would be the candidate's approach to the management of the patient or scenario? Is this patient going to be seen alone or in the company of other colleagues? Are you going to involve other specialists, and what would be their role? Is the care going to be shared with others, or are you only going to take an advisory role? Don't just use the term 'multidisciplinary' loosely, but say what each member of the team would contribute to assessment and treatment.

7. TREATMENT/ADVICE

It is always a good plan to organize treatment into medical or biological, psychological and social in order to achieve a reasonable balance between ideal and realistic management and to focus on the practical. In describing management, candidates should be as specific as they would be in a real-life situation. If they are suggesting prescription of any medication or another modality of treatment, they should say exactly what they mean and why they have chosen that particular option.

GENERAL NOTES

We have consistently found that candidates perform better when they are adequately prepared and systematic in their approach. Most examiners want to see that the candidate has structured the answer in a logical and practical way. Candidates should avoid the temptation to jump to conclusions because they have practised and rehearsed a particular vignette similar to the one presented in an actual examination.

On a general note, we have consistently found that little things usually determine a candidate's performance and these should not be taken for granted. It is important to show that you know what you are talking about and to avoid unnecessary repetition or waffle. Examiners can usually see through this. Do not speak too fast or too quietly or mumble under your breath in the hope that you can muddle through like this. You will not get far.

Attempt to look at the whole picture within a particular scenario and be safe in your approach. Using buzz words is acceptable, but only when they are appropriate. By and large, your answers should bring together aspects of your history, further information, relevant investigations, management approaches and treatment options. Practise as much as possible, fine-tune your structure and make sure you cover most of the topics that may come up. Plan to devote at least one-third of the allocated time to management. It is important not to use up all your time seeking more information. If you think you have finished your answer, close your case gracefully and avoid waffling or marking the time, particularly if you really have nothing more to say.

It is our hope that the suggestions on the following pages will help candidates preparing for this section of the different examinations towards a successful outcome.

2

Psychiatric emergencies

A 24-year-old woman with no previous psychiatric history was seen at the local accident and emergency department after taking an overdose of 20 tablets of paracetamol. This followed a row with her 23-year-old boyfriend. She is now medically fit and the physicians want you to see her before she is discharged.
What would you do?

SUGGESTED PROBES

1. Are there factors, symptoms or signs that would increase her risks?
2. Would you admit her to a psychiatric ward?
3. She is asking to be discharged, but is ambivalent about her future and would not rule out a further suicide attempt. She has the capacity to make decisions about her own care. What would you do?

PMP PLAN

TASKS TO DO

The following five areas are relevant to this vignette but are not necessarily all-inclusive. The list is also not exhaustive:

a) Assess the risk of further self-harm, suicide and domestic violence as separate categories.
b) Assess the psychosocial background, stressors and coping resources.
c) Highlight the risk of physical complications if the overdosing continues.
d) Identify psychiatric disorder, including depression, substance misuse and personality disorder.
e) Demonstrate a multidisciplinary approach to problems, including contingency planning.

ISSUES

- Assessment of the degree of risk that this woman poses
- Suggestion of treatment and follow-up plan to forestall future occurrence of self-harm behaviour.

CLARIFY

- What is the reason for self-harm and what is the risk of suicide?

SEEK MORE INFORMATION

PATIENT

- Circumstances surrounding the overdose
- Intention at the time of overdose and at present
- Full history, history of mental illness or deliberate self-harm
- Risk of suicide and domestic violence.

RELATIVES OR PARTNER

- Elicit corroborative information.

MEDICAL RECORDS/NURSE OR UNIT COORDINATORS

- Rule out previous contact with psychiatric services.

DIFFERENTIAL DIAGNOSIS/DIFFICULTIES

- *Emotional or psychiatric disorder.* Acute stress reaction, adjustment disorder (including brief depressive reaction), mild depressive episode, recurrent depressive disorder, borderline personality disorder (emotionally unstable type), substance misuse or abuse disorder, crisis resolution
- *No mental illness.*

APPROACH TO TREATMENT

- Be empathic but firm.
- Make decisions, bearing in mind risk and safety issues.
- Assess suicidal behaviour using scale, e.g. SAD PERSONS scale.
- Carry out a detailed risk assessment.

- Consider immediate, short-term and long-term management/treatment plans.
- Decide the treatment setting (inpatient or outpatient).

WHAT TREATMENT/ADVICE

NURSING

- Ensure the patient has closer monitoring and supportive care.

MEDICAL

- Ensure medical fitness, inpatient or outpatient treatment of identified mental disorder, antidepressant if there is evidence of depression (not likely).

PSYCHOLOGICAL (INCLUDING SUPPORTIVE PSYCHOTHERAPY)

- Consider treatment for addiction, psychotherapeutic approaches to personality difficulties.

SOCIAL

- Seek input from social services, assistance with housing if domestic violence is a recurrent problem; consider halfway house or women's refuge.
- Consider problem-solving approaches.
- Refer for couple counselling, e.g. to 'Relate' in the UK.

FULL ANSWER

Given that this 24-year-old woman has taken a significant overdose of paracetamol tablets and is now ready for discharge, I would consider seeing her as a priority, because of the need to decide whether it is safe enough for her to return home. The main issue is the need to assess the degree of risk that she poses with a view to advising on treatment and on a follow-up plan in order to forestall future occurrence of this self-harm behaviour. First, however, I would like to clarify with the referrer whether they have any particular concerns. Although this lady is said not to have had previous psychiatric contact, I would contact her GP or family doctor for any relevant medical history and history of depression or self-harm. I would also look through the computerized record system of the local psychiatric team or ask ward staff to check whether she has been admitted before, noting the reasons for such an admission, the treatment given and the outcomes.

I would proceed to the accident and emergency department promptly to assess this lady and would take a full psychiatric history and carry out a mental state examination. I would focus on assessing the immediate risk of suicide, subsequent risk of deliberate self-harm, and current social or related problems. I would find out about the circumstances surrounding the overdose and specifically enquire about her intention at the time. I would find out whether she planned the overdose or if it was an impulsive act to cope with her distress, her expectation when she took the tablets, and whether she performed any final act such as writing a suicide note. I would also ask whether she took any precautions against being found or tried to seek help afterwards. I would ask whether she regretted her action or whether she would have preferred to die. I would also ask whether she continues to harbour thoughts of further self-harm or suicide.

Next, I would look for the presence of any mental illness, such as depression and personality difficulties, and assess patient resources, i.e. the ability to cope under stress in the past. I would ask about problems in her relationship and find out about domestic violence and substance misuse. I would enquire about problems other than relationship difficulties (employment, finance, legal, losses and social isolation). I would ask about friends or relatives who might be able to offer support and establish the patient's ability to access professional help in the future. I would like to assess whether there is a continuing risk of suicide and whether the patient intended to die. I would ask whether she still intends to die, and whether the problems that provoked her overdose are still present. I would decide whether she is suffering from a mental illness and if there are adequate resources to manage her in the community, should I decide she is able to leave.

In view of her presentation, my working diagnosis is acute stress reaction precipitated by relationship difficulties. It may well be possible that this lady is suffering from a depressive illness or personality difficulty. I would bear mind the possibility of an adjustment disorder, mild depressive episode, recurrent depressive disorder and borderline personality disorder (emotionally unstable type) as part of the differential diagnosis. I would also consider the possibility of alcohol and substance misuse disorder as a comorbid problem, underlying her various difficulties. At the same time I would consider other factors such as relationship difficulties, poor impulse control and general inability to cope. It may also be possible that this woman has no mental illness at all.

My approach to treatment would be guided by the outcome of my risk assessment and information and support from her friends and family, in particular her boyfriend, with whom she is living. Treatment would also depend on whether she presents a low or higher risk of further self-harm or suicide. If the perceived risk of further self-harm or suicide were low and she had adequate support from friends and family, I would discharge her and arrange for community follow-up, preferably in the outpatient clinic, where couple counselling and stress management treatment can be carried out. I would ensure there is no immediate risk of harm from domestic violence. If there were any evidence of depression I would treat with the appropriate antidepressant once I was reassured that her blood results, particularly liver function tests, were normal. If there were issues with the harmful use of alcohol and/or illicit drugs, I would refer her to the local drug and alcohol team for assistance.

On the other hand, should the risk of further self-harm or suicide be high and/or if there were evidence of a mental illness, I would consider admitting her to the hospital, either informally or formally, for further assessment and treatment. This would be a temporary measure to manage the present crisis (crisis resolution). Once she was admitted, my immediate treatment plan would include closer monitoring by nursing staff due to the risk of self-harm and suicide, detailed risk assessment and the institution of an appropriate antidepressant, if indicated. Since she has been declared medically fit, I would tailor further physical laboratory investigations (FBC, U and Es, TFTs, LFTs and urine drug screen) to specific needs. In the shorter term, psychological assessment and treatment would be offered to deal with emotional and practical issues in her relationship. I would also consider referring for a cognitive behavioural approach to manage depressive symptoms. I would refer her for couple counselling with an agency such as 'Relate' in the UK. I would try to engage her and find out the cause of her difficulties. I would also consider input from social services and a halfway house or women's refuge in the short term, and seek assistance with the local housing department if domestic violence were a recurrent problem.

I would refer appropriately if there were any work to be done concerning problematic substance misuse. In the longer term I would arrange to see this woman in the outpatient clinic for further support and monitoring. This would be with the aim of reducing the risk of further self-harm, which is known to be high within the first week following an episode. I would refer for psychotherapeutic approaches to address any personality difficulties, if they were a prominent problem.

ANSWERS TO SUGGESTED PROBES

1. Factors that would increase her risks of self-harm and suicide are:
   - definite intent to end her life
   - past history of self-harm and/or suicidal behaviour
   - past and current history of depression
   - elaborate plan made to end life and plans to stop being found out
   - isolation, living alone and severe psychosocial difficulties
   - alcohol, substance and drug misuse
   - access to lethal items or weapons
   - poor impulse and anger control.
2. I would *not* admit to hospital if I considered her at low risk of further self-harm and/or suicide. I would seek to manage and support her as an outpatient instead. I *would* consider admitting her to hospital in the following circumstances:
   - if she continues to present a high risk of suicide and/or self-harm
   - if there is further risk of domestic violence
   - if she suffers from moderate to severe depression
   - if she is unable to guarantee her own safety
   - for crisis management if her situational crisis continues without support.
3. The fact that she is asking to be discharged and has the capacity to make decisions about her own care but is ambivalent about her future and a further suicide attempt would create a difficult situation. Because of her ambivalence, I would suggest further assessment in hospital to look for depression or any other psychiatric illness that could be treated. If she has a low or moderate risk of self-harm and suicide and is willing to receive help from a home treatment team, I would give consideration to managing her in the community with appropriate support. (Note that not every mental health service has a dedicated home treatment team.) If she insists on leaving the hospital and is considered at high risk of suicide, I would consider assessing further for compulsory admission under the relevant legislation. This would only be done as a last resort to prevent further self-harm or suicide.

BUZZ WORDS AND USEFUL TERMINOLOGY

Risk assessment, borderline personality disorder, home treatment team, crisis resolution or intervention, crisis admission, women's refuge.

REFERENCES AND SUGGESTED READING

Boyce P, Oakley-Brown M, Hatcher S 2001 The problem of deliberate self-harm. Current Opinion in Psychiatry 14(2):107–111

Guthrie E, Kapur N, Mackway-Jones K et al 2001 Randomised controlled trial of brief psychological intervention after deliberate self-poisoning. British Medical Journal 323:135

Hawton K, Kingsbury S, Steinhardt K et al 1999 Repetition of deliberate self-harm by adolescents: the role of psychological factors. Journal of Adolescence 22:369–378

Patterson W M, Dohn H H, Bird J et al 1983 Evaluation of suicidal patients: the SAD PERSONS scale. Psychosomatics 24:343–349

Royal College of Psychiatrists 1994 The general hospital management of adult deliberate self-harm: a consensus statement on standards for service provision. Royal College of Psychiatrists, London

2

PSYCHIATRIC EMERGENCIES

2.2 36-YEAR-OLD MAN WHO ATTACKED STAFF ON THE WARD

You have been contacted on the phone about the management of a 36-year-old man who was admitted to the ward a week ago. He has attacked a female member of staff, biting her on the face. He has been restrained but continues to be agitated.
What would be your line of action for his management?

SUGGESTED PROBES

1. At what stage would you consider putting this patient in a seclusion room or into secure confinement?
2. What would be your main concerns if seclusion were implemented?
3. If, at some point, it became apparent that intravenous medication were necessary, what precautions would you take?

PMP PLAN

TASKS TO DO

The following five areas are relevant to this vignette but are not necessarily all-inclusive. The list is also not exhaustive:

a) Show appreciation of the need for urgency, bearing in mind risk and safety issues.
b) Consider relevant differential diagnoses to guide assessment and management.
c) Include immediate (safe, rapid tranquillization and seclusion, if necessary), short-term and long-term management of the patient in your plan.
d) Attend to the safety of staff and residents, and consider appropriate medical treatment, if necessary.
e) Discuss the need for a review of policy and contingency planning.

ISSUES

- Safety of patient, staff and other residents
- Immediate, short-term and long-term treatment of the underlying cause of aggressive behaviour.

CLARIFY

- Has the situation been contained?
- Has appropriate help (including rapid response/emergency team, security, or police if necessary) been summoned?
- Does the patient have access to weapons, and has the safe removal of other patients been achieved?

SEEK MORE INFORMATION

STAFF

- Diagnosis
- Circumstances leading to the incident
- History of similar behaviour
- Current problems and treatment plans.

PATIENT

- Mental state
- Rule out intoxication, paranoid and persecutory ideas and/or delusions, command hallucinations
- When the patient is more settled, ask him what led to the situation.

DIFFERENTIAL DIAGNOSIS/DIFFICULTIES

- Substance misuse, alcohol withdrawal/intoxication, epilepsy
- Paranoid schizophrenia, agitated depression, manic episode, acute psychotic episode.

APPROACH TO TREATMENT

- Attend quickly.
- Ensure safety, de-escalate the situation, administer rapid tranquillization.
- Manage subsequently based on the diagnosis.

WHAT TREATMENT/ADVICE

IMMEDIATE

- De-escalate the situation; give rapid tranquillization.
- Support staff, talk to the patient and offer support or ask the nurse in charge to give support.
- Implement a seclusion policy if acceptable locally and only if necessary.

SHORT-TERM

- Treat any underlying condition appropriately.
- If detoxification has been too rapid, reduce the rate and, if necessary, give an increased dose of medication.

LONG-TERM

- Decide on longer-term treatment of the condition.
- Prevent future occurrences.
- Review ward policy.
- Offer an anger management programme to the patient.

FULL ANSWER

This is a psychiatric emergency that needs prompt attention. The main issue that I would be concerned with is the need to maintain the safety of patient, staff and other residents. Next I would consider the immediate, short-term and long-term treatment of the underlying cause of the aggressive behaviour. I would advise staff to remove other patients from the scene and summon the necessary help while I quickly found my way to the unit. I would immediately clarify with the staff whether the situation is contained and whether appropriate help and support has been sought (i.e. hospital security, police). My immediate priority would be to ensure the safety of the patient, other patients admitted on the ward and staff members. If the use of any potential weapon were involved, I would find out whether the weapon has yet been removed. On getting to the ward, if the patient is under control and restraint, I would ensure that he is safe. I would try to talk him down and to establish whether communication would help to contain the situation. Otherwise, I would consider rapid tranquillization with a benzodiazepine such as lorazepam in the first instance. If it became necessary to use intramuscular drugs, I would ensure that this was the last option and that the patient was medically fit enough (cardiopulmonary) to withstand the treatment. If we were to contemplate transfer to a psychiatric intensive care unit or the intravenous use of drugs, I would ensure that resuscitation facilities, including an oxygen cylinder and defibrillator, were close by in case of cardiopulmonary arrest. I would ask for a pulse oximeter to monitor oxygen saturation. I would aim to give the intravenous medication very slowly and would administer the lowest optimal dose as required. It might also be necessary to remove this patient to a special observation or special care area, seclusion room or secure confinement such as a psychiatric intensive care unit.

Once the situation was contained, I would seek more information from staff on the circumstances leading to the assault and the biting of the member of staff. I would find out more about his diagnosis, behaviour in terms of antecedents, details of the behaviour and how it was immediately managed, and the view of the staff on the precipitant (response to hallucination, detoxification from drug or state of intoxication). I would also find out about the treatment given so far and future treatment plans. I would ensure that I saw the member of staff who was assaulted (victim) for reassurance and to obtain her view of the event. I would see that she received appropriate medical attention and encourage her to go home, accompanied by another staff member if necessary. I would also find out whether this patient was suffering from any communicable diseases such as hepatitis B infection and/or HIV, to ensure that the member of staff was given the necessary treatment to forestall disease development. I would seek advice from the local accident and emergency department, and would refer the staff member to the hospital occupational health department immediately.

After I had gathered the necessary information, my thoughts would be that this man's behaviour might be either related to his primary diagnosis, or completely unrelated. It is possible that the incident was due to a mental illness of the psychotic type (response to auditory hallucination, including command hallucination and/or abnormal persecutory ideas and delusions), substance misuse (including alcohol intoxication and withdrawal state), agitated depression, manic episode or perhaps an epileptic attack. There might also be an ongoing and unresolved dispute with the staff member he assaulted. Bearing in mind the underlying cause of the problem, my approach to treatment would be to assess the risk and safety issues. This assessment, along with my discussions with ward staff, would form the basis of my advice on how any future occurrences could be prevented. There might also be a need to review ward policy, but this would be best discussed with the ward manager and the appropriate consultant.

In my overall management, I would consider treatment and management aimed at the patient, the treatment of the staff involved, and also the well-being of other residents on the ward. In the immediate term, I would act to ensure safety on the ward and to contain the situation as I have already stated. In the short term, I would consider treating the underlying causes of the problem in this patient, using appropriate psychotropic medication or psychological intervention, as deemed necessary. If there were a need to increase the dose of medication, I would do that in such a way that unnecessary side-effects were avoided. In the longer term, there might be a need to treat this patient's anger management if his behaviour is totally unrelated to a specified mental illness. I would also address the issue of illicit substance and alcohol misuse/abuse, if these were problems. In the longer term, I would consider measures aimed at reducing the risk of a recurrence of the incident. I would talk to other residents who might have witnessed the incident, or perhaps ask the nurse in charge, who might be better known to the patient, to reassure staff and residents. The ward staff might also benefit from external incident debriefing and reassessment of procedures to prevent and manage any future incident.

ANSWERS TO SUGGESTED PROBES

1. I would consider putting this patient in a seclusion room if he continued to be agitated and threatening, and to put himself and others at risk, despite attempts to de-escalate the situation by non-drug means, or after giving the maximum amount of medication for rapid tranquillization according to local guidelines and protocol.

2. If seclusion were implemented, my main concerns would be the need to:
   - maintain the safety of the person in seclusion, making sure the place is well ventilated
   - ensure access to fluids and conveniences
   - make provision for the safe monitoring of the patient by staff
   - ensure that the seclusion period did not go beyond what was necessary.

3. If the intravenous administration of drugs became necessary, I would ensure that:
   - it was the last option and that the patient was medically fit (cardiopulmonary)
   - resuscitation equipment was to hand, including oxygen cylinder, pulse oximeter to monitor oxygen saturation, and defibrillator
   - the lowest optimal dose of medication was given
   - intravenous medication was given very slowly
   - there was adequate medical backup in case of cardiopulmonary arrest.

Note: intramuscular injection is safer and nearly always possible. The authors have never had to give intravenous injections for restraint. While such situations are uncommon, trainees should nevertheless be aware of what to do. The medical fitness of the patient is very important and candidates should be aware that cardiopulmonary arrest is a possible complication.

BUZZ WORDS AND USEFUL TERMINOLOGY

Rapid tranquillization, control and restraint, command hallucination.

REFERENCES AND SUGGESTED READING

Cheung P, Schweitzer I, Tuckwell V et al 1997 A prospective study of assaults on staff by psychiatric inpatients. Medicine, Science and the Law 37(1):46–52

Cookson J 1998 Management of a newly admitted patient with acute psychiatric disturbance. In: Lee A. Recent Topics from Advances in Psychiatric Treatment, vol. 1. Gaskell, London, pp 2–6

MacPherson R, Anstee B, Dix R 1998 Guidelines for the management of patients with acute disturbance. In: Lee A. Recent Topics from Advances in Psychiatric Treatment, vol. 1. Gaskell, London, pp 7–13

Quintal S A 2002 Violence against psychiatric nurses: an untreated epidemic? Journal of Psychosocial Nursing and Mental Health Services 40(1):46–53

2.3 19-YEAR-OLD GIRL CUTTING HERSELF WITH A RAZOR AT THE HOSPITAL GATE

A 19-year-old female is sitting at the gate of the hospital cutting herself with a razor blade. Security staff who seem to know her think she has a mental illness and have contacted the accident and emergency department. They have asked you for an urgent psychiatric assessment.

What are your differential diagnoses and how would you manage her?

SUGGESTED PROBES

1. This woman is known to the neighbouring services and has been 'blacklisted' due to assaultative behaviour. What would you do?
2. Three days after admission, this patient is better but her local services refuse to accept her back. What would you do?
3. You conclude that she suffers from borderline personality disorder. What are your short-/long-term treatment options?

PMP PLAN

TASKS TO DO

The following five areas are relevant to this vignette but are not necessarily all-inclusive. The list is also not exhaustive:

a) Adopt a strategy that minimizes risk to self and others, including summoning and using appropriate help and resources (e.g. security, police and experienced nursing staff).
b) Demonstrate the ability to prioritize actions in dealing with issues on a practical level, liaising with other services if necessary.
c) Consider both organic and non-organic states in your diagnosis.
d) Use the appropriate legal framework, if the patient lacks insight, in the midst of obvious risk and safety concerns.
e) Include practical problem-solving, medication and psychosocial approaches in your management plans, and consider immediate, short- and long-term management.

ISSUES

- Safety of the patient and others (the woman is in a public place)
- Determining the underlying factors and presence of a mental disorder.

CLARIFY

- Is the patient known to local or nearby services?
- Is there a threat to others, and to any specific person?
- Does the patient have access to and the use of weapons, and why was she 'blacklisted'?
- Is there any serious injury that needs immediate medical or surgical intervention?

SEEK MORE INFORMATION

SECURITY STAFF

- How long have they known her?
- Behavioural problems in the past
- Previous management, who by and where?

PATIENT'S RECORD

- Check if known to any service.

PATIENT

- History, mental state examination, risk assessment
- Physical assessment including drug screen, blood test and/or testing for alcohol.

DIFFERENTIAL DIAGNOSIS/DIFFICULTIES

- *Organic mental illness.* Substance misuse disorder with intoxication with drug or alcohol, withdrawal state from drugs and alcohol, delirium from organic disorder such as epilepsy or a space-occupying lesion
- *Functional mental illness.* Depressive disorder, psychotic illness including schizophrenia and drug-induced psychosis, learning disabilities, borderline personality disorder with predominant features of deliberate self-harm, adjustment disorder, acute stress reaction, and last but not least, a delusional disorder.

APPROACH TO TREATMENT

- Ensure safety.
- Consider immediate actions, short-term measures and long-term management plan.

BIOLOGICAL AND MEDICAL

- Treat identifiable mental disorder, including drug and alcohol addiction.
- Use antidepressants and mood stabilizers.
- Refer to other relevant services.

PSYCHOLOGICAL TREATMENT

- Instigate anger management, cognitive behavioural therapy (CBT), dialectical behavioural therapy (DBT), group therapy, therapeutic community.

SOCIAL AND OTHER MANAGEMENT

- Assess risk before discharge.
- Arrange appropriate accommodation.
- Arrange for home treatment, assertive outreach treatment.
- Transfer patient back to her own local services if she lives out of the catchment area.

FULL ANSWER

Given the presentation and the fact that this woman is in a public place, I would immediately be concerned about safety, both that of the patient and that of others. The other issue is to determine the most likely underlying factors or problems and the presence of a mental disorder. I would consider the possibility of a functional psychiatric illness such as a psychotic one, including schizophrenia, depression, acute stress reaction and adjustment disorder. Her behaviour might also be explained by illicit substance or alcohol use (intoxication or withdrawal state), or an underlying personality difficulty. As part of the differential diagnosis, I would also consider delirium from an organic disorder such as epilepsy or a space-occupying lesion.

In managing this woman, I would bear in mind that this is in a way a psychiatric emergency that needs prompt attention. Nevertheless, I would adopt a strategy that minimizes risk to the patient and others. Accordingly, I would summon help from appropriate people such as experienced nursing staff, security, and the police if necessary. I would instruct staff to make the area safe for members of the public who might be coming through the gate. Before getting too close to her, I would clarify whether she is carrying any potential weapon; if she were, I would make sure she were disarmed. I would approach her with caution, in a way that would not leave her feeling vulnerable and/or intimidated. I would also make sure that she does not have a serious injury that needs immediate medical or surgical intervention. I would treat any medical wound and give a tetanus toxoid, if necessary.

I would then encourage her to come into the accident and emergency department or an appropriate area designated for psychiatric assessment. While this was being carried out, I would ask a member of staff to check available records to find out whether she is known to any local mental health services. If so, I would ask for more relevant information from the professionals that have been involved in her care in the past. After this, I would clarify with her why she was sitting and harming herself at the hospital gate and would ask the cause of her distress. I would seek more information from her on her previous psychiatric contact, diagnosis, medication and her key (main) worker, if she has one. I would ask for the name and contact details of her GP and relatives, in order to obtain corroborative information when appropriate. I would conduct a thorough assessment of her mental state, looking in particular for evidence of an affective disorder such as depression and bipolar illness, psychotic illness, adjustment disorder or an alcohol- or drug-related problem. In addition, I would specifically enquire about this girl's intention and why she has resorted to harming herself. I would find out about her past history of self-harm behaviour and ask her if she still wishes to harm or kill herself. I would also ask about any current relationship, financial, domestic, accommodation, employment and legal problems or loss events. I would also use the opportunity to ask her if she has any further thoughts of self-harm or plans to harm other people.

Having conducted a thorough assessment of her previous problems and present difficulties and formulated a risk assessment, my approach to treatment would be to decide whether she has a psychiatric illness or not, and if there is an immediate risk of suicide or subsequent risk of deliberate self-harm. If there were an immediate risk of suicide or harm to others, I would consider admitting her to the psychiatric unit for further assessment and management. If there were no such problem, but there remained a risk of further self-harm, I would still consider admitting to hospital. Alternatively, if she has an adequate support network and has no ongoing difficulties in the absence of a severe mental illness, it might be appropriate not to admit her to hospital but to follow her up in the community. If the information gathered on this patient from the psychiatric records and from talking to relatives or carers suggests the possibility of a personality difficulty or disorder, I would be careful about opting for hospital admission. I would not consider hospital admission unless absolutely necessary as it might create a culture of dependency, and in the long run, be counterproductive for this patient. Regular community follow-up by a named staff member might be a more appropriate strategy to prevent 'splitting'. This would be part of a package of a comprehensive range of interventions suitable for patients with personality disorder. Biological options include antidepressants and mood stabilizers in the short term, and mood stabilizers such as carbamazepine and sodium valproate in the long term. Psychological options include anger management and cognitive behavioural therapy in the short term, and dialectical behavioural therapy in the long term. Social options include assertive outreach, home treatment team and practical problem-solving (such as housing) in the short term, and a therapeutic community in the long term.

Should she have an underlying psychiatric or alcohol- and drug-related problem, this would be treated using a broad range of biological, psychological and social interventions. I would treat any depression and anxiety with suitable antidepressants; these might also be useful in treating symptoms of mood instability, irritability, anxiety and impulsivity, which are common in patients with borderline personality disorder. If there were any evidence of drug and alcohol problems, I would refer the patient to the drug and alcohol services in the long term. If the patient has a learning difficulty, I would seek advice from the local learning disability team in the first instance. In addition, she might need referral to the social service department for practical problem-solving to deal with the necessary social issues such as accommodation and finance.

ANSWERS TO SUGGESTED PROBES

1. If the patient is known to neighbouring services and had been 'blacklisted', I would find out why and would clarify the nature of her assaultative behaviour. This information, which would help in her risk assessment, would be shared among staff to determine the best way and the best setting to manage her.
2. If, 3 days after admission, the patient were better but her local services refused to accept her back, I would make them aware of their responsibility to offer treatment and appropriate follow-up while wanting to know and understand why she was blacklisted. I would manage her in the acute phase, assess and manage the risks, and then

transfer her to the local psychiatric service for long-term care and follow-up.

3. The short-term and long-term treatment options for borderline personality disorder are described in my full answer.

BUZZ WORDS AND USEFUL TERMINOLOGY

Borderline personality disorder, acting out, therapeutic community.

REFERENCES AND SUGGESTED READING

Boyce P, Oakley-Brown M, Hatcher S 2001 The problem of deliberate self-harm. Current Opinion in Psychiatry 14(2):107–111

Hawton K, Kingsbury S, Steinhardt K et al 1999 Repetition of deliberate self-harm by adolescents: the role of psychological factors. Journal of Adolescence 22:369–378

Isacson G, Rich C L 2001 Management of patients who deliberately harm themselves. British Medical Journal 322(7280):213–215

Royal College of Psychiatrists 1994 The General Hospital Management of Adult Deliberate Self-harm: a Consensus Satement on Standards for Service Provision. Royal College of Psychiatrists, London

2.4 21-YEAR-OLD MAN WHO BECAME VIOLENT BETWEEN PSYCHOTHERAPY SESSIONS

You are the specialist registrar in a psychotherapy department. You have been seeing a 21-year-old man who has a history of childhood trauma and who was unhappy about the way he felt his father had treated him. He found the therapy session difficult during your last meeting. While he is settling down to see you the week before his final two sessions, he has an angry outburst and bangs ferociously on the table, saying he no longer wants to see you, but he eventually sits down.

How would you manage the situation?

SUGGESTED PROBES

1. What action(s) would you take in the immediate term to ensure safety and minimize risks?
2. What information do you need to establish the possible causes of this behaviour?
3. While he is settling down to see you, his mother rings asking that you please extend your sessions by another 2 weeks. What management approach would you adopt and how exactly would you manage?

PMP PLAN

TASKS TO DO

The following five areas are relevant to this vignette but are not necessarily all-inclusive. The list is also not exhaustive:

a) Pay attention to safety and act in a way that minimizes risks.
b) Seek the appropriate information and carry out a proper risk assessment, risk quantification, risk analysis and management.
c) Discuss the possible causes of this behaviour and have an understanding of its psychodynamic formulation.
d) Discuss the feasibility of continuing the work, and settings, approaches, goals and target outcomes. Good candidates will also cover the renegotiation of the terms on which future sessions are based.
e) Consider other treatment options, to include medication, psychosocial intervention and practical problem-solving, as well as drug treatment, if necessary, and seek supervision from senior colleagues.

ISSUES

- Safety and the management of a potentially volatile situation
- Procedure, if the situation is found to be manageable
- Management of any mental illness, alcohol or drug misuse, risks of harm to self and others.

CLARIFY

- What are the safety issues? Are potential weapons involved?
- Is there enough support/backup, an alarm bell, a safety exit?

SEEK MORE INFORMATION

PATIENT

- Feelings about the sessions
- Feelings of abandonment
- Thoughts of self-harm and/or suicide.

DIFFERENTIAL DIAGNOSIS/DIFFICULTIES

- *Functional.* Axis I diagnosis—mental illness particularly depression, post-traumatic stress disorder (PTSD) with flashbacks, psychosis; or Axis II diagnosis—consider antisocial behaviour and personality difficulties or issues related to psychotherapy, such as content of difficult sessions, anger, transference issues, issues with ending therapy
- *Organic.* Intoxication and withdrawal reactions from drug and alcohol.

APPROACH TO TREATMENT

- Determine whether it is safe to continue. Only continue if the situation is safe and under control.
- If unsafe, call for help and get out!
- Seek advice from your supervisors.
- Renegotiate the terms of future sessions.

WHAT TREATMENT/ADVICE

- Continue treatment if it is safe, and stick to the original plan.
- Offer anger management.

- Refer to the drug and alcohol team, if indicated.
- Refer to the acute mental health service.
- Treat with an antidepressant, if appropriate.

FULL ANSWER

I think this would be a difficult situation to be in. I would be very concerned about safety issues and how to manage this potentially volatile situation. The other issue is how to proceed if the situation were found to be manageable. The safe management of any mental illness and alcohol or drug misuse, and risk of harm to self and to others would be equally important in the long term, considering that this man is nearing the end of his therapy. First of all, I would want quickly to consider the risks involved and whether it was safe for us to continue the session. I would be concerned about my own safety, the safety of the patient, and that of other staff in the clinic. If I thought the situation were too dangerous, I would terminate the session immediately and seek assistance with the use of a panic button or alarm. If I were reassured about safety, I would try to de-escalate the situation by not being confrontational. I would quickly check whether this man is intoxicated or not, and it would be sensible to do this tactically. I would make sure there were no potential weapons or missiles to hand. I would clarify with the patient whether he is happy to continue with the session or not.

Once he had settled down, I would want to find out what is making him angry. I would consider whether his anger might be due to the presence of a mental illness, personality difficulties, or the use of alcohol and illicit substances or drugs, or whether it stemmed purely from issues related to the psychotherapeutic sessions. I would explore his feelings about the last session and whether he had seen his father since then. I would also find out whether he is having flashbacks or is depressed. I would ask whether he has been self-harming, or coping by using drugs and/or alcohol. I would enquire about his mood and about any thoughts of self-harm or suicide. I would find out whether he felt he was going to be abandoned as the therapy was coming to an end, and what he had wished to happen. I would seek more information from him about how he has been finding the sessions, and I would explore for profound negative transference and whether he thinks I was acting like his father, with whom he is angry. I would ask whether he harbours any ill feelings against his father, others and me.

Having asked all these questions, I would hope to develop an understanding of why this man behaved the way he did. I would consider finding the session difficult as one of the problems. It might also be that the man was becoming depressed and feeling unable to cope. I would also consider poor anger control, substance misuse disorder, PTSD, and severe anxiety and panic disorder in the attempt to explain his behaviour. My approach to treatment would first be to negotiate the terms of future engagements with him. I would seek advice from my seniors and supervisors. I would let him know that I cannot work with him if he makes me and others feel unsafe, and if I am not able to guarantee his safety and the safety of others. If he continued to make threats of self-harm or of harming others, I would carry out a risk assessment, and consider the possibility of further assessments in hospital or support by the home treatment team, where available. I would refer to the appropriate catchment area psychiatrist for adequate follow-up.

I would continue with the psychotherapy sessions once the issues of risk and safety were addressed and on condition that the client is willing and agrees with the terms and conditions of treatment. While we would try to explore his difficulties further, we would stick to the original plan and timetable. Rather than giving more sessions, we would explore how he is going to deal with the end of therapy without behaving in any negative way, if that were a major concern. I would consider whether counter-transference has contributed to the way the patient has behaved. If there were ongoing relationship difficulties, anger control difficulties, family disharmony and lack of support, or an alcohol and/or substance misuse disorder, I would refer him to the appropriate services.

I would use this opportunity to seek appropriate supervision and advice from my senior or consultant on the way forward for this man if he were to continue or restart therapy.

ANSWERS TO SUGGESTED PROBES

1. To ensure safety and minimize risks in the immediate term, I would:
   - take a calm and reassuring approach and try to calm him down, by not arguing with him or becoming confrontational
   - shout for help, use the panic button or alarm to alert security and other staff
   - make the necessary moves to get out of the room and alert others.

2. I have already covered the question of what information I would need to establish the possible causes of this behaviour in my full answer.

3. In response to his mother, I would politely explain that extending the sessions would not be in her son's best interests, and indeed, would make termination of the sessions more difficult. I would reassure her that we would look into how to manage the ending of the sessions and also into the kind of support he would have post-session.

BUZZ WORDS AND USEFUL TERMINOLOGY

Transference, countertransference, acting out, boundaries.

REFERENCES AND SUGGESTED READING

Ursano R J, Silberman E K 1988 Individual psychotherapies. In: Talbott JA, Hales RE, Yudofsky SC (eds) Textbook of Psychiatry. American Psychiatric Press, Washington DC, pp 855–859

Ursano R J, Ursano A M 2000 Brief individual psychodynamic psychotherapy. In: Gelder MG, López-Ibor Jr JJ, Andreasen NC (eds) New Oxford Textbook of Psychiatry, vol. 2. Oxford University Press, Oxford, pp 1421–1432

2.5 38-YEAR-OLD MAN WITH PSYCHOSIS WHO DRILLED A HOLE THROUGH HIS WALLS

You are asked to see a 38-year-old man who has previously assaulted his CPN and made threats to kill a police officer. No charges have been pressed against him. He has accused his neighbours of plotting against him and has drilled holes through the adjoining walls to 'smoke them out'. He has refused to see his CPN or social worker and will not take medication. What would you do?

SUGGESTED PROBES

1. What factors would guide your decision on where this man should be managed?
2. If you decided that this man needs clozapine, what precautionary measures would you take?
3. This man is considered as posing a high risk of harm to others. Are there statutory legal measures to ensure he uses medication and complies with treatment in the community?

PMP PLAN

TASKS TO DO

The following five areas are relevant to this vignette but are not necessarily all-inclusive. The list is also not exhaustive:

a) Assess the risks involved and take the necessary precautions to ensure safety.
b) Take a detailed history, carry out a mental state and risk assessment, and arrange for treatment and supervision.
c) Show understanding of the appropriate mental health law to enable treatment in an appropriate secure setting. (This will differ from one jurisdiction to another.)
d) Discuss the need to prosecute offenders who commit serious crime.
e) Consider medical, psychological and social factors and the treatment of substance misuse in your treatment plans, as well as appropriate accommodation and adequate monitoring strategies.

ISSUES

- Consideration of the risks the patient poses to self and others (e.g. further deterioration, aggression to others and property, and risk of fire)

• How to go about assessment of patient while giving consideration to the safety of patient and others.

CLARIFY

• What is the situation at home?
• Are there concerns about the safety of the patient and others, particularly the neighbours?
• What is the potential for the use of weapons and what is the risk of fire?
• Is backup available for assessment (supporting staff)?

SEEK MORE INFORMATION

MENTAL HEALTH SERVICE

• History, previous treatment plans and compliance, daytime activities
• Substance misuse
• Persistent psychosocial stressors
• Severity of psychotic symptoms
• Command hallucinations
• Risk assessment
• Expression of harm to self or others.

PSYCHIATRIC NOTES

• Review.

PATIENT

• Once it is safe, a brief history of his account of events, looking for paranoid ideas and delusions, command auditory hallucinations, threatening visual hallucinations, passivity phenomenon, drug intoxication or withdrawal
• Compliance with treatment and patient's insight
• Any particular or named target?

DIFFERENTIAL DIAGNOSIS/DIFFICULTIES

• *Functional.* Paranoid schizophrenia, delusional disorder, drug-induced psychosis and schizoaffective disorder, acute manic episode and other schizophreniform psychosis
• *Organic.* Not likely, given the present history.

APPROACH TO TREATMENT

- Ensure safety and involve others, e.g. police, relatives.
- Seek legal means to transfer him to an appropriate facility with adequate security.

WHAT TREATMENT/ADVICE

- Consider immediate, short-term and long-term management plans.

MEDICATION

- Administer rapid tranquillization.

PSYCHOLOGICAL

- Consider treatment such as illness awareness therapy, compliance therapy, treatment for substance misuse.

DISCHARGE PLANNING

- Take a multidisciplinary approach for appropriate follow-up and monitoring relapse indicators.
- Agree a workable crisis and contingency plan.

PSYCHOSOCIAL

- Arrange daytime activities and support for carers.

LEGAL FRAMEWORK

- Facilitate compliance and contact with services.

FULL ANSWER

I would consider this situation an emergency and I would want to clarify as far as possible when anybody, including his family members, last saw the man. I would find out about his home situation, the concerns of his family and neighbours, and other issues regarding the safety of the patient (such as suicide and self-neglect) and others, particularly the neighbours. Since it has been reported that he has been drilling holes to 'smoke people out', there would be a great risk of fire, which might endanger lives. I would suggest that the local services give assistance to the immediate neighbours, to enable them to move out while we tried to reach the man. Due to the potential for the use of weapons and the possible risk of fire and injury to the staff who visit this man at home, I would seek assistance from the police in assessing him. I would explore the possibility of obtaining a warrant to enter his home forcefully with police assistance, should he become threatening and refuse to open his door. Ideally, I would see him with other relevant mental health workers who know him in order to facilitate his assessment and possibly admission to a psychiatric intensive care unit (PICU) or other secure facility. In England and Wales, an approved social worker (ASW) would be able to complete an application for detention under the Mental Health Act 1983, following recommendations from two medical practitioners.

While I was making these arrangements, I would quickly seek more information on this man, who is well known to the services. I would talk to his key worker or CPN about the crisis and contingency plan. I would check his diagnosis, previous risk assessment and whether he has any propensity to violence and fire-setting. I would ask for his psychiatric notes to examine his treatment history, previous treatment plans and compliance, substance misuse, persistent difficult psychosocial stressors and attendance at daytime activities. Once I had this information, I would proceed to assess him with the necessary backup. I would hope that he would allow access to staff but, if not, we would use police power (enforceable under Section 135 of the Mental Health Act 1983 in the UK) to enter his property. (Readers and candidates in other jurisdictions are advised to seek appropriate legal advice and consult the relevant references. Community Treatment Orders are applicable in parts of the USA, Canada, Australia and New Zealand.)

Once we had gained access to the patient, I would use the opportunity to examine him for any evidence of self-neglect, attempts at setting a fire, and any damage he has done to the walls. If it were possible, I would ask him a few questions about his thoughts and perceptions, and examine his basis for concluding that his neighbours were conspiring against him. As regards his mental state, I would look for evidence of distractibility, response to visual or auditory hallucinations, evidence of thought disorder, passivity phenomenon and command hallucinations. I would find out whether he was using alcohol and illicit substances, particularly cannabis and amphetamines, and would look for evidence of drug intoxication or withdrawal. I would check whether he is targeting any specific person(s) and whether he has any plans (elaborate or not) of self-harm or harm to others. I would ask him about his compliance with treatment and examine his insight into his condition.

Paranoid schizophrenia, delusional disorder, drug-induced psychosis, schizoaffective disorder, acute manic episode and other schizophreniform psychosis would be on the list of differential diagnoses that I would be considering. My general approach to his treatment and management would be to consider safety at all times. I would request police assistance to transfer him to hospital under the appropriate legal framework. I would consider the risks he has posed in the past, his present threat of harm to others, the risk of absconding, the opportunity for close monitoring and the availability of support from staff in deciding which facility to admit him to. Ideally, I would aim to admit him to a secure unit, but a PICU or locked ward might be sufficient.

I would consider immediate, short-term and long-term treatment and management plans. My immediate treatment would be to nurse him in a safe environment and treat him regularly with antipsychotics until he settles down. I would observe closely for any side-effects of the medication and also advise close supervision to prevent self-harm and harm to others. Once he had settled down and started engaging, we would use the opportunity to address medication awareness, compliance issues and substance misuse. Other psychological treatments would include compliance therapy, coping skills, and anger and stress management. I would ensure that discharge planning was multidisciplinary in approach, and would involve his family and carers. During the discharge process, the issues of medication, further psychological treatment, compliance, treatment for substance misuse, appropriate monitoring and follow-up by medical and non-medical staff would be discussed. We would document clearly the known relapse indicators, agreed crisis plan, framework (including legal) to facilitate compliance, contact with services in the future, and any advanced directives on care if the patient lacked the capacity to make decisions. We would facilitate daytime activities and necessary support for carers.

ANSWERS TO SUGGESTED PROBES

1. The factors that would guide my decision on where this man should be managed include his current risk of absconding, the risk of harm to others, a current and past history of aggression, and the degree of his insight. I would consider him a risk and would seek to manage him on a PICU at the very least, and would also consider a medium secure unit (MSU) in the UK.

2. If I decided that this man needed clozapine, I would ensure that:
   - he currently has normal blood levels
   - he has no history of agranulocytosis, neutropenia or bone marrow disorder
   - he has no medical conditions such as severe uncontrolled epilepsy, active liver disease or cardiac disorder (heart failure), or severe renal impairment
   - he has no bleeding disorder.
3. As for statutory legal measures to ensure he uses medication and complies with treatment in the community, there are none. In the UK, the Provision of Aftercare under Supervision (Section 25) of the Mental Health Act 1983 can be a useful legal framework or way of achieving some objectives that may encourage this gentleman to comply with treatment plans. This section of the Act requires that patients allow access to professional carers, and may stipulate that they reside at a particular place. The dedicated or key staff may, however, encourage patients to continue to take medication. The Supervision Order does not allow forceful treatment against a patient's wishes, but allows services to convey a patient who is suspected of relapsing and is at risk of self-harm or neglect, or poses a risk of harm to others to a safe place for further assessment.

BUZZ WORDS AND USEFUL TERMINOLOGY

Aftercare arrangements, risk assessment and evaluation, contingency planning, relapse prevention, relapse indicators.

REFERENCES AND SUGGESTED READING

Buchanan A 1999 Risk and dangerousness. Psychological Medicine 29:465–473

McIvor R 1998 The community treatment orders: clinical and ethical issues. Australian and New Zealand Journal of Psychiatry 32:223–228

Swanson J W, Holzer C E, Ganju V K et al 1990 Violence and psychiatric disorder in the community: evidence from the epidemiologic catchment area surveys. Hospital and Community Psychiatry 41(7):761–770

2.6 50-YEAR-OLD SEMICONSCIOUS WOMAN WHO HAS A CK OF 1500 UNITS/LITRE

A 50-year-old lady who has been maintained on clozapine for the last 2 years was readmitted a week ago. She presented with symptoms of depression and was started on citalopram in a 20 mg dose. Your senior house officer has contacted you, stating that the patient has been feeling more unwell for the last few days. Creatine kinase (CK) level is 1500 units/litre. She is now acutely ill and semiconscious. She had similar symptoms when she was on a depot antipsychotic 14 years ago.

What are your differential diagnoses and what will be your management approach?

SUGGESTED PROBES

1. What are the criteria for the diagnosis of neuroleptic malignant syndrome (NMS)?
2. While examining her, you find that her temperature is 39.4°C. What do you do?
3. You decide to restart the patient on medication. What do you give and why?

PMP PLAN

TASKS TO DO

The following five areas are relevant to this vignette but are not necessarily all-inclusive. The list is also not exhaustive:

a) Demonstrate skill in appreciating and managing safety and risk issues.
b) Decide on appropriate further investigation and necessary referrals.
c) Discuss the various differential diagnoses and the most likely one (NMS).
d) Demonstrate knowledge of the options for safe management and monitoring, including the use of appropriate medication.
e) Discuss post-acute treatment and reinstatement of treatment with antipsychotics following NMS.

ISSUES

- Immediate transfer of the patient to the care of physicians for acute medical support

- Establishment of the root cause of her physical condition and the institution of appropriate treatment to stabilize her
- Careful reintroduction of neuroleptics (and other psychotropics) to reduce the risk of a repeat incident.

CLARIFY

- What is the patient's cardiopulmonary status?
- Is there a life-threatening condition that necessitates immediate transfer to an intensive care unit?

SEEK MORE INFORMATION

REVIEW OF TREATMENT

- Current dose of clozapine
- Current haematological status: red, amber or green?
- Suggestion of NMS while on depot medication.

PHYSICAL EXAMINATION

- Altered mental state, confusion, agitation, slurred speech, diaphoresis, autonomic imbalance, bradycardia, rigidity, low haematological status, infection, pyrexia, neurological symptoms
- Primary features of NMS: hyperthermia, extreme generalized rigidity, autonomic instability and altered mental state.

INVESTIGATION AND/OR TRANSFER TO ICU

- Serial CK, ESR, LFTs, RFTs, FBC with white cell count and differentials, TFTs, urine toxicology, ECG, pulse oximetry, CT and viral studies.

DIFFERENTIAL DIAGNOSIS/DIFFICULTIES

- *Organic.* NMS, serotonin syndrome, catatonia, medication-induced acute dystonia, drug-induced movement disorder, malignant hyperpyrexia, viral encephalitis including HIV, toxaemia (carbon monoxide, strychnine), tetanus. Rarely, psychedelic, anticoagulant or alcohol withdrawal, syndrome of Karl Ludwig Kalbaum or acute lethal catatonia
- *Functional.* Most likely not due to functional illness.

APPROACH TO TREATMENT

- Consider safety as paramount.
- Maintain a high index of suspicion for NMS.
- Carry out an immediate medical assessment and institute appropriate treatment.

WHAT TREATMENT/ADVICE

IMMEDIATE

- Discontinue antipsychotics and antidepressants.
- Transfer to medical ICU.
- Support ventilation and stabilize autonomic function.
- Rehydrate.
- Use vecuronium/midazolam to relax muscles and reduce agitation.
- Treat with a direct-acting dopamine agonist, e.g. bromocriptine, pergolide or dantrolene sodium, to reduce fever.
- Instigate external cooling treatment.
- Rule out or treat any infection.

SHORT-TERM

- Monitor more closely.
- Support using benzodiazepines and supportive psychotherapy.
- Consider ECT if severe psychosis continues.

LONGER-TERM

- Reintroduce medication (antipsychotic rechallenge): clozapine after the acute phase (2 weeks after NMS started), starting with lower doses of medication (usually another class of antipsychotic).

FULL ANSWER

My immediate concern in the management of this lady would be to ensure that she is safe and treated medically as appropriate. I would seek to establish the diagnosis and manage appropriately. I would clarify her cardiovascular status and appraise the findings on examination of her vital signs. As she is semiconscious, this might be a life-threatening condition and I would seek her immediate transfer to the ICU under the care of physicians for acute medical support. I would then make an attempt to find out the root cause of her physical condition, so as to institute appropriate treatment, before considering a careful reintroduction of neuroleptics (and other psychotropics) to reduce the risk of a repeat incidence. Given that she has just had changes made to her medication and has a background history of similar episodes while on depot antipsychotics 14 years ago, I would have a high index of suspicion for neuroleptic malignant syndrome (NMS). This diagnosis would be supported by a raised CK (far beyond the upper limit of 200 units/litre of most reference ranges). I would look specifically for the primary features of hyperthermia, extreme generalized rigidity, autonomic instability and altered mental state. I would also bear in mind other differential diagnoses, which include catatonia, serotonin syndrome, medication-induced acute dystonia or movement disorder, malignant hyperpyrexia and heat stroke. I would consider other possibilities such as a viral encephalopathy, including HIV infection, toxaemia including carbon monoxide and strychnine poisoning, tetanus, and symptoms of withdrawal from salicylates, psychedelics and rarely anticoagulants.

With this background in mind, I would seek more information and carry out an urgent physical examination, looking for altered mental state, confusion, agitation, slurred speech, and diaphoresis or sweating. I would also look for evidence of autonomic imbalance, such as labile blood pressure and pulse rate. I would look for rigidity, slurred speech and hyper-reflexia during a neurological examination. I would look for evidence of infection and poisoning. If all these suggested NMS, I would refer to the physicians immediately for further investigation and assessment. They would be able to carry out serial CK tests, looking particularly at the muscle-derived component. They would also carry out LFTs, RFTs, TFTs, FBC with white blood count and differentials, urine toxicology, ECG and C-reactive protein, ESR and other studies as suggested by the differential diagnosis I have already mentioned. They would also be able to use a pulse oximeter to monitor oxygen saturation, carry out viral studies, and perform a CT scan to rule out intracranial organic pathology.

In my approach to treatment I would consider safety to be paramount and have a high index of suspicion for NMS, while bearing in mind other possibilities. My immediate treatment plan would be to discontinue all psychotropics (the antipsychotic clozapine and the antidepressant citalopram) and refer immediately. I would transfer the patient to the ICU immediately in order to support her ventilation, in case her condition started to deteriorate. This might be suggested by rigidity of the chest wall or by respiratory failure. The aim of medical treatment would be to stabilize autonomic function and rehydrate with intravenous fluids. External cooling techniques such as tepid sponging might be used to reduce the temperature as fast as possible, in addition to giving bromocriptine (a dopamine agonist) 5–6 mg daily, pergolide or dantrolene sodium to reduce the fever. I would suggest that medication such as midazolam or vecuronium be administered to reduce rigidity. I would continue to liaise with the acute medical services while these treatments were being administered. I would also advise that a registered mental health nurse monitor the patient closely on the acute ward while she is recovering.

Once acute treatment under the physicians was completed, benzodiazepines could also be used to reduce agitation and to sedate the patient. If she continued to show symptoms of severe psychosis, I would consider ECT, as antipsychotics cannot be used in the post-acute treatment phase. I would ensure that there was no infection; if there were infection, I would treat it accordingly. Once the condition was completely stabilized and serially monitored investigations (particularly CK) were normal, I would consider rechallenging with an antipsychotic after 10–14 days. In this particular case I would still rechallenge with clozapine because there is little option for the use of other antipsychotics. The use of a typical antipsychotic, apart from having induced NMS in this lady in the past, carries a higher risk of inducing NMS than an atypical antipsychotic. The reason why the patient is on clozapine in the first instance is probably that she was not improving on other medications or could not tolerate them. Therefore there is no guarantee that other atypical antipsychotics would be able to control her symptoms as clozapine can. I would ensure that her haematological profile was normal before I rechallenged with this medication. I would reintroduce it very gradually and slowly, using small doses as far as possible. I would continue to monitor her physical and mental states closely during the period of antipsychotic reintroduction, and once the patient was stable I would continue treatment as usual.

ANSWERS TO SUGGESTED PROBES

1. The criteria for a diagnosis of NMS are presence of severe muscle rigidity and hyperthermia (pyrexia), plus two or more of the following:
   - diaphoresis
   - dysphagia
   - tremor

- incontinence
- altered level of consciousness, ranging from confusion to coma and mutism
- bradycardia
- labile blood pressure
- presence of autonomic imbalance
- leucocytosis
- elevated CK–MB.

All these symptoms will not be due to other drugs such as phencyclidine or a neurological condition such as viral encephalitis. Neither can this condition be accounted for by any other mental disorder such as depression.

2. If the patient's temperature increased to 39.4°C, I would call for medical help and consider immediate transfer to an ICU. I would immediately apply external measures (tepid sponging) to reduce the high temperature while waiting for help. While she is on the medical ward or ICU, the physicians would ensure adequate hydration and ventilation. I would give either dantrolene sodium at a dose of 1 mg per kg body weight every minute, or bromocriptine or pergolide.

3. If I decided to restart the patient on medication, I would still consider clozapine, for the reasons I have given in my full answer.

BUZZ WORDS AND USEFUL TERMINOLOGY

Antipsychotic rechallenge.

REFERENCES AND SUGGESTED READING

Pi E H, Simpson G M 2000 Medication-induced movement disorders. In: Sadock B J, Sadock V A (eds) Comprehensive textbook of Psychiatry, vol. 2, 7th edn. Lippincott, William & Wilkins, Philadelphia, pp 2266–2267

Illing M, Ancill R 1996 Clozapine-induced neuroleptic malignant syndrome: clozapine monotherapy rechallenge in a case of previous NMS. Canadian Journal of Psychiatry 41(4):258

Kohen D, Bristow M 1996 Neuroleptic malignant syndrome. Advances in Psychiatric Treatment 2:151–157

Parks-Veal P 1990 Neuroleptic malignant syndrome. Hospital Pharmacy 25:121–123, 133

Taylor D, Paton C, Kerwin R 2003 The Maudsley Prescribing Guidelines, 7th edn. Martin Dunitz, London

3
General adult psychiatry

A 29-year-old shopkeeper who recently went through a divorce from his wife of 7 years, has been referred to you. He says he has been drinking water excessively to flush out toxins from his body. He is worried that his ex-wife may have been poisoning him for years. The patient is not suffering from diabetes mellitus. The GP dismisses his story of toxaemia and thinks he needs psychiatric help.

How would you go about assessment and management?

SUGGESTED PROBES

1. What features in this presentation suggest a diagnosis of adjustment disorder?
2. At what point would you consider admission for this patient?
3. The patient becomes confused 24 hours after admission. What is your main concern?

PMP PLAN

TASKS TO DO

The following five areas are relevant to this vignette but are not necessarily all-inclusive. The list is also not exhaustive:

a) Show an appreciation of the complications that may arise from excessive water-drinking and address the issue.
b) Consider safety and risk issues and management of possible self-harm and harm to others in light of the recent divorce.
c) Include a range of functional (psychotic and non-psychotic) disorders that may be responsible in your discussion.
d) Discuss the range of investigations required.
e) Discuss in detail the management of one possible (and/or most likely) cause of the disorder.

ISSUES

- Determining if the symptom of excessive water consumption is due to any organic condition or a functional illness
- Determine what is the underlying psychiatric condition if problem not due to organic condition.

CLARIFY

- Is there any immediate risk of medical complication?
- What are the risk issues (to self and others, in particular his ex-wife in light of the recent divorce)?

SEEK MORE INFORMATION

GP

- Results of U and Es, creatine kinase and LFTs
- Any history of encephalitis, flu-like illness, head injury or syndrome of inappropriate antidiuretic hormone secretion (SIADH).

RELATIVES/EX-WIFE

- Corroborative information.

PATIENT

- Full history of onset and progress of problems, coping mechanism following recent divorce, history of alcohol or drug misuse
- Why he believed his ex-wife was poisoning him
- Mental state: look for thought and perceptual abnormalities. Ensure the patient is not confused and that he is generally well. Examine insight
- Further investigation: appraise the results of investigations or order an FBC, U and Es, RFTs, LFTs and other tests only if necessary
- Refer to endocrinology for hormonal assay.

DIFFERENTIAL DIAGNOSIS/DIFFICULTIES

- *Functional.* Acute psychotic episode, paranoid schizophrenia, delusional disorder, monosymptomatic hypochondriacal delusion, psychotic depression, anxiety disorder, adjustment disorder, obsessive-compulsive disorder, and psychogenic polydipsia (as may be caused by some of the conditions listed above)

- *Organic.* Diabetes insipidus/mellitus, brain tumour, epilepsy, SIADH, meningoencephalitis, head injury.

APPROACH TO TREATMENT

- Exclude the need for urgent medical attention, given that excessive water consumption can result in hyponatraemia and consequently rhabdomyolysis, renal failure, compartment syndrome, confusion and death.
- Assess risk and consider safety issues (including the safety of the patient's partner in light of their recent divorce).
- Decide on the treatment setting and type of treatment.

WHAT TREATMENT/ADVICE

- Include immediate, short- and long-term management.
- Consider a range of biological and psychosocial interventions.
- Gear treatment towards addressing any emergency situation that may have arisen from the excessive water consumption and then address the underlying problem.
- Treat psychosis and depression.

FULL ANSWER

Given the history of excessive water consumption in this 29-year-old shopkeeper, my immediate thought would be to establish the possible causes of this presentation and pay particular attention to immediate/imminent risk and safety issues. Hence, I would like to clarify with the GP whether he is aware of any imminent physical complications and risk issues. I would ensure that the patient is not suffering from water intoxication and acute fluid overload, which might be life-threatening. I would pay attention to the possibility of self-harm in this man and also harm to his ex-wife due to the recent divorce.

I would seek more information from the GP on the patient's past medical and psychiatric history, including psychosis and depression. If he has a history of depression or psychosis, I would find out whether toxaemia has been a subject of his delusions in the past, and if so, the way it presented and was managed. I would like to know about investigations to date, and to clarify with the GP why he or she is dismissive of this man's story of toxaemia. If at all possible, I would talk to the patient's relatives for corroborative information and their own understanding of developments.

Finally, once I was confident that there are no imminent physical complications, I would arrange to see this man with one of my colleagues or offer an urgent outpatient appointment with the aim of taking a full psychiatric history, performing a detailed mental state examination and appraising the results of any investigation that has been carried out. In the history, I would pay particular attention to the onset of the problems in relation to the recent divorce. I would ask the patient if he thought his wife had divorced him because she thought he was unclean. I would explore how he fixed on the idea of toxins in his body and also examine how fixed his belief is. I would find out who he thinks is responsible for putting these toxins into him and whether he has decided to do anything about it. I would carefully examine for abnormal perceptions, such as 'voices' that are suggesting he has toxins in his body. I would also like to establish the presence of any psychosocial maintaining factors, such as child custody problems or financial difficulties as a result of the divorce. I would try to identify his coping mechanisms since his divorce and his belief about when the 'toxaemia' problems began. I would rule out the presence of alcohol or illicit drug misuse, as these may be used as a way of coping with distress. I would carry out a limited cognitive assessment to ensure that the patient is not confused and that he is generally well. I would examine whether he has insight into his difficulties.

After a detailed history and mental state examination, my thought would be that this man might be suffering from a functional psychiatric illness such as an acute psychotic episode, paranoid schizophrenia, delusional disorder, monosymptomatic hypochondriacal delusion, psychotic depression, anxiety, adjustment disorder or OCD. Other possibilities include organic disorders such as diabetes insipidus or mellitus, brain tumour, SIADH, meningoencephalitis, epilepsy and head injury. As far as possible, I would rule out an organic cause before considering a functional illness as a differential diagnosis. My initial approach to treating this man would be to make a decision on safety issues, and I would carry out a formal risk assessment, paying attention to issues of self-harm and harm to others. I would attempt to establish a diagnosis, and to decide on the appropriate treatment and the setting of such treatment.

My immediate management plan would be to admit this man for further assessment, investigations and treatment. If a CT or MRI had not recently been carried out, I would order one to rule out a brain tumour, which might be responsible for inappropriate ADH secretion. I would consider restricting his fluid intake, guided by the results of the U and Es, urine osmolarity and advice from the medical (endocrinologist and/or chemical pathology) team. If there were evidence of a functional mental illness, this would be treated accordingly. If this man were suffering from a psychotic illness, I would suggest treatment with atypical antipsychotics and treat any depression with antidepressants. If there were evidence of organic pathology, I would liaise with the appropriate specialist for active medical or surgical intervention. Bearing in mind that this man has recently divorced, I would consider psychological treatment in the form of supportive psychotherapy or cognitive behavioural therapy. I would also consider social interventions such as practical problem-solving to deal with any legal, financial and child custody issues that might have arisen following the divorce. These may be the psychosocial factors causing this man great distress and exacerbating his illness. I would hope that this combination of treatments would control this man's symptoms.

ANSWERS TO SUGGESTED PROBES

1. The feature that suggests a diagnosis of adjustment disorder is onset precipitated by life events/psychosocial stressor in the form of the patient's separation from his wife.
2. I would consider admission in this patient in the event of:
   - non-remission of symptoms
   - unclear diagnosis
   - the presence of risk and safety issues.
3. If the patient became confused 24 hours after admission, my main concern would be that he may have developed an acute medical complication such as water intoxication, hyponatraemia, rhabdomyolysis, renal failure, compartment syndrome or epileptic fit, or be slipping into coma and death.

BUZZ WORDS AND USEFUL TERMINOLOGY

Psychogenic polydipsia, SIADH.

REFERENCES AND SUGGESTED READING

Strain J J, Newcorn J, Cartagena-Rochas A 2002 Adjustment disorders. In: Gelder M G, López-Ibor Jr J J, Andreasen N C (eds) New Oxford Textbook of Psychiatry, vol. 1. Oxford University Press, Oxford, pp 774–775
Korzets A, Ori Y, Floro S et al 1996 Severe hyponatremia after water intoxication. American Journal of Medical Science 312(2):92–94
Kulkarni J, McLachlan R, Copolov D 1985 The medical and psychological investigation of psychogenic polydipsia. British Journal of Psychiatry 146:545–547
Singh S, Padi M H, Bullard et al 1985 Water intoxication in psychiatric patients. British Journal of Psychiatry 146:127–131

3.2   52-YEAR-OLD WITH LITTLE OR NO RESPONSE TO TWO DIFFERENT ANTIDEPRESSANTS

You have just resumed duty as the specialist (or senior) registrar on an acute psychiatric ward. Your predecessor has handed over to you a 52-year-old woman who has not responded to two antidepressant treatments for recurrent depressive disorder over the last 7 months.
What would be your line of management?

SUGGESTED PROBES

1. What further information would you seek to enable you to proceed?
2. How would you approach the problem?
3. What further treatment(s) would you give?

PMP PLAN

TASKS TO DO

The following five areas are relevant to this vignette but are not necessarily all-inclusive. The list is also not exhaustive:

a) Show awareness of risk and safety issues.
b) Demonstrate a systematic approach in the management of treatment-resistant depression.
c) Demonstrate knowledge of possible causes and establish whether there are factors maintaining illness.
d) Show awareness of treatment guidelines, including uses and complications of combination therapy.
e) Show awareness of the need for multidisciplinary involvement.

ISSUES

- Review treatments so far and ascertaining patient has actually got a treatment-resistant depression
- Deciding on further treatment options including change or augmentation of current therapy.

CLARIFY

- Are there any safety concerns?

SEEK MORE INFORMATION

MEDICAL NOTES AND DRUG CHART

- Past and present symptomatology; the presence of medical problems such as thyroid, cardiac or other physical disease
- Review of physical examination, investigations and use of depressogenic medication, e.g. thiazide diuretics and other antihypertensives
- Detailed medication history
- Compliance with medication.

MEDICAL AND NURSING STAFF

- Medication compliance, mental state and interaction on the ward
- Use of illicit drugs.

OCCUPATIONAL THERAPIST/PSYCHOLOGIST

- Engagement in sessions, presentation and views on diagnosis and management.

PATIENT

- History to establish the presence of any psychosocial maintaining factors or substance misuse and also to carry out a detailed current mental state examination
- Any discharge anxieties, social isolation or financial problems.

DIFFERENTIAL DIAGNOSIS/DIFFICULTIES

- *Functional.* Treatment-resistant depression, recurrent depressive disorder, schizoaffective disorder, simple schizophrenia
- *Organic.* For example, mood disorder secondary to endocrine disorders such as thyroid disorders, Cushing's disease and hyperparathyroidism.

APPROACH TO TREATMENT

- Take a multidisciplinary approach.

WHAT TREATMENT/ADVICE

BIOLOGICAL

- Trial of alternative antidepressants bearing in mind the various stages of treatment-resistant depression as shown on Table 3.1.

Table 3.1 Stages of treatment-resistant depression

Stage	Intervention
1	Failure of at least one adequate trial of one major class of antidepressant
2	Stage 1 plus failure to respond to adequate trial of antidepressant from a different class
3	Stage 2 plus failure to respond to lithium augmentation
4	Stage 3 plus failure to respond to monoamine oxidase inhibitor
5	Stage 4 plus failure to respond to electroconvulsive therapy

PSYCHOLOGICAL

- Use cognitive behavioural therapy, either in a group or individually.

SOCIAL

- Give practical help and advice, and problem-orientated treatment.
- Offer assistance with relationships, family and children (if she still has children living at home or causing a problem).

FULL ANSWER

This lady's presentation is very suggestive of a depressive illness that has not responded well to treatment. In managing this case, I would first like to clarify whether there are any safety concerns that need immediate attention. Second, I would seek more information from the patient's medical notes on her past and present symptoms, and the presence of medical problems such as thyroid, cardiac or other physical disorders that might cause depression. I would find out whether she is taking any medication that might cause depression. I would review physical examinations and investigations (such as thyroid function tests) that have already been carried out. Next, I would talk to nursing staff regarding her compliance with medication, and ask about her appetite, sleep, interaction with other patients and staff, and level of engagement during one-to-one sessions with her key nurse. I would seek the views of the occupational therapist and psychologist involved in her care on her presentation and management. I would interview the patient to rule out any psychosocial factor that could have precipitated and maintained the illness. In addition, I would rule out the possibility of drug and alcohol misuse, which may still take place whilst the patient is in hospital.

Once I had reviewed relevant aspects of her presentation, I would look into the medication history, paying attention to her past antidepressant treatment, the dose and duration of each treatment. I would enquire about side-effects to establish whether they had contributed to possible poor compliance. I would consider enlisting the help of the hospital pharmacy to generate a detailed medication history. Having looked at and ruled out the possibility of an alternative diagnosis, comorbid problems such as the use of drugs or alcohol, poor medication compliance and psychosocial maintaining factors, I would consider a broad range of biopsychosocial intervention. As far as biological treatment is concerned, I would use a different class of antidepressant at an adequate dose and for an adequate length of time, usually about 6–8 weeks. Should this fail, I would augment her treatment with one of several medications such as lithium or tri-iodothyronine. L-tryptophan can also be used for augmentation. I would look out for the possibility of serotonin toxicity. If my augmentation strategy failed, I would consider the use of monoamine oxidase inhibitors. If these also failed, the next stage would be to consider electroconvulsive therapy. If there were any urgency, such as in the presence of very severe dehydration, severe psychotic depression or psychomotor retardation or agitation, I would consider ECT at a much earlier stage. If this lady were unwilling to consent to ECT, appropriate sections of the Mental Health Act would be implemented, once I believed that such treatment was in the patient's best interests and was urgently needed. In England and Wales, the administration of ECT requires the patient's consent or application of Section 58 (second opinion). If there is a need for urgent treatment, an application can be made under Section 62, which would provide for the continuation of emergency treatment up to the point at which the crisis that made urgent treatment necessary is brought to an end.

Psychologically, I would consider combining her pharmacological treatment with cognitive behavioural therapy, either in a group or individually. Socially, any marital, occupational or financial difficulties could be explored and practical help and advice given. If there were marital or family problems, treatment in the form of marital or family therapy would also be considered.

ANSWERS TO SUGGESTED PROBES

See the full answer above.

BUZZ WORDS AND USEFUL TERMINOLOGY

Psychosocial stressors.

REFERENCES AND SUGGESTED READING

Cowen P J 1999 Pharmacological management of treatment-resistant depression. In: Lee A. Recent Topics from Advances in Psychiatric Treatment, vol. 2. Gaskell, London, pp 52–59

Moorey S 1998 Psychological treatment of depression. In: Stein G, Wilkinson G (eds) Seminars in General Adult Psychiatry, vol. 1. Gaskell, London, pp 243–271

Stimpson N, Agrawal N, Lewis G 2002 Randomised controlled trials investigating pharmacological and psychological interventions for treatment-refractory depression. British Journal of Psychiatry 181:284–294

3.3 34-YEAR-OLD PATIENT WITH BIPOLAR ILLNESS FOUND HAVING SEX IN PUBLIC

The forensic medical officer (or police surgeon) has referred to you a 34-year-old female who was arrested after being found having sex in a public place. She is known to suffer from bipolar affective disorder and there have been several episodes of similar behaviour in the past. One of her children is in care and the other two have been adopted. You suspect she is having a relapse of her illness.

How would you go about assessment and management?

SUGGESTED PROBES

1. What factors will increase her risk?
2. During admission the patient thinks she has HIV and asks for further investigation. What would you do?
3. A week into her admission she complains about three male staff indecently assaulting her. How will you manage?

PMP PLAN

TASKS TO DO

The following five areas are relevant to this vignette but are not necessarily all-inclusive. The list is also not exhaustive:

a) Understand the risk of inappropriate sexual behaviour in patients with mental illness including bipolar affective disorder.
b) Carry out a systemic evaluation of risk and assessment.
c) Discuss the need for appropriate treatment to reduce the risks.
d) Consider the mental health law and legal framework that may be useful in treatment.
e) Show an awareness of a multimodal and multidisciplinary approach to treatment and risk management including follow-ups.

ISSUES

- Determination as to whether this sexual behaviour is due to deterioration in her mental illness
- Assessment of the risk that this patient poses
- Institution of appropriate management, monitoring and follow-up plans to forestall future occurrence and minimize risks.

CLARIFY

- Is there a history of mental illness or learning difficulties in the participating partner?
- Is coercion or exploitation involved?
- Have any charges been brought against the patient or her participating partner?

SEEK MORE INFORMATION

GP

- History of mental illness
- About responsible mental health services previously involved
- Previous treatment for repeated sexually transmitted disease (STD) and unwanted pregnancies.

MENTAL HEALTH SERVICE

- Diagnosis and treatment
- Follow-up arrangements
- Compliance
- When the patient was last seen, what were the scenario(s) and relapse indicators?

PATIENT

- Identification of the participating partner (is the partner mentally ill or known to mental health services?)
- Coercion, exploitation, protected or non-protected sex, use of contraceptives, male and female condom, pregnancy and STD
- Symptoms of mania: elation of mood, over-familiar, sexual disinhibition, thought disorder, pressure of thought, flight of ideas
- Delusions of love, overvalued ideas of love, grandiose delusion, extent of vulnerability, use of illicit drugs, prostitution
- Living alone or taking care of any children?

DIFFERENTIAL DIAGNOSIS/DIFFICULTIES

- *Functional.* Bipolar illness, schizoaffective disorder
- *Organic.* Learning disability.

APPROACH TO TREATMENT

- Adopt a non-judgmental approach.
- Suggest that staff have concerns about her vulnerability.

- Suggest hospital admission or assessment under the Mental Health Act if necessary.
- Consider gender issues during assessment to prevent further untoward behaviour or spurious allegations.

WHAT TREATMENT/ADVICE

IMMEDIATE

- Rule out physical injuries, STDs, pregnancy.
- Treat mood disorder; re-establish on a mood stabilizer, use antipsychotics and benzodiazepines, if necessary.

SHORT-TERM MEASURES

- Instigate nursing observation on the ward.
- Reduce contact with male patients and staff, to avoid unwarranted allegations or complaints.
- Give supportive psychotherapy. Psychological work includes insight orientation work, illness and risk awareness, and compliance therapy.
- Offer substance misuse counselling if addiction is a problem.

LONG-TERM MEASURES

- Think about discharge planning.
- Consider medication compliance, depot antipsychotics, further closer support and monitoring (including enhanced Care Programme Approach (CPA) in England) outpatient department appointments, and assertive outreach treatment team referral.
- Consider the legal framework for supervision after discharge (Section 25 in England and Wales).
- Give contraceptive advice; sterilization should be suggested. Sexual health promotion.
- Arrange supported accommodation, if the patient is living alone.

FULL ANSWER

In attending to this woman's case, I would first of all want to ensure that she is safe and to clarify whether the sex was consensual or not. I would ask about the exact location of the incident, and whether the patient appeared unwell at the time. I would find out who she was having sex with and whether this person was arrested too or is known to the mental health services. I would find out whether their liaison is consensual or whether there is any coercion by the participating partner, a threat to the patient's life or any form of exploitation. I would also clarify with the police whether any charge was brought against the patient or her partner. One of the main issues that I would be concerned with is determining whether this sexual behaviour is due to a deterioration in her mental illness. I would also assess the risk that this lady poses, with a view to instituting appropriate management, monitoring and follow-up plans to forestall future occurrence and minimize risks.

I would seek more information from the GP or from any mental health services that might be involved, and also from the patient. I would ask the GP whether this woman has had episodes of repeated sexually transmitted diseases or unwanted pregnancies in the past, and under what circumstances these came about. I would ask the mental health service managing her about the kind of treatment she is undergoing, what the follow-up arrangements are, and when she was last seen. I would find out about her compliance with treatment plans, her relapse indicators and the kinds of situation she has put herself in the past. If the patient were still at the police station, I would arrange to see her with a female officer. Otherwise, I would see her on the psychiatric unit with another colleague, preferably a female staff member, to reassure her, make her more comfortable and protect myself against possible unwanted and unsubstantiated accusations. I would make an effort to ascertain the identity of the person she was having sex with and to find out if there was any element of coercion or exploitation on the part of that person. I would enquire whether she has been having protected sex, whether she is using any contraception or whether the participating partner used a condom. I would look for evidence of elation of mood, over-familiarity, sexual disinhibition, thought disorder, flight of ideas, ideas and delusions of love, overvalued ideas of love and grandiose delusions, and assess the extent of her vulnerability including risk to children and the use of illicit drugs. I would also tactically establish whether she has been prostituting herself for money to maintain herself or to buy illicit drugs. I would find out about any possible pregnancy or sexually transmitted disease and look for any symptoms that might suggest these. If they were present, I would refer to my colleagues at the genitourinary medicine department for assistance.

While I have been told this lady has a diagnosis of bipolar affective illness I would also remember that there might be an associated learning disability. In my approach to treatment I would try to engage her and put to her our concerns about her vulnerability, bearing in mind that she might expose herself to unwanted pregnancies, STDs, physical and emotional abuse and a further deterioration in her mental state. I would suggest hospital admission for further assessment and treatment. If she refused this offer, I would consider the risk of her returning to further chaotic and risky living. If this were high, I would assess her under the relevant mental health law (assessment order and treatment order, Sections 2 and 3 respectively of the Mental Health Act 1983 in England and Wales). While doing this I would also consider the setting in which this lady might be best managed, a single-sex unit if at all possible.

Once a suitable unit had been identified, her immediate management and treatment plan would include the ruling out of any physical injury, STD or pregnancy, and I would ask a gynaecologist to see her as soon as possible, particularly if the sexual intercourse was not fully consensual. In the immediate term I would treat her mood disorder and re-establish her on a mood stabilizer using lithium, carbamazepine, sodium valproate or any other suitable one. If necessary, antipsychotics and benzodiazepines would be used to treat a manic or hypomanic episode. I would carry out investigations including FBC, U and Es, TFTs, RFTs and ECG. I would measure the lithium, carbamazepine or sodium valproate levels in the blood to see whether they were adequate and to ensure compliance. I would also examine for evidence of depression and suicidality. I would ensure she has adequate sleep and give medication for sedation if necessary.

As part of the management I would also arrange for nursing observation, preferably on a one-to-one basis, and would offer her supportive psychotherapy and the opportunity to speak to staff about her distress and concerns. As far as possible I would seek to reduce contact with male staff to avoid unsubstantiated allegations about sexual harassment or assaults. If the patient settled well on the ward in the short term, we would be thinking of carrying out psychological treatment focusing on insight, illness and risk awareness, assertiveness, compliance with medication, and drug misuse if there is any. I would expect this lady to continue to improve with adequate monitoring and support, treatment with medication and psychological support. In the long term, while considering discharge, I would discuss with her the need for further closer monitoring and, in particular, support from the outpatient clinic, with a view to ensuring compliance and monitoring mental state. There would be a referral to the local assertive outreach team, if one were available, and I would consider using an appropriate legal framework for supervision after discharge, such as under Section 25 (After-Care Under Supervision/Supervised Discharge) of the Mental Health Act and the enhanced Care Programme Approach (CPA) in England.

I would also make sure that she receives the necessary contraception advice, including an offer of permanent sterilization if appropriate. Sexual health promotion would be incorporated into her care to enable her to make informed choices as to appropriate contraception and to give her the opportunity to explore acceptable boundaries in different types of interpersonal relationship. In order to continue to monitor her and give her support, it might be useful to consider the use of supported accommodation if her living on her own is thought to be too risky. By putting this immediate, short-term and long-term management in place, we would try to reduce the risk of future inappropriate behaviour in this woman.

ANSWERS TO SUGGESTED PROBES

1. The factors that would increase her risk are:
   - sexual disinhibition dominating her presentation during illness
   - her vulnerability in consenting to sex with another vulnerable male with possible mental health problems
   - lack of insight, loss of self-esteem, living alone
   - poor financial status
   - use of alcohol and drugs and the need to finance habits
   - having multiple partners
   - poor compliance with medication and default on follow-ups.

2. If this patient thought that she might have HIV, I would take her concerns very seriously. I would find out whether she has any other STD and would refer her straight away to the STD clinic, which would advise her on the need for an HIV test according to the local protocol. The issue of informed consent for such testing would be paramount and we would seek the opinion of other colleagues in coming to a conclusion as to whether this woman has the capacity to make that judgment or not. In the management of the outcome of the testing, I would be guided by the advice from the STD clinic.

3. If the patient complained about three male staff members indecently assaulting her, I would take her very seriously, even though this allegation is likely to prove unfounded or unsubstantiated. I would document clearly and seek the advice of the legal department. I would follow the local agreed protocols on accusation of staff. I would ask female staff to carry out close observation in order to protect the male staff from further allegations. Due to practical problems in providing female staff at all times, it might be necessary to

move this lady to another unit, preferably a female-only one. This type of facility might not exist locally, which could be a problem. If there were issues with compliance and no response to medication, I would seek to nurse this patient in a special unit or an intensive care area, where she could be monitored and her compliance checked properly.

BUZZ WORDS AND USEFUL TERMINOLOGY

Compliance, relapse indicators, relapse prevention, psychoeducation, vulnerability, assessment and treatment order, sexual health promotion.

REFERENCES AND SUGGESTED READING

Colom F, Vieta A, Martinez-Aran A et al 2003 A randomised trial on the efficacy of group psychoeducation in the prophylaxis of recurrences in bipolar patients whose disease is in remission. Archives of General Psychiatry 60(4):402–407

Goodwin G M 2003 Evidence-based guidelines for treating bipolar disorder: recommendations from the British Association for Psychopharmacology. Journal of Psychopharmacology 17(2):149–173

Raja M, Azzoni A 2003 Sexual behaviour and sexual problems among patients with severe chronic psychoses. European Psychiatry 18(2):70–76

3.4   57-YEAR-OLD FEMALE EXCESSIVELY AND REPEATEDLY FOLDING HER CLOTHES

You have been asked to see a 57–year-old widow who has become engrossed in repeatedly folding and refolding the clothes in her bedroom. She rearranges them until a particular order is achieved and then starts again. She no longer goes out during the day, even to cash her benefits. How would you go about assessment and treatment?

SUGGESTED PROBES

1. What role is there for systematic desensitization?
2. If this patient failed to respond to treatment, what conditions and symptoms would you be concerned about?
3. If you had the choice between medication and behavioural treatments, what would you offer the patient?

PMP PLAN

TASKS TO DO

The following five areas are relevant to this vignette but are not necessarily all-inclusive. The list is also not exhaustive:

a) Give a differential diagnosis including depression, obsessive-compulsive disorder (OCD) and the possible role of bereavement in her presentation.

b) Seek more information on the nature of her symptoms and the temporal sequence of the problem in relation to her bereavement.

c) Consider the risk of self-harm and/or suicide and exhaustion, and admission to hospital if necessary.

d) Include biological and psychological aspects in your approach to treatment. A good candidate would discuss the issue of the acceptability of treatment options, compliance and treatment failure.

e) Demonstrate a knowledge of objective measures of treatment response and of the literature to support your treatment approaches.

ISSUES

- Ascertaining diagnoses after detailed assessment.
- Institution of appropriate management with consideration given to risk issues.

CLARIFY

- What is the nature of the symptoms, their temporal sequence and their relationship to the patient's bereavement?
- How are the symptoms impacting on and disrupting the patient's life?
- What is the past psychiatric history?

SEEK MORE INFORMATION

GP

- Medical history, presentation and treatment for psychiatric illness in the past.

MENTAL HEALTH SERVICES

- If she is known to any, her presentation, diagnosis and treatments.

PATIENT

- Symptoms suggestive of OCD, depression and anxiety, possible psychotic symptoms and pathological grief (abnormal bereavement reaction). Family history of OCD and Tourette's
- Look for evidence of self-neglect.

DIFFERENTIAL DIAGNOSIS/DIFFICULTIES

- *Functional.* OCD, psychotic depression, generalized anxiety disorder, bereavement and monosymptomatic delusions, and other schizophrenia-like illness and hypochondriasis
- *Organic.* Head injury, memory difficulties, organic orderliness in the context of presenile dementia, partial complex seizures, hypoparathyroidism and acute intermittent porphyria.

APPROACH TO TREATMENT

- Assess the patient's degree of insight and motivation for treatment.
- Involve her family in the assessment.
- Engage the patient.

- Educate and admit her for further assessment and treatment if indicated.
- Assess risks.

WHAT TREATMENT/ADVICE

MEDICAL

- Prescribe an antidepressant: a selective serotonin re-uptake inhibitor (SSRI).
- Treat with atypical antipsychotics if symptoms are part of a psychotic illness.
- Consider a combination of SSRIs and exposure and response prevention (ERP) treatments.
- Consider augmentation in refractory cases using buspirone, clonazepam, fenfluramine, gabapentin, lithium and L-tryptophan.
- Consider adding clomipramine to an SSRI.
- Consider inpatient treatment.

PSYCHOLOGICAL

- Arrange for ERP, cognitive behavioural therapy (CBT) for depression and anxiety, and bereavement counselling if indicated.

SOCIAL

- Give assistance towards obtaining benefit, vocational activities and day care services.

FULL ANSWER

My immediate concern would be to find out the cause of the patient's problems and to exclude any risk or safety concern. I would want to clarify the duration of her symptoms, map out the sequence of events, find out if the symptoms have any relationship to her bereavement and what impact they have had on her life, and assess whether there is a significant risk of self-harm and self-neglect. Prior to seeing this woman, I would seek more background information and ask the GP for a relevant medical and psychiatric history, in particular relating to anxiety, depression, obsessive-compulsive disorder and psychosis, and eating disorder. I would also find out about past treatment and treatment response. If she were known to the local mental health service, I would find out exactly what her presentations and diagnosis have been, and the treatments that were given.

I would arrange to see her at home with one my colleagues and/or her GP. I would explore whether a family member who knows her well (such as her son, daughter or other close relative or friend) could be present during the assessment to give a corroborative account. Seeing her at home would give us the opportunity to see her current living conditions and any evidence of neglect or other impact her illness has had on her. On seeing her, I would take a brief history, carry out a mental state examination and review her for any significant physical condition that might be relevant, such as the presence of liver disease or a cardiac condition. The latter would be important should the need to prescribe an antidepressant or other psychotropic arise. In my history I would be particularly interested in any past psychiatric issues and treatment for depression, phobia, anxiety or 'nerves'. I would find out if there is a family history of such conditions or of OCD. I would find out how soon after she lost her husband the symptoms started and how she has coped.

I would specifically look for symptoms suggestive of OCD and find out about the nature of the recurrent thoughts that precede the compulsive act of folding and refolding. I would ask for her opinion about what she is thinking and doing: whether she thinks these are her own thoughts and acts, whether she finds them pointless and senseless or whether she rationalizes them. I would explore whether she makes efforts to resist the acts and feels anxious when she tries to resist, and whether acting relieves the anxiety. I would try to establish the significance of her arranging clothes in a particular order, and whether she feels threatened or perceives a potential harm if the clothes are not in a particular order, and whether she feels that her compulsive acts prevent some objectively unlikely event. If that were the case, I would consider OCD first of all in my differential diagnosis. OCD may be either primary or secondary to an underlying depressive disorder or psychotic illness. I would also consider the possibility of generalized anxiety disorders, monosymptomatic delusions, hypochondriasis, other schizophrenia-like illnesses and an abnormal bereavement reaction. The condition may also be due to an organic orderliness in the context of a presenile dementia, head injury and memory difficulties, partial complex seizures, hypoparathyroidism, and acute intermittent porphyria.

In my approach to treatment and management, I would seek to involve the family and also educate them. I would consider the risk of suicide or self-harm, self-neglect and exhaustion, which may be associated with her repeated actions, and also the possibility that this lady may be severely depressed. The decision as to whether to manage her as an outpatient or inpatient would be guided by the severity of her illness, the risk of harm and suicide, the availability of family support and the wishes of the patient. If this patient were considered to be at high risk of self-neglect, exhaustion or suicide, I would consider admitting her to hospital, either formally or informally. This would also enable closer monitoring and management of her risks. I would consider pharmacological and psychological treatments (including bereavement counselling) and the social support that can be given. Before commencing treatment, I would use the Yale–Brown Obsessive-Compulsive Scale (Y–BOCS Symptoms Checklist), an objective validated instrument for assessing the degree of her OCD symptoms as a baseline. I would couple this with continuous clinical assessment of mental state and function.

As regards pharmacological treatment, I would consider the use of clomipramine or an SSRI that has been found to significantly reduce symptoms in up to 60% of patients suffering from OCD after 10 weeks of treatment. I would give 200–300 mg of clomipramine for up to 10–12 weeks before determining the response to ensure that an adequate dose has been given. I would consider the use of other SSRIs such as fluoxetine, fluvoxamine, paroxetine, sertraline and citalopram if necessary, or if the patient does not tolerate clomipramine. (Caution needs to be exercised in patients with cardiovascular problems or closed-angle glaucoma.) This would also be useful in the treatment of concurrent anxiety and/or a depression component to her illness and presentation. I would only use antipsychotics if there were an underlying psychotic illness or symptoms. If, following treatment, the presentation suggested a treatment-refractory condition, I would consider using augmentation therapy with buspirone, clonazepam, fenfluramine, gabapentin, lithium and L-tryptophan. I would also consider adding clomipramine to an SSRI under expert supervision and guidance in an inpatient treatment setting.

Concerning psychological treatments, I would explore graduated or graded exposure combined with self-imposed response prevention techniques (exposure and response prevention (ERP)). I would assess the patient's degree of insight into the irrationality of the behaviour as this might influence her willingness to cooperate in ERP. I would explain at the outset that the treatment would provoke anxiety, but that she would need to persevere with it. I would then refer her to a therapist who is skilled in the use of this method. Usually, the patient would be asked to choose a cue that provokes mild to moderate anxiety. In this case that would be the clothes. The exposure to these clothes would be coupled with refraining, for 1 or 2 hours, from performing the usual anxiety-relieving compulsion, the refolding of clothes. I would also encourage a detailed written ERP homework assignment, which the woman should carry out several times daily in order to break the connection between the stimulus (the clothes) and the provoked anxiety. Some researchers have suggested a 75–80% significant symptom reduction in patients who engage in treatment.

If depression formed a major component of her illness, cognitive behavioural therapy might also be useful. I would explore the need to offer bereavement counselling to this lady after many of her OCD symptoms have settled. Others measures that would form part of her treatment include social support. I would refer to the team social worker to see what assistance could be given to the patient and/or her carer with a view to obtaining the appropriate benefits and social supports. I would suggest that she is allocated a CPN or care coordinator to check on her from time to time. I would also facilitate a referral to a day programme where she could have access to useful day vocational activities.

ANSWERS TO SUGGESTED PROBES

1. Systematic desensitization is not a treatment for OCD. It is used in the treatment of phobias.
2. According to Foa (1978), 15% of the patients who did not respond to treatment have:
   - a strong conviction about the rationality of their obsessive beliefs
   - prominent major depression
   - a comorbid tic disorder
   - an underlying medical condition.

   The medical conditions that may predispose to OCD are:
   - head trauma
   - cerebrovascular accident
   - neurodegenerative disorder such as Huntington's disease
   - infections such as HIV and encephalitis lethargica
   - Tourette's syndrome (just in case you mention or are asked about Gilles de la Tourette's syndrome or if this forms part of the probes from the examiner, it is useful to know that the point prevalence for Tourette's disorder is about 0.05–5.2 per 10 000 and the lifetime prevalence in the general population for OCD is between 1% and 3%. The prevalence is about three to four times higher in males than females)

- partial complex seizures
- hypoparathyroidism
- acute intermittent porphyria.

3. As regards treatment, while I would be guided by the wishes of the patient, I would prefer to use a combination of both biological and cognitive behavioural therapy. The various medications that have been found useful are clomipramine, fluoxetine, fluvoxamine, paroxetine, citalopram, sertraline and venlafaxine.

BUZZ WORDS AND USEFUL TERMINOLOGY

Engage, rituals, compulsions, refractory condition.

REFERENCES AND SUGGESTED READING

Clomipramine Collaborative Study Group 1991 Clomipramine in the treatment of patients with obsessive-compulsive disorder. Archives of General Psychiatry 48:730–738

Foa E B, Chambless D L 1978 Habituation of subjective anxiety during flooding in imagery. Behaviour Research and Therapy 16(6):391–399

Karno M, Golding J M, Sorenson S B 1988 The epidemiology of obsessive-compulsive disorder in five US communities. Archives of General Psychiatry 45:1094–1099

Koran L M 1999 Obsessive-compulsive and Related Disorders in Adults: a Comprehensive Clinical Guide. Cambridge University Press, Cambridge

Stern R, Drummond L 1991 The Practice of Behavioural and Cognitive Psychotherapy. Cambridge University Press, Cambridge

A 26-year-old male with what appears to be the first episode of a manic illness is admitted to your ward. Staff have noticed that he suffers from episodes of uncontrollable aggression, which seem to become more apparent shortly after visits from friends or family members. He has to be given up to 80 mg daily of haloperidol, as well as other psychotropic medications, with limited benefit.

How would you manage this patient?

SUGGESTED PROBES

1. What are the alternatives to haloperidol in the management of this patient?
2. You have discovered he has a history of bipolar affective disorder and that he has only responded to high doses of antipsychotics like haloperidol. What would you do, i.e. what precautionary measures would you take?
3. Six weeks into treatment with haloperidol, the patient starts feeling quite agitated and 'can't keep still'. What is the most likely diagnosis and how would you manage?

PMP PLAN

TASKS TO DO

The following five areas are relevant to this vignette but are not necessarily all-inclusive. The list is also not exhaustive:

a) Take a systematic approach to assessment and management.
b) Consider the various reasons why the patient is not responding: for example, his physical condition, a psychological problem or a reaction to social stressors. A good candidate would also consider the possibility of patient being given illicit drug by visiting friends or relatives.
c) Demonstrate an awareness of the various risk issues: for example, harm to self, harm to others and risk of cardiac complications from the use of a high-dose antipsychotic.
d) Demonstrate knowledge of the various alternatives to haloperidol in the management of this patient.

e) If you decide to continue high-dose haloperidol, you should demonstrate that you can be trusted to practise safely, i.e. by taking the necessary precautionary measures such as ECG monitoring and/or seeking a second opinion.

ISSUES

- Determination of the diagnosis and whether there is a link between the aggressive behaviour and visits from friends and family
- Management at a facility or place that is safe for the patient and the staff.

CLARIFY

- Are there any immediate safety concerns? Uppermost would be the safety and health of this patient (self-harm, physical exhaustion and cardiac arrest from high-dose antipsychotics) and others (other clients and staff).

SEEK MORE INFORMATION

Seek more information at the earliest opportunity from the nursing staff, ward doctor, psychologist, occupational therapist and others who might have been involved in the patient's care.

NURSING STAFF

- The patient's mental state
- Reviews of reason for non-response, i.e. poor medication compliance or use of illicit drugs.

WARD DOCTOR

- The circumstances leading to admission
- Patient symptomatology
- Results of physical examination and investigations
- The patient's past psychiatric, medical and medication history.

REVIEW

- Outcome of interview with relatives or any other collaborative information.

PATIENT

- Review the patient, preferably accompanied by staff
- Presentation, in particular current symptoms/signs suggestive of a manic episode, such as mood elation of at least 1 week's duration, hyperactivity, development of many new interests, decreased need for sleep and disinhibited behaviour
- Other relevant medical/past psychiatric history and possible illicit drug use
- Any investigations already done; consider further investigations.

DIFFERENTIAL DIAGNOSIS/DIFFICULTIES

- Manic episode in the context of bipolar affective disorder
- Manic episode secondary to various physical or drug-related conditions (see Box 3.1).

APPROACH TO TREATMENT

- Pay immediate attention to any risk or safety issues.
- Review available information.
- Decide on the reason for failure to respond to such a high dose of antipsychotic. If cause can be identified, treat appropriately. Consider:
  - wrong diagnosis: treat underlying problem
  - physical problem: refer to appropriate medical specialties
  - drug use: withdraw offending drug

Box 3.1 Drugs and organic conditions that can cause manic episodes

Drug use/medical condition	Drug withdrawal	Organic brain disorder
Psychostimulants	Fenfluramine	Cerebrovascular disease
Amphetamine	Baclofen	Head injury
Cocaine	Clonidine	Cerebral tumour
Recreational drugs		Epilepsy
Cannabis		Multiple sclerosis
Alcohol		Dementia
Medication		
Steroids		
Endocrine/metabolic conditions		
Thyrotoxicosis		

- poor medication compliance: consider the intramuscular route, at least until the patient develops insight and appreciates the need to take medication.
- If the lack of response is not due to any of the above, there may be the need for a comprehensive review of treatment and management plan.

WHAT TREATMENT/ADVICE

MEDICAL

- Treatment options include a decreased dose of haloperidol or gradual substitution with another psychotropic like olanzapine (dispersible or velotabs).
- Alternatively, continue haloperidol with regular ECG monitoring and consider a second opinion.
- Exclude organic mood disorder.
- Consider mood stabilizers like lithium, or sodium valproate treatment.
- Consider adding a benzodiazepine.
- Consider the use of other protective antimanic agents like lamotrigine, gabapentin and clozapine or risperidone.

PSYCHOTHERAPEUTIC

- Use approaches like family therapy to address any psychosocial problems.
- Consider cognitive behavioural therapy in the longer term (i.e. after an acute episode) for relapse prevention.

FULL ANSWER

The issues that I would like to address in this situation are determining the diagnosis and whether there is any link with the aggressive behaviour and the visits from friends and family. I would also consider this man's management at a facility or place that is safe for the patient and the staff. The presentation in this 26-year-old man demands prompt attention, given the various risks involved and also the need to get him better as soon as possible. With regard to risk, I would consider risk to the patient in terms of physical exhaustion, accidental injury and also sudden death from a high dose of antipsychotic medication. There is also the risk of harm to staff or other patients due to his uncontrollable episodes of aggression.

To begin with, I would like to clarify with staff whether they have any other concerns and also try to analyse his behaviour functionally in terms of the antecedent, details of the behaviour and what happened afterwards. Next, I would attend the ward to assess this man after seeking more information, especially from the nursing staff, focusing on the details of his mental state, behaviour on the ward and whether staff have any concerns over medication non-compliance. I would also obtain collaborative information from other relevant members of the team, for example, a psychologist or occupational therapist who might have been involved in his care. It would also be useful to talk to the ward doctor to have more idea of the circumstances leading to his admission, the patient symptomatology, results of physical examination and investigations, and details of the patient's past psychiatric, medical and detailed medication history. I would also consider talking to his relatives or checking the notes for any information that might have been taken from them. When I saw this patient, preferably accompanied by a staff member given his history of aggression, I would ask him to describe the circumstances leading to his admission in chronological order, and his symptoms then and now, and would also observe him during the interview looking for evidence of a manic illness such as elation of mood of at least 1 week's duration, hyperactivity, a reduced need for sleep, and disinhibited behaviour. I would also assess for the presence of psychotic symptoms; in case it is related to his aggressive outburst, I would enquire about the use of illicit drugs and also his insight into the nature of his illness.

Prior to making any alteration in or adjustment to this man's medication, I would bear in mind that his presentation might truly be a manic episode in the context of a bipolar affective disorder, which unfortunately has not responded to a high dose of haloperidol. I would also consider the possibility that the manic episode might have been secondary to various physical or drug-related problems. With regard to physical problems, I would consider organic brain disorders such as epilepsy or head injury, or medical conditions such as thyroid disease or other endocrine and metabolic conditions. It is also possible that episode was due to the use of psychoactive substances like amphetamine and cocaine or withdrawal from drugs such as clonidine or fenfluramine.

My approach to treating this man would be first to pay attention to risk and safety issues, then review the available information and try to come to a conclusion as to why he failed to respond to a high dose of haloperidol. For example, is this man suffering from a psychiatric illness other than a manic episode, such as an agitated depressive state, or is his presentation secondary to drug use or a drug withdrawal state? I would also consider the possibility of poor medication compliance. Should this be the case, I would consider using an intramuscular route for his medication, at least until he develops insight and appreciates the need to take medication. Alternatively, if I were able to confirm that he did have a manic episode and that poor response was not due to any of these reasons, I would consider making a series of adjustments to his medication including the addition of a mood stabilizer like sodium valproate, carbamazepine or lithium. Should this not help, I would add a benzodiazepine such as lorazepam. Other putative antimanic agents that I would consider using include lamotrigine, gabapentin and clozapine. If necessary, I would give consideration to psychotherapeutic approaches such as family therapy, psychosocial intervention and cognitive behavioural therapy in treating this man's problem. However, I would bear in mind that cognitive behavioural therapy might be more appropriate after the acute phase of this illness, to prevent relapse and to facilitate the early identification of any subsequent episodes. Should this man's poor response be due to a medical problem, I would refer to the appropriate specialties. Should it be due to a drug-related problem such as amphetamine or cocaine use, it might be appropriate to refer him to the drug user and alcohol liaison team for the assessment and treatment of his addiction.

ANSWERS TO SUGGESTED PROBES

1. The alternatives to haloperidol in the management of this patient have already been described.
2. With the patient's history of bipolar affective disorder and the fact that he has only responded to high doses of antipsychotics like haloperidol, I would consider continuing the haloperidol but would ensure that he has regular ECG monitoring and consider seeking a second opinion.
3. The report of inability to keep still 6 weeks into treatment on haloperidol raises the possibility of akathisia. In order to support this diagnosis, I would observe for the presence of fidgety movements or swinging of the legs, rocking from foot to foot while standing, pacing to relieve restlessness, or inability to sit or stand still for at least several minutes. Nevertheless, I would bear in mind that this complaint may well have arisen in the context of agitation as part of his manic episode or anxiety, or might well be histrionic behaviour. Given the distressing nature of these symptoms, however, which have been known to drive patients into suicidal behaviour and could have a bearing on medication

compliance in the future, I would have a low threshold for making a diagnosis of akathisia in this patient who is on a rather high dose of neuroleptic. I would therefore consider the following measures in succession:

- reducing the dose of antipsychotic medication
- switching to a low potency antipsychotic such as olanzapine, quetiapine or clozapine
- using an antimuscarinic agent like benzatropine
- using propranolol, a benzodiazepine, cyproheptadine or clonidine.

BUZZ WORDS AND USEFUL TERMINOLOGY

Risk assessment, multidisciplinary approach to assessment and management.

REFERENCES AND SUGGESTED READING

American Psychiatric Association 2002 Practice guideline for the treatment of patient with bipolar disorder. American Journal of Psychiatry 159(4) supplement:1–50

Calabrese J R, Kimmel S E, Woyshville M J et al 1996 Clozapine for treatment-refractory mania. American Journal of Psychiatry 153(6):759–764

Cookson J 1998 Mania, bipolar disorder and treatment. In: Stein G, Wilkinson G (eds) Seminars in General Adult Psychiatry, vol. 1. Gaskell, London, pp 51–101

Pi E H, Simpson G M 2000 Medication-induced movement disorders. In: Sadock B J, Sadock V A (eds) Kaplan & Sadock's, Comprehensive Textbook of Psychiatry, vol. 2, 7th edn. Lippincott, Williams and Wilkins, Philadelphia, pp 2265–2271

3.6 35-YEAR-OLD MAN WITH SCHIZOPHRENIA NOT RESPONDING TO THREE DIFFERENT ANTIPSYCHOTICS

A 35-year-old man with paranoid schizophrenia has been referred to you by the inpatient general adult psychiatrist. The patient has been treated with at least two different classes of antipsychotic but with very limited improvement in his psychotic symptoms. In your role as one of the doctors on the rehabilitation team, with the capacity to manage the patient for a much longer period, the referring psychiatrist wonders if you could take him for further assessment, treatment and rehabilitation back into the community.

How would you proceed with assessment and management?

SUGGESTED PROBES

1. Would you consider rehabilitation work in this patient? If so, what would be the focus and aims of your rehabilitation programme?
2. The patient develops tardive dyskinesia 3 months into treatment with haloperidol. How would you manage him?
3. You decide to change him to clozapine, which appears to be effective in controlling his symptoms. However, he is unhappy about dribbling saliva on his pillow every morning. How would you manage this?

PMP PLAN

TASKS TO DO

The following five areas are relevant to this vignette but are not necessarily all-inclusive. The list is also not exhaustive:

a) Take a comprehensive and systematic approach to assessment and management.
b) Enquire about his present and past symptoms, diagnosis and factors that may perpetuate resistant schizophrenia.
c) Appreciate the need to take or enquire about a detailed medication history.
d) Attempt to elicit possible predisposing, precipitating and perpetuating factors to the illness and give consideration to other diagnostic possibilities.
e) Take a multidisciplinary/multimodal approach to assessment and management.

ISSUES

- Establishing that this man does actually have treatment-resistant schizophrenia and the reason behind the treatment failure
- Detailed assessment of treatment given so far and what new treatment is likely to help
- Decision on other treatment options, including adjunctive therapies, to ensure optimal functioning.

CLARIFY

- Are there any acute symptoms?
- Is there any safety concern that might make it rather unwise to manage this patient in the more relaxed environment of the rehabilitation unit?

SEEK MORE INFORMATION

REFERRER

- Legal status
- Patient's current symptoms, past psychiatric, medical and drug history, problems with compliance or use of non-prescribed medication, most especially illicit substances, request for initial clinical (part 1) summary of the patient if available
- What his specific rehabilitation needs are considered to be.

MEDICAL RECORDS

- Review of outpatient notes with particular attention to present and past symptoms, aetiology of illness, risk and safety issues
- Detailed medication history, preferably in collaboration with the hospital pharmacist, particularly if the patient has a long history of psychiatric illness. Attention should be paid to the drug doses (within the British National Formulary (BNF) therapeutic limit in the UK) and duration of treatment (a minimum of 6–8 weeks).

PATIENT

- Thorough review of history, mental state, physical examination and investigations
- Patient's insight and whether he consented to the treatment given previously, his compliance and what he derived from the treatment

- Core beliefs/psychotic symptoms and his rationale for the beliefs. Are these beliefs shakeable?
- Strengths and weaknesses, especially in terms of functional ability. There may be a need to request an occupational therapy assessment.

KEYWORKER/NAMED NURSE

- Mental state on the ward, including level of interaction with staff and other clients
- Any evidence of abnormal experience of beliefs
- Any concern over poor medication compliance, risk and safety.

DIFFERENTIAL DIAGNOSIS/DIFFICULTIES

- *Diagnosis.* Wrong diagnosis, delusional disorders, schizoaffective disorders, comorbid substance misuse problem and organic problems such as endocrine disorders
- *Compliance.* Poor medication compliance
- *Subtherapeutic dose or duration of antipsychotic treatment.*
- *Psychosocial problems.*

APPROACH TO TREATMENT

- Ask for the latest risk assessment and other relevant documentation, such as the occupational therapy report.
- Accept the request to admit the patient to your unit, preferably after seeking the view of the liaison nurse from your team, who would hopefully assess the patient on the acute inpatient unit prior to transfer.
- Give consideration to a broad range of biopsychosocial interventions, including the use of atypical medications, cognitive behavioural therapy, family education therapy and social support (see Table 3.2).

FULL ANSWER

The presentation of this man raises the possibility of a treatment-resistant schizophrenic illness. The issues that I would like to address include establishing that this man does actually have a treatment-resistant schizophrenia and the reason behind the treatment failure. I would also carry out a detailed assessment of the treatment given so far and decide on which new treatment is likely to help this man's condition. I would then decide on other

Table 3.2 Management of treatment-resistant schizophrenia

	Biological	Psychological	Social
Immediate	Review history, physical examination and investigations	BPRS	Assessment of social situation
Short-term	Atypical antipsychotic Consider clozapine (might take up to 1 year for maximum benefit) Consider augmenting clozapine with: Sulpiride Lamotrigine Risperidone Omega 3-triglycerine Amisulpiride	CBT Family therapy Drug and alcohol team if comorbid substance misuse Social skill training Rehabilitation	Psychosocial support
Long-term	Subject to CPA? Depot if compliance a problem	Cognitive remediation Anxiety management Compliance therapy	Gentle rehabilitation to the community MIND* National Schizophrenia Fellowship* Therapeutic employment

*MIND and National Schizophrenia Fellowship are registered mental health charities offering support and advice for users in the UK.

treatment options, including adjunctive therapies, to ensure optimal functioning.

To begin with, I would like to clarify whether there are acute symptoms that require treatment before a takeover by our rehabilitation team is even considered. I would also enquire about safety concerns that might make it inappropriate to manage this patient in the more relaxed environment of a rehabilitation unit. I would ask what his specific rehabilitation needs are considered to be. This would help us to gauge whether the rehabilitation unit would be able to meet those needs.

I would then proceed to seek more information from the referrer, medical records, patient's keyworker or named (responsible) nurse, and also from the patient himself. I would ask the referring consultant about this patient's current symptoms, and his past psychiatric, medical and drug history. I would ask whether there are any problems with his compliance to medication and if he uses non-prescribed drugs, especially illicit substances. Next, I would request the initial clinical (part one) summary, the discharge summary and the risk assessment on this patient. Alternatively I would visit the ward to review his medical records, paying particular attention to his symptoms, risk and safety issues and likely predisposing, precipitating and maintaining factors for his presentation. I would take the opportunity presented by the ward visit to talk to this patient's keyworker or named nurse, enquiring specifically about his mental state on the ward, including level of interaction with staff and patients and the presence of psychotic symptoms. I would also peruse the occupational therapy report, if there were one, to have an idea of this man's level of functioning in various activities of daily living. This report would also give an insight into his strengths, which would help me to decide on what to use positively in rehabilitation.

I would see the patient on the ward to take a relevant history and seek his own insight into his illness. I would explain to him that I am from the rehabilitation unit and why I have come to see him. I would find out if positive symptoms, such as hallucination and delusions, or negative symptoms dominate his presentation, as this may influence the treatment options and approach. As far as possible, I would try to identify the patient's core beliefs about his psychotic symptoms, his rationale for these beliefs and whether they are shakeable. I would assess whether he had willingly consented to previous treatment, his compliance with medication and the benefit he thinks he derived from the treatment. What are the patient's strengths and weaknesses, especially in terms of functional ability? I would ask him about his psychosocial situation and consumption of alcohol or illicit drugs to see whether these have any relevance to his illness. I would also ask about the support he has in the community and his social network. I would find out about his perception of the impact of his illness on his life, his plans for the future, what help or treatment he thinks he needs, and what he thinks should be done. I would let him know that our team would be responsible for his day-to-day treatment, if we decided to take over his care.

Having taken the above history, I would consider the possible reasons for his treatment resistance. I would therefore seek to exclude other diagnostic possibilities and maintaining factors: for example, physical illness such as endocrine disorders (hypothyroidism or hyperthyroidism) or a brain tumour, and psychological problems such as psychotic depression and psychosocial problems. I would also consider the possibility of a delusional disorder and psychotic illness exacerbated by illicit substance use.

I would consider accepting the patient for further assessment and rehabilitation, preferably after seeking the view of the liaison nurse from our team, who would hopefully assess the patient on the acute inpatient unit prior to transfer. The initial assessment would be geared towards the review of available information (history, mental state assessments, physical examination, psychological and occupational therapy assessments and investigations), further information-gathering from patient and relatives, and a request for other relevant investigations. I would try to gain an understanding of the family history and dynamics, in particular relating to psychotic illness and a high level of expressed emotion within the family, which may respectively be predisposing and perpetuating factors in this man's illness. I would review the various drugs used in treating this man since admission to the hospital. Should it become apparent that he has a history of previous treatment, I would consider liaison with the pharmacist to obtain a more elaborate medication history. Attention would be paid to the doses and duration of treatment on these medications and the patient's response to such treatment.

Having considered all these issues, a treatment plan that would include a broad range of biological, psychological and social intervention would be formulated. This might include switching the patient to an atypical antipsychotic, if this has not already been done. If his treatment has included an atypical antipsychotic, I would consider the use of clozapine, after explaining to the patient the benefits and side-effects of the medication, the need for regular blood tests, and the likely outcome if he takes, refuses or discontinues treatment. I would ensure that the dosage is within the therapeutic range of at least 0.35 mg/litre, in accordance with the guidelines given by the Clozaril Patient Monitoring Service. I would also bear in mind that it might take up to 3–6 months or even 1 year before maximum benefit could be achieved. Should the response to clozapine be unsatisfactory, I would consider augmentation with mood stabilizers such as lamotrigine, ensuring that regular blood checks are done to prevent toxicity from clozapine, as lamotrigine decreases the metabolism.

Along with these biological interventions, I would consider the use of cognitive behavioural therapy, family therapy and psychosocial support. Treatment would also include occupational therapy assessment and interventions to promote independent living. Should there be concerns over the use of illicit drugs, I would consider referring this man to the drug and alcohol team. Part of the overall treatment plan would be to make arrangements for his care, should he relapse and need acute treatment.

ANSWER TO SUGGESTED PROBES

1. I certainly would consider rehabilitation in this man, most especially during his short- and long-term management. Such rehabilitation would focus on five main areas, namely:
   - the need for comprehensive and long-term therapy
   - individually tailored treatment programmes based on his needs
   - reduction in possible limitations the patient might suffer as a result of the illness
   - getting his family actively involved in treatment
   - maximizing his strengths and helping him redevelop his abilities.

2. Given the history of treatment with an antipsychotic and the possibility of a recent increase in that medication, it would not be unusual for the patient to develop tardive dyskinesia. To begin with, I would like to clarify that there are no other odd movements in the trunk or extremities, which are also not uncommon in tardive dyskinesia. I would check the duration of this side-effect and also its progression and the impact on the patient's self-esteem and function. Perhaps it has left him with feelings of depression or contemplating the need to keep on taking the medication. Next, I would exclude the possibility of neurological or general medical conditions such as Huntington's disease, Sydenham's chorea, spontaneous dyskinesia and hyperthyroidism. If the history suggests he has noticed this problem well before starting antipsychotic medication, it would certainly be worthwhile exploring some of these diagnostic possibilities further.

   Once I was convinced that he was suffering from tardive dyskinesia secondary to antipsychotic treatment, I would take the following steps in succession:
   - Withdraw any antimuscarinic medication.
   - Consider gradually withdrawing the antipsychotic.
   - Give clozapine, olanzapine or quetiapine, as it is essential that this man continue on his medication.
   - Try other measures such as vitamin E, clonazepam, nifedipine, sodium valproate, ondansetron, propanolol,

botulinum toxin (for tardive dystonia) and tetrabenazine (although the increased risk of depression limits its use).
3. I would first reassure him that the dribbling might wear off, but also share his concern about this side-effect of clozapine, which some patients find difficult and troublesome. Should the problem persist, the options would include hyoscine 300 μg sucked and swallowed at night. Pirenzepine is another alternative, but this drug is not licensed for use in the UK at the present time.

BUZZ WORDS AND USEFUL TERMINOLOGY

Treatment-resistant schizophrenia, drug review, biopsychosocial intervention.

REFERENCES AND SUGGESTED READING

Cree A, Mir S, Fahy T 2001 A review of treatment options for clozapine-induced hypersalivation. Psychiatric Bulletin 25:114–116

Pi E H, Simpson G M 2000 Medication-induced movement disorders. In: Sadock B J, Sadock V A (eds) Comprehensive Textbook of Psychiatry, vol. 2, 7th edn. Lippincott, Williams & Wilkins, Philadelphia, pp 2265–2271

Taylor D, McConnell H, Duncan-McConnell D, Kerwin R 2001 Clozapine — management of adverse effects: the Maudsley Prescribing Guidelines, 6th edn. Martin Dunitz, London, p 204

4

Addiction and substance misuse disorders

4.1 PATIENT ADMITTED FOR ALCOHOL DETOXIFICATION AND WHO IS ASKING FOR HELP TO QUIT SMOKING

You are the registrar on a drug and alcohol unit. While walking in the corridor of your hospital, you are stopped by one of your patients, who is currently undergoing inpatient detoxification from alcohol. He is very concerned about his excessive cigarette consumption and is asking for your help to stop smoking.

What help would you offer him and how would you go about it?

SUGGESTED PROBES

1. Do you think this is the right time for him to stop smoking?
2. How would you assess his motivation?
3. What factors would make his success in quitting smoking less likely?

PMP PLAN

TASKS TO DO

The following five areas are relevant to this vignette but are not necessarily all-inclusive. The list is also not exhaustive:

a) Discuss the need to prepare the patient adequately for treatment.
b) Arrange liaison with or referral to a smoking cessation clinic, if one is available.
c) Include biological, psychological and social means in achieving goals in your approach.
d) Demonstrate knowledge of common antismoking agents, including amfebutamone (bupropion) and the medium in which they are presented.
e) Discuss what would happen if the plan fails or if the patient finds things difficult.

- Decision as to whether it is appropriate for a patient undergoing detoxification to commence a smoking cessation programme
- Giving the patient adequate information on the various treatment options. Engagement on a smoking cessation programme.

CLARIFY

- Why has the patient decided to stop smoking at this particular time?
- What does he think are his chances of success?

SEEK MORE INFORMATION

PATIENT

- Current dependence on nicotine, using the Fagerström test questionnaire
- Success or failure of previous treatment programmes, reason for relapse, previous and current support networks
- Motivation and readiness for change.

DIFFERENTIAL DIAGNOSIS/DIFFICULTIES

- Not relevant.

APPROACH TO TREATMENT

- Complete the current detoxification and then assess the patient's readiness to change.

WHAT TREATMENT/ADVICE

HEALTH EDUCATION

- Educate about the benefits of stopping smoking, the difficulties that may arise, relapse prevention and dealing with relapses.

MEDICAL

- Offer nicotine replacement therapy (NRT), in the form of sprays, patches or chewing gums.
- Prescribe bupropion, but rule out epilepsy or seizures and hepatic disorder. Explain the side-effects, which include dry

mouth, weight loss, insomnia and, rarely, cardiac death. Give 150–250 mg b.d. for 2 weeks. After stopping smoking, the patient would continue on bupropion for another 3 months.

- Treat with an antidepressant: nortriptyline or amitriptyline.
- Use a combination of bupropion and NRT.
- Consider naltrexone.

PSYCHOLOGICAL

- Refer to smoking cessation clinic, supportive counselling, group counselling.
- Think about relapse prevention.
- Advise on weight gain.
- Reassure and advise on exercise, diet and lifestyle.

SOCIAL

- Consider referring to Nicotine Anonymous.

FULL ANSWER

I would want to thank this patient, and let him know that I appreciate him coming to let me know about his concerns regarding smoking. The main issue for me in this situation would be to decide whether it is appropriate for him to commence a smoking cessation programme at the same time as undergoing detoxification, or whether it should be deferred. The other issue is the need to assess his motivation to stop smoking and to give adequate information on the various treatment options before preparing him for engagement on a smoking cessation programme. As the meeting took place on the corridor, I would arrange for us to meet on the ward for further discussion and assessment, as well as for confidentiality and convenience. Once I had ensured that the setting was appropriate, I would clarify with the patient the main reason why he has decided to stop smoking. I would ask him to be sure that there is no pressure on him to quit at this time. I would explore the general, economic, social and health reasons why he has made this choice. I would find out whether he is strongly motivated and check what stage he is at in his detoxification programme. I would find out whether he has a good detoxification history and has tried to give up smoking before. I would seek more information on the reasons why he relapsed. I would generally suggest that, in order to optimize his chances of being substance-free, he should finish alcohol detoxification before commencing another programme to quit smoking. One of the concerns would be that immediate discontinuation of smoking would result in a relapse in his alcohol use.

Once the alcohol detoxification had finished, I would assess his level of dependence on nicotine using the Fagerström test questionnaire, which is simple and easy to administer. This would rate him on a scale ranging between very low and very high dependence. I would encourage him to set a date for stopping smoking, and to make a list of his smoking paraphernalia and make sure he gets rid of it. I would advise him to inform peers, colleagues, family and employers, if he likes, and to enlist their support. I would encourage him to tell his friends who smoke not to smoke in his house or to avoid smoking when he is present, if possible. I would enquire whether a partner, close friend or employer could give support. It might be helpful to involve them in the treatment programme if the patient agrees. It might also be useful if he could find a partner to work with, who also is willing and motivated to quit smoking. Using motivation techniques, I would try to encourage the patient to cut down his cigarette intake before treatment starts. This would also help me to assess how motivated he is.

My approach to his treatment would involve medical, psychological and social means, and I would also offer psychoeducation. As part of the latter, I would discuss with him the benefits of stopping smoking as regards his health, finances and lifestyle. I would educate him as to what he is likely to face and the risk of relapse. I would explain to him that he might feel some withdrawal symptoms, which are usually helped by nicotine replacement therapy (NRT). In order to maximize his chances of quitting smoking, I would refer him to the local smoking cessation clinic after I started him on a medical treatment option that is acceptable to him. The choice would depend on his preference and on patient factors, particularly if there were contraindications to any of the medication. To enhance his understanding, I would provide him with information leaflets and self-help brochures, if these were available.

For the medical treatment, I would suggest NRT, which can be offered in the form of sprays, patches or chewing gum. Another option would be to use bupropion after ruling out epileptic fits or seizures and hepatic disorder. I would explain the side-effects of bupropion, which include dry mouth, weight loss, insomnia and, rarely, cardiac death. I would give 150–250 mg twice a day for 2 weeks. I would advise the patient not to smoke during treatment. After he achieved smoking cessation, I would continue bupropion for another 8–12 weeks. I would also consider treatment with an antidepressant, either nortriptyline or amitriptyline, if the measures I have described did not work. The combination of bupropion and NRT has also been found to be effective, but I would watch for side-effects of this medication. It is, however, questionable whether this would increase the chances of him quitting smoking. I would stop the attempt to quit if he continued to smoke after 7 days, with the intention of trying the programme again in the future. If prompt cessation were not possible, I would advise harm reduction strategies by suggesting that the patient reduce the amount of cigarettes smoked daily. The use of naltrexone, an opioid antagonist, might be considered, since it has been shown to lead to a reduction in the number of cigarettes smoked, and would have the added advantage of helping with his alcohol dependence.

This treatment would be coupled with psychological aspects, which could be offered in groups at the smoking cessation clinic or the local day hospital. An attempt would be made to address relapse prevention, and the factors that might reduce his chances of success would be examined. These would include failure in the present alcohol detoxification programme, with subsequent relapse into the harmful use of alcohol or illicit drugs, including cannabis. Lack or withdrawal of pledges to support him, environmental and social factors such as a partner, workmates or friends who smoke, and the failure of others who are trying to quit smoking might also adversely affect him. I would look into concurrent psychosocial stressors, depression and the presence of any other mental illness.

This patient might need reassurance on the possibility that smoking cessation could be followed by weight gain. I would mention that only about 10% of quitters have very large and significant weight increases, and would provide the necessary advice on exercise, diet and lifestyle. I would consider referring him to Nicotine Anonymous for further support, if the service were available locally.

ANSWERS TO SUGGESTED PROBES

1. I do not think that this is the right time for this man to stop smoking. I would generally advise him to finish the alcohol detoxification first and to make sure he is well prepared to quit smoking before initiating smoking cessation treatment. I would ensure that he is completely free from alcohol and has a normal liver function status before initiating treatment with medications that are potentially hepatotoxic.

2. I would assess his motivation by examining:

- his stage of change, i.e. precontemplation →
  contemplation → determination → action
- his reasons for wanting this change.
3. The factors that would reduce his chances of success in
  quitting smoking are:
  - failure in the present detoxification programme and
    relapse into the harmful use of alcohol
  - the use of illicit drugs, including cannabis
  - concurrent psychosocial stressors
  - lack or withdrawal of pledges of support
  - environmental and social factors, such as a smoking
    partner, workmates or friends
  - failure of others trying to quit smoking
  - depression and other mental illness.

BUZZ WORDS AND USEFUL TERMINOLOGY

Relapse prevention, motivation, engagement, replacement therapy, psychoeducation, smoking cessation clinic.

REFERENCES AND SUGGESTED READING

Heatherton T F, Kozlowski L T, Frecker R C, Fagerström K O 1991 The
Fagerström test for nicotine dependence: a revision of the Fagerström
tolerance questionnaire. British Journal of Addiction 86:1119–1127
McEwen A, West R 2001 Smoking cessation activities by general practitioners
and practice nurses. Tob Control 10:27–32
Medicine Control Agency 2000 Zyban (Bupropion Dihydrochloride): a Safety
Update. Medicine Control Agency, London
Prochazka A V, Weaver M J, Keller R T et al 1998 A randomised trial of
nortriptyline for smoking cessation. Archive of Internal Medicine
158:2035–2039
Romberger D J, Grant K 2004 Alcohol consumption and smoking status:
the role of smoking cessation. Biomedicine and Pharmacotherapy
58:77–83
West R I, McNeill A R 2000 Smoking cessation guidelines for health
professionals: an update. Thorax 55:685–691

4.2   18-YEAR-OLD PREGNANT WOMAN WHO IS INJECTING HEROIN

An 18-year-old woman has been referred to your outpatient clinic for anxiety. In the course of your interview you discover that she is injecting heroin and is currently 22 weeks pregnant. She is living with her partner, who sells illicit drugs. He has assaulted her recently and threatened to kill her and her baby if she leaves him. She is asking for any help you can offer in terms of medication and with her domestic situation.

What would be your approach to management, and what help and treatment would you offer her?

SUGGESTED PROBES

1. What are the likely medical complications that can be associated with this lady's condition?
2. You manage to get this lady into a safe house, but unfortunately she leaves after 2 weeks without telling anyone. What would you be concerned about?
3. She decides she wants maintenance replacement therapy. What would you give her?

PMP PLAN

TASKS TO DO

The following five areas are relevant to this vignette but are not necessarily all-inclusive. The list is also not exhaustive:

a) Make a full assessment of the patient's drug use. Give counselling about the risks to her fetus and to herself. Discuss and counsel on HIV, and hepatitis C and B.
b) Understand the need to engage the patient and adopt a harm minimization approach.
c) Involve the statutory agencies, such as social services and the child protection team. Ensure antenatal care.
d) Demonstrate skill in the assessment and treatment of an intravenous drug user, including stabilization on methadone if possible.
e) Discuss medical, psychological and social interventions in an addicted intravenous drug user who is pregnant.

ISSUES

- Safety of the intravenous drug user, whose life is being threatened
- Harm minimization
- Child protection.

CLARIFY

- What are the patient's main worries: her own health and safety and those of the baby, or fear for her life? Don't be surprised if her priority is where to get her next heroin ('fix')
- Who is responsible for making her pregnant?
- Are any other forms of aggression involved, such as emotional abuse and sexual coercion?

SEEK MORE INFORMATION

GP

- Relevant medical history, treatment for depression and anxiety, prescription of benzodiazepines.

PATIENT

- History of pregnancy (including antenatal care); any other children
- Past psychiatric, drug and alcohol history, relevant medical history
- Complications of drug use, such as hepatitis B, hepatitis C and HIV infection
- Assessment of current mental state—look for depression and anxiety symptoms. Assess stage of change and motivation to do so. Assess factors that would make changes difficult for her.

INVESTIGATIONS

- Screen for hepatitis B and C and HIV infection
- Prenatal screen for fetal viability and/or abnormality using 3-D fetal ultrasonography.

SPECIALIST REFERRALS

- Refer to midwifery team and obstetricians.

SOCIAL SERVICES

- Advise on child protection procedures, support for rehousing or women's refuge.

DIFFERENTIAL DIAGNOSIS/DIFFICULTIES

- Not relevant.

APPROACH TO TREATMENT

- Remember that engagement of the service user is very important for success.
- Consider immediate, short- and long-term treatment, bearing in mind the biopsychosocial options.
- Involve the local drug addiction services.
- Seek the advice and support of social services.

WHAT TREATMENT/ADVICE

See Table 4.1.

IMMEDIATE

- Keep the patient safe.

SHORT-TERM

- Advise on the need to seek a court injunction if there are further concerns over safety.
- Liaise with other professionals, including the obstetrician.

LONG-TERM

- Involve the child and family team, social worker and drug worker.
- Instigate methadone maintenance, psychological treatment.
- Address rehousing.

FULL ANSWER

I think this must be a difficult situation for an 18-year-old to be in. I would be very sensitive and empathic, and try to engage this lady as far as possible. I would clarify what her main worries are, and why she has sought help at this time. I would find out

Table 4.1 Strategy for management of an intravenous drug user

	Biological	Psychological	Social
Immediate	Routine investigation Ensure fetal viability	Nursing support	Move the patient to a safe house
Short-term	Stabilize on methadone and withdraw slowly Buprenorphine can also be used for detoxification and maintenance but is rarely used Refer to midwives and obstetricians	Relapse prevention work Engage with drug prevention worker Discuss harm minimization	Inform social services Seek court injunction against violent partner
Long-term	Low-dose methadone maintenance if unable to withdraw completely	Monitor for postnatal depression or puerperal psychosis post-delivery Transfer to mother and baby unit post-delivery	Women's refuge, safe house Assistance with rehousing Child protection procedures if necessary

whether she fears for her own safety or that of her baby, and whether any other children are involved. I would ask her if one of her main concerns is where to get her next heroin ('fix'). I would clarify whether there has been any domestic violence against her in the past or recently, and whether she has informed the police at any time. I would ask her about other forms of aggression, such as emotional abuse and sexual coercion. I would find out who is responsible for her pregnancy and whether it was planned or not. I would establish whether she is concerned about the lack of a continuous supply of drugs if she leaves the partner who allegedly assaulted her.

I would seek more information about her drug use and estimate how much opiate she is using and how she funds her habit. I would also like to know whether she is currently known to the local drug services, has undergone any detoxification programme in the past, or is currently on methadone maintenance. If she has completed a successful detoxification in the past, I would find out her longest abstinence period and the reasons for relapse. I would also check this lady's psychosocial situation, including finances, debts and social networks. I would carry out a thorough assessment of her mental state, looking for evidence of comorbid mental illness such as depression. I would ask her if she has been prescribed benzodiazepines for her anxiety by her GP. I would also carry out a brief physical examination to look for complications of illicit drug use, such as abscesses from intravenous drug use and liver problems from viral hepatitis or excessive alcohol consumption. I would like to find out more about her pregnancy, in particular the care she has received so far and whether or not she has been tested for hepatitis B, C and HIV infection. I would carefully ask her whether she is known to the local social services department. At this stage, I would like to find out what her intentions are and reassure her that I want to help her as far as I can.

Having carried out a comprehensive assessment, my initial approach to managing this woman would be to evaluate the various risk issues, such as harm to herself or the baby, risk of miscarriage, risk of violence from her partner, whether she leaves him or stays, and the risk of becoming homeless or lacking support should she leave him. I would also consider the risk of treatment failure should she continue to live with her partner whilst on treatment. I would seek advice from an approved social worker on the issue of child protection and also on accommodation for this young lady, who could be at risk of relapse and domestic violence should she continue to live with a drug dealer. I would involve the local drug services at this stage to seek their advice and also their cooperation in post-treatment follow-up and care.

My treatment plan would be to move the patient into a safe house or admit her to a ward for detoxification, or for stabilization on low-dose methadone if detoxification proved difficult or threatened her pregnancy. Once she was on the ward and before commencing treatment, I would request the necessary tests, such as screens for hepatitis B, hepatitis C and HIV infection to rule out any complications of drug use. I would make sure she had pretest counselling for HIV testing. I would refer her to the midwives and obstetrician for assistance in the assessment and management of her pregnancy, and to obtain the necessary advice. This might include a prenatal screen for fetal viability and/or abnormality, using 3-D fetal ultrasonography. Concerning medical treatment, it might be more appropriate because of the stage of her pregnancy to give equivalent doses of methadone for her heroin use and withdraw this gradually over a period of up to 28 days if necessary. The aim would be to maintain her on as low a dose as possible, but high enough to prevent any adverse withdrawal reaction that might threaten her pregnancy. It might be necessary for her to continue methadone maintenance treatment. In some cases buprenorphine might be used for detoxification and maintenance. I would hope that, with this plan, the patient would be able to reduce her opiate use completely or significantly before discharge.

Before she was discharged, I would discuss harm minimization strategies with her. I would warn her that, since she has been relatively free from opiates, her tolerance would have reduced remarkably. I would warn her that a return to heroin use might lead to accidental and potentially fatal opiate overdose. I would refer her back to the local drug and alcohol team for further management, which would include regular follow-up and urine testing to rule out the use of heroin. At this stage, I would also ensure appropriate liaison with the obstetrician throughout the pregnancy and also with the paediatrician closer to delivery, to warn them of possible respiratory depression and opiate withdrawal symptoms in the child on delivery. The other medical and supportive treatment would be around and after delivery of her child. Bearing in mind the outcome of my assessment, my long-term management plan would be to decide whether to go for absolute detoxification or to continue harm minimization through a methadone maintenance programme. This could be done in the outpatient clinic or on a residential rehabilitation programme. In addition, I would assess the need to transfer this lady to a mother and baby unit, depending on her mental state. If she were free from illicit and non-prescribed drugs for an appreciable period, such as 6 weeks after delivery, I would assess for symptoms of depression, anxiety or puerperal psychosis and treat accordingly.

Aside from methadone substitution, psychological treatment strategies to include relaxation, stress and anger management, compliance therapy, motivational interviewing techniques and relapse prevention would be considered as part of the overall treatment. Their aim would be to address the situation and/or state of mind that might be predisposing this woman to seek the immediate gratification afforded by illicit drug use. She would also benefit from counselling and, where the opportunity existed, I would consider her for long-term residential rehabilitation, preferably at a facility with resources for accommodating a mother and young child. Ideally, it would be better for her not to return to her drug-using and dealing partner to increase her chances of abstaining from illicit drugs. Should domestic violence become an issue, the options would include a safe house, women's refuge or perhaps a court injunction against her partner.

I would also refer the woman to the relevant social services department with a view to putting a child protection procedure in place as part of the social care package. This would be very important, given the risk of this lady returning to her partner or to a chaotic lifestyle and her drug-seeking behaviour. I would explain to her why she is being referred and allay any fears she might have over the services denying her parental responsibility. It would be the duty of the local authority staff to carry out a detailed needs and risk assessment, and if the child were considered to be at risk, to call a child protection conference attended by her partner, GP, midwives, health visitors, substance misuse staff, housing department staff, child and family services and the local community mental health service, if the patient were known to them. The decision taken would depend on the outcome of the needs and risk assessment, the risk to the newborn child, the mother's acceptance of suggested treatment programmes, the likelihood of compliance and the availability of local resources to meet her needs. It might be necessary to put the child on the 'at risk' register, to arrange a foster placement with relatives or professional carers while the mother is pursuing treatment, or, in a situation where she is found unfit to look after her child, to start the process of alternative care including long-term fostering and permanent adoption.

Note: child protection procedures and laws differ from region to region and country to country. Sadly, some countries do not have statutory services for narcotic addiction or child protection laws.

ANSWERS TO SUGGESTED PROBES

1. Medical complications that could arise in this lady are:
   - fatal accidental opiate overdose
   - infections, including cellulitis, subcutaneous abscesses, septicaemia, HIV, hepatitis B or C, and infective endocarditis
   - deep vein thrombosis.
2. If she abandoned treatment my concerns would be:
   - a return to intravenous opiate use, with the risk of a potentially fatal accidental overdose due to her very reduced tolerance
   - harm from her partner
   - harm to her unborn baby
   - homelessness and loss to follow-up
   - self-neglect
   - depression and suicide
   - obstetric complications.

3. If she decided she wanted maintenance replacement therapy, I would give her methadone. Lofexidine cannot be used for maintenance therapy in pregnancy or afterwards.

BUZZ WORDS AND USEFUL TERMINOLOGY

Engagement, relapse prevention, accidental overdose, harm minimization, harm reduction, fetal viability, child protection procedure, child protection conference, 'at risk' register.

REFERENCES AND SUGGESTED READING

Department of Health 1999 Drug misuse and dependence. Guidelines on Clinical Management. HMSO, London
King J C 1997 Substance abuse in pregnancy: a bigger problem than you think. Postgraduate Medicine 102(3):135–150
Martin S L, Beaumont J L, Kupper L L 2003 Substance use before and during pregnancy: links to intimate partner violence. American Journal of Drug and Alcohol Abuse 29(3):599–617
Stuart G L, Moore T M, Kahler C W et al 2003 Substance abuse and relationship with violence among men court-referred to batterers' intervention programs. Substance Abuse 24(2):107–122
Ward J, Mattick R P, Hall W 1998 Methadone maintenance in pregnancy. In: Ward J, Mattick R P, Hall W (eds) Methadone Maintenance Treatment and other Opioid Replacement Therapies. Harwood Academic, Amsterdam, pp 397–417

4.3 PATIENT WITH SCHIZOPHRENIA ADDICTED TO HEROIN

As the doctor at a local substance misuse service, you have been asked to see a 20-year-old man who is currently on a psychiatric inpatient unit with a relapse of paranoid schizophrenia. He uses crack cocaine occasionally and up to half a gram of heroin (both by inhalation and intravenously) on a daily basis. The team thinks these have led to his admission and to frequent relapses in the past.

You have been asked for advice on the management of his illicit drug use. How would you proceed?

SUGGESTED PROBES

1. What are the main issues in the management of this patient?
2. What are the active ingredients involved in motivational interviewing?
3. What are the alternatives to methadone in the treatment of this man, and how do they compare to methadone?

PMP PLAN

TASKS TO DO

The following areas are relevant to this vignette but are not necessarily all-inclusive. The list is also not exhaustive:

a) Discuss the link between mental illness and drug misuse, and the need for liaison with the referring team.
b) Demonstrate adequate knowledge of drug assessment and the complications of drug use.
c) Demonstrate knowledge of the stages of change and the importance of assessing for this at the interview.
d) Discuss the risk of relapse and complications from drug use.
e) Show a good knowledge of treatment modalities, including biopsychosocial intervention. Long-term rehabilitation may be necessary.

ISSUES

- Interplay between this patient's illicit drug use and his schizophrenia
- Assessment of whether the patient is at a stage when he is motivated and ready, and has the ability to address his problems
- Treatment with an emphasis on joint management.

CLARIFY

- Are there any suspicions over substance misuse, and any urine or relevant tests?
- Has this patient acknowledged his use of illicit drugs?

SEEK MORE INFORMATION

REFERRER

- Details of illicit drug use and result of urine test.

WARD STAFF

- Is this patient using drugs on the ward? Any positive urine drug screen?
- Behaviour on the ward. Is his mental state upset by illicit drug use?
- Access to illicit drugs on the ward. Are other residents using drugs?
- Risky behaviour (unprotected sex, sharing of needles, injecting drugs, violence and aggression against person or property) on the ward
- Possibility of moving the patient to another ward
- Compliance with schizophrenia medication.

PATIENT

- On referral: does he see his drug use as a problem?
- Detailed drug history and treatment to date
- Complicity with alcohol
- Does this patient fulfil the criteria for substance dependence or is he just a harmful user?
- History of abuse of prescribed medication, alcohol and cannabis
- Insight into his diagnosis (paranoid schizophrenia) and the treatment he is receiving
- Does he think the drug affects his mental state or does he medicate his symptoms using illicit drugs?
- Distressing auditory hallucinations ('voices'), paranoid and persecutory delusions, low mood, restlessness and insomnia
- Psychosocial situation: does he have a supporting partner and, if so, is he or she another drug user or dealer?

DIFFERENTIAL DIAGNOSIS/DIFFICULTIES

- Not relevant.

APPROACH TO TREATMENT

- Arrange to see the client and attempt to engage him whilst on the ward.
- Take a multimodal, i.e. biopsychosocial approach, including joint or shared care of his dual diagnosis between the acute psychiatry and substance misuse services.

WHAT TREATMENT/ADVICE

MEDICAL AND BIOLOGICAL

- Control psychotic illness with antipsychotic medication.
- Instigate methadone substitution.
- Test urine regularly.
- Maintain liaison work.

PSYCHOLOGICAL

- Agree on goals.
- Carry out motivational interviewing.
- Work on relapse prevention.
- Give psychological treatment for 'voices'.
- Give compliance therapy.
- Start on illness and medication awareness programme.

SOCIAL

- Arrange day care.
- Arrange drug rehabilitation (including long-term residential rehabilitation).
- Arrange appropriate accommodation.
- Supervise after discharge for supervision or Community Treatment Order (CTO).

FULL ANSWER

My management of this 20-year-old man would centre on initial assessment and engagement, comprehensive assessment of his drug use, his motivation to change, harm minimization and relapse prevention. One of the issues that I would like to address is the interplay between his illicit drug use and his schizophrenia.

Another issue is to determine whether he is at a stage when he is motivated, ready, and has the ability to address his problems. In offering advice on treatment, I would emphasize the need for joint management between the acute mental health service and the drug misuse service in order to achieve the optimal result.

To begin with, I would clarify with the referring team whether this young man is well enough to discuss his substance misuse problem. I would ask whether there are any suspicions at this time over substance misuse and whether a urine drug screen has been performed. I would find out whether the patient acknowledges his use of illicit drugs, minimizes it, or denies it outright. I would make sure that there were no complications related to his drug use that needed urgent medical attention.

I would seek more information from the referring team on events leading to the current admission, and how they reached the conclusion that he is taking illicit drugs. I would ask about his compliance with his schizophrenia medication. I would enquire about his behaviour on the ward and whether his mental state is disturbed by the use of illicit drugs. I would ask staff how they think he is getting access to illicit drugs on the ward and whether other residents are known to be using too. I would enquire whether this patient is engaging in risky behaviour, such as unprotected sex, sharing of needles, injecting drugs, and violence and aggression (against person or property) on the ward. I would find out if there were any possibility of him being moved to another ward. I would establish whether relevant investigations such as urine testing for heroin and cocaine have been carried out, and if the gentleman is suffering from complications related to his illicit drug use. I would ask specifically about the results of hepatitis B, hepatitis C or HIV screening, if this has already been performed.

On seeing this man, I would clarify with him why he has continued to take heroin and whether he sees his drug use as a problem or not. I would find out if he uses or abuses any prescribed medication, alcohol or cannabis. I would ask him about his current use of heroin and cocaine in terms of level and pattern of use and about his typical day (onset of withdrawal symptoms, relief use, primacy of drug-seeking and drug-using behaviour). I would take a drug use history focusing on the age of his first use, psychosocial precipitants including peer pressure, craving and development of tolerance, how his drug use escalated, the onset of injecting practices, and history of risk-taking behaviour such as sharing needles, sexual activities with strangers and engaging in unprotected sex. I would also ask him about any medical, psychiatric, forensic and social complications of his drug use. I would be interested in any past contact with the drug and alcohol services, and the success or failure of any treatment received. I would pay attention to why he thinks he failed or succeeded, as this might be important for relapse prevention. I would find out about any periods of abstinence and whether this occurred in a protected environment or not.

I would assess his level of insight into his diagnosis of paranoid schizophrenia and the antipsychotic treatment he is receiving. I would ask him about distressing auditory hallucinations ('voices'), paranoid and persecutory delusions, low mood, restlessness and insomnia, and would find out if he thinks the drugs affect his mental state adversely or if he medicates his symptoms by using illicit drugs. I would assess his current mental state and motivation to change, and conduct a thorough physical examination looking for injection sites and the presence of physical complications like injection abscesses. If it had not already been done, I would seek this man's permission to test for hepatitis B, hepatitis C and HIV after pretest counselling. I would ask for a urine test to confirm his use of heroin and any other drugs, and for other relevant investigations such as FBC, LFTs and U and Es. I would then enquire about his psychosocial situation and the presence of stressors and adverse life events that might perpetuate and encourage his continuous use of drugs. I would find out whether he is employed or engaged in any vocational or leisure activity during the day. It would also be important to establish whether he has a supporting partner or not, and whether this partner is another drug user or dealer.

Once I had gathered the necessary information, my approach would be to begin to engage the patient whilst on the acute psychiatric ward. I would aim for joint or shared care of his dual diagnosis between the acute psychiatry and substance misuse services. Obviously, the direction of management would depend on his degree of motivation and cooperation. If he agrees he has a problem and is prepared to engage on a programme, I would ask him what he hopes to achieve. If treatment were acceptable to him, its aim would be to assist him to remain healthy until he is able to abstain from heroin completely, to reduce his use of illicit drugs, to minimize the harm that might result from his choice of route and drug-sharing habit, to reduce the duration of each episode of drug misuse, and to prevent relapse into further drug use or further episodes of mental ill-health. I would emphasize the need for adequate treatment of the psychotic symptoms of schizophrenia, which he might be using illicit drugs to medicate. I would then focus on biopsychosocial measures aimed at tackling his addiction and maintaining optimal mental health.

My immediate treatment plan would be to give psychoeducation to this man, and to decide on the setting and type of treatment to be offered. Psychoeducation would cover issues such as diagnosis, possible complications from his drug use, treatment options, relapse prevention, and advice on how to prevent overdose if he reinstates any use after detoxification or a period of abstinence resulting from prolonged hospital admission. I would emphasize that his tolerance would decrease following a period of abstinence, which might be very dangerous if he reuses. With regard to treatment setting, my immediate thought would be to engage him whilst on the ward and to offer outpatient treatment once he was discharged from hospital. I would consider inpatient treatment, preferably in a drug rehabilitation unit, if in addition to him having a psychiatric diagnosis, there were complicating factors such as misuse of other substances and lack of family support and accommodation that promote his drug use. The presence of complicating medical problems would also signal the need for inpatient treatment.

In terms of treatment, I would consider a broad range of biopsychosocial interventions. As part of the psychological assessment and treatment, I would clarify which stage of change he is at, bearing in mind the various stages of precontemplation, contemplation, determination, action and maintenance, as suggested by Prochaska and DiClemente (1984). I would use motivational interviewing to move him to a more appropriate stage of change where he is able to consider the need to address his problems. I would encourage him to participate in group sessions that address substance misuse and addiction, drug awareness, relapse prevention and assertiveness. If necessary, I would consider compliance therapy, an illness and medication awareness programme and psychological treatment for 'voices', if these are a problem. I would continue to assess his mental state and risk issues, looking for evidence of depression or psychosis that might need further treatment. Where resources are available, I would also consider cognitive behavioural therapy and family interventions, which have been seen to be more effective than routine psychiatric care.

I would consider further medical treatment if there were acute medical concerns, as suggested by the physical examination and detailed laboratory investigations. Once the man was fit, I would suggest a gentle detoxification programme using methadone, a long-acting μ-opioid receptor agonist or another alternative including an alpha$_2$-adrenergic receptor agonist such as clonidine or lofexidine. These groups of medication decrease noradrenaline release into the synaptic cleft and are useful in reducing the characteristic hyperadrenergic withdrawal symptoms of opioids. If this man were a heavy user and unable to cope with complete detoxification, I would suggest methadone maintenance treatment. I would decide on the right dose by titration, starting with a low dose of about 20–30 mg of methadone per day and increasing slowly if there were signs of withdrawal. Approximation based on the estimated level of use per day as assessed over 3–4 days is not usually used nowadays, as it is considered by some to be dangerous. Maintenance could be continued in the community after discharge by a daily pick-up, initially at the methadone clinic or via a local pharmacy. If there were any suggestion that this patient still used street heroin, I would encourage him to use clean needles, which can be obtained at the local needle exchange programme. Other alternatives to methadone maintenance include an opiate receptor partial agonist such as buprenorphine; levacetylmethadol, an opiate receptor agonist; or an opiate receptor antagonist, for example, naltrexone. The latter could be used as an adjunctive treatment to prevent relapse once this man was detoxified. Usually, an interval of about 7–10 days of complete opiate abstinence must elapse before commencing naltrexone. (Naltrexone has been used with clonidine for rapid detoxification, but this controversial treatment is considered dangerous by many clinicians and in any case would not be necessary for this particular patient.)

Social intervention would involve asking the social worker to look into this man's accommodation needs. If he is to remain abstinent from illicit drugs post-detoxification, it is important that he lives in an environment free from undue pressure and away from a drug-promoting culture. In addition, I would recommend a day care and drug rehabilitation programme to consolidate the gains made during admission. It might also be necessary to refer him to a long-term residential rehabilitation unit. Also, given his diagnosis of paranoid schizophrenia, which is a severe and enduring mental illness, I would suggest that this patient be subjected to a legal framework to assist in future follow-up and care in the community. The supervision order under Section 25 (Supervised Discharge) of the Mental Health Act 1983 in England and Wales, or a Community Treatment Order (CTO) in parts of Australia, New Zealand and the USA might be useful in this respect. There would be a need for liaison with the general adult psychiatric services and regular reviews with the other professionals involved in his care.

In very severe conditions, injectable heroin can be prescribed under special licence (from the Home Office in the UK), particularly if one can be reassured about safety and that the patient will not dabble with street drugs. In the UK I would need to complete a standard form, which would then be sent to the regional drug misuse database once my assessment was completed.

ANSWER TO SUGGESTED PROBES

1. The main issues involved in the management of this patient focus on assessment and treatment of his drug use, and include:
   - risk assessment
   - harm minimization and opiate substitution
   - relapse prevention
   - management of his dual diagnosis.
2. The active ingredients of motivational interviewing include:
   - empathy
   - reflective listening
   - development of discrepancy between the patient's goals or values and his/her current problem behaviour
   - avoidance of argument and direct confrontation
   - rolling with resistance
   - supporting optimism for change.
3. The alternatives to methadone for this man include levacetylmethadol hydrochloride, buprenorphine and lofexidine.

   Lofexidine belongs to the same class (opioid receptor agonist) as methadone but has a longer half-life, so that supervision can be only one or two visits per week. The drawbacks are that patients are often not allowed to take it home and its use is usually limited to specialist clinics. If the dose is increased too rapidly, it may cause sedation, orthostatic hypotension, poor concentration and overdose. It is relatively easy to use and can be prescribed for rapid detoxification.

   Buprenorphine, on the other hand, is a partial µ-opioid agonist. Its advantages over methadone include the fact that it is safe in overdose, attenuates drug 'highs' in patients using 'on top', and has low levels of psychological reinforcement and minimal withdrawal symptoms during detoxification.

   Levacetylmethadol hydrochloride (LAAM) is a new synthetic opiate substitute as addictive as methadone, but one dose can act for up to 72 hours. It blocks euphoric effects so that so there are no 'highs'. LAAM is taken orally so eliminates the dangers of needle use.

BUZZ WORDS AND USEFUL TERMINOLOGY

Harm minimization, engagement, relapse prevention, motivational interviewing, opiate substitution, reduced tolerance, dual diagnosis, shared care, care programme approach.

REFERENCES AND SUGGESTED READING

Barrowclough C, Haddock G, Tarrier N et al 2001 Randomised controlled trial of motivational interviewing, cognitive behaviour therapy, and family interventions for patients with comorbid schizophrenia and substance use disorders. American Journal of Psychiatry 158:1706–1713
Law F D, Nutt D 2002 Drugs used in the treatment of the addictions. In: Gelder M G, López-Ibor Jr J J, Andreasen N C (eds) New Oxford Textbook of Psychiatry, vol. 2. Oxford University Press, Oxford, pp 1337–1340
Marlatt G A, George W H 1984 Relapse prevention work: introduction and overview of the model. British Journal of Addiction 79:261–273
Prochaska J, DiClemente C 1984 Stages of change in the modification of problem behaviours. Progress in Behaviour Modification 28:183–218
Rollnick S, Miller W R 1991 Motivational Interviewing: Preparing People to Change Addictive Behaviour. Guilford, New York
Unnithan S, Gossop M, Strang J 1992 Factors associated with relapse among opiate addicts in an outpatient detoxification programme. British Journal of Psychiatry 161:654–657
Winstock A R, Strang J 2002 Opiates: heroin, methadone and buprenorphine. In: Gelder M G, López-Ibor Jr J J, Andreasen N C (eds) New Oxford Textbook of Psychiatry, vol 1. Oxford University Press, Oxford, pp 523–530

4.4   32-YEAR-OLD BUILDER WITH EXCESSIVE ALCOHOL CONSUMPTION AND VIOLENT BEHAVIOUR

A 32-year-old builder has been referred to you, who has been paying frequent visits to his general practice in the last 2 weeks and complaining of feeling suicidal. He has been using up to 156 units of alcohol weekly and demanding diazepam to 'calm down'. The local drug and alcohol team, to whom he has threatened violence, will only offer him treatment when he is sober and not suicidal.

How would you manage this patient?

SUGGESTED PROBES

1. If this man continues to take alcohol, what neurological complications are likely?
2. After securing funding for residential rehabilitation, the patient changes his mind, saying his partner would be unable to cope in his absence. What would you do?
3. The patient has asked you to prescribe disulfiram. What factors would you consider before doing this?

PMP PLAN

TASKS TO DO

The following five areas are relevant to this vignette but are not necessarily all-inclusive. The list is also not exhaustive:

a) Focus your discussions on substance misuse disorder and the threat of self-harm, suicide and aggression.
b) Discuss risk assessment and motivation for treatment.
c) Discuss immediate, short-term and long-term goals and treatment plans.
d) Discuss the different modalities (biological, psychological and social) and approach to treatment.
e) Show a good understanding of the different pharmacological agents that can be used and the rationale for their uses.

CLARIFY

- What is the patient's current state and what are the risks of him ending his own life, becoming aggressive or developing physical complications from excessive alcohol consumption?
- Is he fit to be admitted to a psychiatric ward?

SEEK MORE INFORMATION

GP

- Patient's full history, mental state examination and review of relevant physical findings
- Knowledge of his excessive alcohol consumption, and previous medical and psychiatric complications
- Interrelationship between alcohol consumption and his moods
- Consumption of other drugs of addiction
- Reason for requesting benzodiazepines
- Previous treatment and success
- Assessment of moods and plans to self-harm and/or harm others.

DIFFERENTIAL DIAGNOSIS/DIFFICULTIES

- *Functional.* Alcohol dependence, mental and behavioural disorders secondary to excessive and harmful use of alcohol, poly-substance drug misuse disorder. A recurrent depressive disorder is likely to be comorbid.

APPROACH TO TREATMENT

- Consider safety issues as paramount.
- Assess risks.
- Plan treatment: immediate, short- and long-term using a biopsychosocial management approach.

WHAT TREATMENT/ADVICE

See Table 4.2.

MEDICAL

- Consider safety; admit for crisis management and to reduce risk of suicide.
- *Immediate.* Consider safe detoxification; monitor for withdrawal symptoms.

Table 4.2 Treatment plan for alcohol dependence

	Biological/medical	Psychological	Social
Immediate	Benzodiazepine detoxification, thiamine injections for 5 days P.r.n. benzodiazepines if necessary	Supportive psychotherapy	Assess social circumstances
Short-term	Multivitamins Assess mood after detoxification	Motivational interviewing, group therapy	Practical problem-solving
Longer-term	Acamprosate Naltrexone Disulfiram Antidepressant	Relapse prevention programmes	Alcoholics Anonymous Social skills Vocational training

- *Short-term.* Assess for mood disorder when the patient is sober. Prescribe antidepressant if necessary.
- *Long-term.* Consider pharmacological methods such as disulfiram, or a neurobiological agent such as acamprosate or naltrexone; the latter has been found to be useful in some patients.

PSYCHOLOGICAL

- Consider relapse prevention, motivational interviewing, anger management, drug awareness, stress management.

PSYCHOSOCIAL

- Arrange for long-term rehabilitation, including options for day and residential care.
- Refer to groups such as Alcoholics Anonymous (AA).

FULL ANSWER

I think this 32-year-old man presents a complex scenario and, for the sake of clarity, I would want to deal with the problems one by one. The main issues for me in this case would be the need to keep this man safe, assess him for his mood and alcohol misuse disorder, institute an appropriate management plan and put in place the necessary follow-up arrangements, including referral to the local alcohol and substance misuse team. I would quickly want to clarify how things stand at present, and the risk of him ending his life, becoming aggressive and developing physical complications from excessive alcohol consumption. As admission may be an option, I would assess his fitness to be attended to on a psychiatric ward. I would refer him to other acute medical services if there were urgent medical issues such as severe liver disease and head injury.

While I was doing this, I would want to seek more information from his GP on his excessive alcohol consumption, and on any previous medical and psychiatric complications. I would arrange to see the patient and take a full history, carry out a mental state examination and review the relevant physical findings. I would be particularly interested in his alcohol consumption and alcohol history. I would enquire about the interrelationship between his consumption of substances and his moods. I would also find out about his consumption of other drugs of addiction, his reason for requesting benzodiazepines, previous treatments and their success or failure. I would establish whether this man meets the criteria for alcohol dependence and assess his mood for a depressive disorder once he was weaned off alcohol. I would make an assessment of his moods and thoughts and of his plans to self-harm or to harm others. I would use a validated rating scale such as Beck's Depression Inventory or Hamilton Rating Scale to assist in the objective assessment and monitoring of his mood. I would specifically ask if there are psychosocial stressors that the excessive consumption of alcohol might be helping him cope with.

I would consider alcohol dependence, mental and behavioural disorders secondary to excessive and harmful use of alcohol, recurrent depressive disorder and poly-substance misuse disorder in my differential diagnosis. The assessment of risk and safety issues would be paramount in my approach to the management of this case. I would plan treatment in the immediate, short term and long term with the multidisciplinary team, bearing in mind biopsychosocial interventions. In managing and treating this man, I would ensure that he was medically fit enough to be admitted to a psychiatric ward, consider safety issues, and admit him for crisis management aimed at general harm reduction and also specifically preventing suicide. Once he was admitted and before treatment commenced, I would carry out routine baseline investigations including FBC, U and Es, LFTs, RFTs and TFTs. I would also order a CT or MRI if there were any suggestion of brain injury. Neuroimaging might also reveal alcohol-induced brain damage. If this man has had multiple blackouts that have not been investigated, I would also consider an EEG. I would carry out a cognitive assessment using a Mini Mental State Examination (MMSE) as a screening tool. I would refer him for a formal neuropsychological assessment if necessary.

Concerning treatment, I would institute a safe plan to achieve detoxification from alcohol using one of the benzodiazepines in the immediate term. If there were evidence of severe liver disease I would opt for oxazepam. I would monitor for possible seizure attacks and prescribe thiamine injections to prevent Wernicke's psychosis. I would watch for anaphylaxis if intravenous thiamine were required. In the short term, I would assess him for a mood disorder when he was sober and prescribe an antidepressant if necessary. In the long term, I would also consider the use of neurobiological agents such as acamprosate and naltrexone to reduce craving, and would review the need for continuous use of antidepressants.

I would also suggest cognitive and behavioural interventions to address his mood and drinking behaviour and to manage his suicidality. This would be with the aim of identifying predisposing factors, establishing the interaction between his addiction and mental health, and understanding the relapse indicators to enhance recognition of the suicide risk. During the admission, I would carry out psychological interventions such as relapse prevention, motivational interviewing and drug awareness, and also consider stress management strategies if stressors appeared to push him to drink more and more. In this regard, I would offer practical problem-solving to deal with stressors in his life that might be perpetuating his drinking difficulties. I would offer practical assistance to deal with any psychosocial stressors such as legal and offending problems, interpersonal and relationship difficulties, financial problems, childcare, accommodation and debts.

In order to increase the chances of success, I would suggest post-discharge longer-term rehabilitation to consolidate the gains of the admission. I would offer residential rehabilitation after assessing his motivation to engage in the programme. I would also consider the options for day rehabilitation if this seemed appropriate, or if the patient found longer-term rehabilitation unacceptable or unfeasible. I would encourage him to join self-help groups such as Alcoholics Anonymous in the UK to consolidate his gains from hospital admission and detoxification.

ANSWERS TO SUGGESTED PROBES

1. Neurological complications that may follow continuous excessive alcohol consumption include:
   - *Wernicke–Korsakoff syndrome.* Nystagmus, ophthalmoplegia (abducens and conjugate palsies), ataxia of gait and global confusional state (in acute Wernicke's encephalopathy)
   - *Korsakoff syndrome.* Marked memory disorder amnesia (diencephalic) with preservation of other cognitive functions, confusion, disorientation and confabulations (non-deliberate recitation of imaginary events to fill gaps in memory). Atrophy of mammillary bodies can also be seen on MRI
   - *Cerebellar degeneration.* Ataxia of stance and gait, some intellectual deterioration
   - *Peripheral neuropathy.* Numbness in feet, pins and needles, burning sensations, intense hyperaesthesia and pain. Also sensory ataxia, foot drop, dependent oedema and dystrophic changes of the skin and nails
   - *Amblyopia.* Dimness in central vision for green and red, peripheral neuropathy. More acute blindness may occur

in methyl alcohol consumption, particularly in areas where commercial alcohol is adulterated

- *Marchiafava–Bignami disease.* Ataxia, dysarthria, epilepsy, impairment of consciousness, and in more slowly progressive form, spastic paralysis and dementia
- *Central pontine myelinosis.* Usually acute and often fatal; presents with obtundation, bulbar palsy, quadriplegia and loss of pain sensation in limbs and trunk. May present with vomiting, confusion, disordered eye movement and coma. Some patients present with 'locked-in syndrome'.

(Candidates would be well advised to familiarize themselves with the clinical features of these complications, as examiners may want to probe their relevance and candidates' knowledge further.)

2. If the patient declined residential rehabilitation, I would ask him why. I would establish why he thinks his partner would be unable to cope, to see if we could give any assistance.

   I would invite the partner to see me, try to explain the benefits of residential rehabilitation, and suggest available assistance.

   If, despite this explanation, a residential rehabilitation were not feasible or possible, I would suggest and facilitate day rehabilitation programmes with support from the alcohol treatment service.

3. In deciding whether to prescribe disulfiram or not, I would consider:
   - contraindications to its use, including concomitant use of drugs or medication with potentially dangerous interaction, such as the imidazoles: for example, metronidazole
   - the patient's motivation and ability to stick to the treatment plan without drinking alcohol while using disulfiram
   - the availability of a friend, partner or relative who is willing to supervise medication use
   - the absence or presence of medical conditions such as heart failure, severe liver disease, cerebral thrombosis and diabetes, as an alcohol reaction to disulfiram could be fatal.

BUZZ WORDS AND USEFUL TERMINOLOGY

Harm minimization, engagement, relapse prevention, motivational interviewing, opiate substitution, reduced tolerance.

REFERENCES AND SUGGESTED READING

COMBINE Study Research Group 2003 Testing combined pharmacotherapies and behavioural interventions in alcohol dependence: rationale and methods. Alcoholism Clinical and Experimental Research 27(7):1107–1122

Conner K R, Li Y, Meldrum S et al 2003 The role of drinking in suicidal ideation: analyses of Project MATCH data. Journal of Alcohol Studies 64(3):402–408

Cornelius J R, Salloum I M, Day N L 1996 Patterns of suicidality and alcohol use in alcoholics with major depression. Alcoholism Clinical and Experimental Research 20(8):1451–1455

Schuckit M A, Daepen J B, Tipp J E et al 1998 The clinical course of alcohol-related problems in alcohol dependent and non-alcohol dependent drinking women and men. Journal of Alcohol Studies 59:81

4.5 PRE-ADMISSION ASSESSMENT IN A 42-YEAR-OLD WITH EXCESSIVE ALCOHOL CONSUMPTION

You are the registrar in a local drug and alcohol service. You are asked to carry out a pre-admission assessment of a 42-year-old man who has an extensive history of excessive alcohol consumption, intravenous drug use and a depressive disorder. He has been referred for detoxification as he has been drinking 312 units of alcohol a week.

How would you go about your assessment and what would be your strategy for management?

SUGGESTED PROBES

1. What are the purposes of a pre-admission assessment in this case?
2. What would guide your decision to manage as an outpatient or inpatient?
3. You find that this man is depressed but, unfortunately, there is a waiting list of 6 weeks on your unit. What advice would you give?

PMP PLAN

TASKS TO DO

The following five areas are relevant to this vignette but are not necessarily all-inclusive. The list is also not exhaustive:

a) Show an understanding of the purpose of a pre-admission assessment.
b) Assess the risk of medical and psychiatric complications, self-harm and suicide.
c) Discuss the issue of motivation for treatment, and the factors that would affect the decision to accept the patient for admission.
d) Discuss appropriate routine investigations, to include neurological and liver function tests.
e) Focus your strategy for management on immediate, short-term and long-term goals, and include biological, psychological and social approaches in your treatment plans.

ISSUES

- Decision as to whether this man, a poly-substance abuser, is fit and suitable for treatment at this time

- Decision as to whether the service is adequately resourced to offer the appropriate safe management.

CLARIFY

- What is the patient's suitability for treatment at this time?
- What is his mental state, and what are the medical risks and risk of suicide or aggression?
- Is he at immediate risk of medical complications?

SEEK MORE INFORMATION

REFERRER

- Previous detoxifications and outcomes.

GP AND PHYSICIANS

- History of medical illness and complications
- Current treatment
- Medical fitness.

PATIENT

- Motivation for change
- Available support
- Acceptance of proposed medical, psychological and social care plans
- Other commitments or distractions, relationships/divorce/childcare/court cases
- Aftercare plans and need for long-term rehabilitation.

DIFFERENTIAL DIAGNOSIS/DIFFICULTIES

- Not relevant, given this man's extensive history of excessive alcohol consumption, intravenous drug use and depressive disorder.

APPROACH TO TREATMENT

- Consider the risk of relapse, deterioration in the patient's mental state, risk of suicide and aggression, and how these risks are going to be managed.
- Involve the multidisciplinary team in planning admission and treatment.

WHAT TREATMENT/ADVICE

See Table 4.3.

MEDICAL DETOXIFICATION

- Watch out for medical complications.
- Attend to mental health needs and give antidepressants if required.
- Ensure that the patient has a normal liver function so that antidepressants, particularly selective serotonin re-uptake inhibitors (SSRIs), may be used safely.

PSYCHOLOGICAL

- Plan relapse prevention, motivational interviewing techniques, drug awareness and coping strategies.
- Refer him to residential and day rehabilitation programmes, as well as support groups such as Alcoholics Anonymous and Narcotics Anonymous.

SOCIAL

- Arrange social and vocational skills training, problem-solving, long-term rehabilitation and a halfway house.
- Improve his positive social network through befriending and/or attendance at a day hospital.

FULL ANSWER

I think the main issue at hand in addressing a pre-admission assessment in this man is to determine his suitability for treatment at this time. Another issue is to establish whether our drug and alcohol service is sufficiently well resourced to offer him the appropriate safe treatment or if it will be necessary to refer him elsewhere, given the magnitude and complexity of his habit. It would also be necessary to determine whether there are factors contraindicating treatment and whether he is prepared to accept the treatment on offer in line with the policy of the unit. The assessment would also enable us to agree on a strategy for his entire treatment and rehabilitation.

First of all, I would want to clarify whether there are any medical risks such as liver failure or cardiac complications, or psychological risks, such as self-harm and/or suicide and aggression to others. I would also clarify whether he has other commitments or

Table 4.3 Strategy for treatment and management in alcohol and drug dependence

	Biological/medical	Psychological	Social
Immediate	Benzodiazepine detoxification Thiamine injections P.r.n. rectal diazepam	Supportive psychotherapy Closer monitoring	Needs assessment
Short-term	Multivitamins Assess mood after detoxification	Motivational interviewing Group therapy Drug awareness	Practical problem-solving Coping skills
Long-term	Acamprosate Naltrexone Disulfiram Antidepressant	Relapse prevention programmes Rehabilitation Day rehabilitation (not preferred in this particular case)	Alcoholics Anonymous Halfway house Social skills Vocational training Improve positive social networks

issues that might be sources of distraction, such as court cases, childcare problems, and difficulties with relationships and/or divorce.

I would arrange to see the man to seek more information on his current drinking, moods and social situation. I would prefer to carry out an outreach visit with another colleague to enable me to appreciate his psychosocial situation better. In my assessment, I would explore his current drinking patterns in terms of quantity and quality, and as far as possible reassure myself of the diagnosis of alcohol dependence which is by far the most likely. I would find out about previous treatment, including previous detoxifications and their outcomes, and whether this man has previously engaged in a longer-term rehabilitation programme. I would find out if there are any psychosocial pressures that are exacerbating his problems. I would assess his motivation for change, what problems he thinks may confront him on his way to recovery, and the support that would be available to him at this time. In addition, I would examine this man's mood for a possible depressive illness and ask him whether he has any thoughts of harming himself or others. I would ask him if he has a history of complications from excessive alcohol use, such as blackouts, epileptic fits, Wernicke's psychosis, head injury, bleeding gastric ulcers and severe liver disease.

I would seek specific assistance in managing any active medical conditions and would liaise with other specialists for his treatment. I would discuss the patient with other colleagues during our multidisciplinary referral meeting. I would discuss with him the components and stages of the proposed treatment, which would include medical and psychological aspects, and a longer-term rehabilitation programme. I would suggest he discuss the proposed treatment with his GP, family and relevant others before coming to a conclusion about what to do. This period would also be useful in dealing with any medical condition that might complicate treatment. I would ask him if he accepts the proposed treatment plan before committing our service to accepting him for treatment. I would involve a multidisciplinary team in my approach to his treatment. I would plan for an inpatient detoxification first, and assess his mental state properly for depression and other mental illnesses when he is more sober. Before admission, I would carry out a risk assessment and consider the risk of medical complications, self-harm, suicide, violence, aggression and harm to others. We would also discuss how these risks are going to be managed.

Concerning treatment, this would be divided into medical, psychological and social management and would address the immediate, short and long term, as well as follow-up of this gentleman. He is likely to have developed neuroadaptation and physical dependence on alcohol, given his history of excessive consumption and significant poly-substance misuse. My immediate treatment plan would be to detoxify the man from alcohol in hospital, where he could be monitored for compliance and complications. I would also attend to any medical and mental health needs that arose. I would prescribe for him a reducing regimen of one of the benzodiazepines, chlordiazepoxide or diazepam (or oxazepam in patients with significant liver function abnormalities), and monitor for any withdrawal reaction and medical complications such as Wernicke's encephalopathy. If there were a significant risk of seizures, I would add an anticonvulsant such as sodium valproate or carbamazepine (not favoured for liver diseases). I would prescribe a high-potency multivitamin preparation containing thiamine to prevent acute encephalopathy secondary to acute thiamine deficiency (Wernicke's). Due to the possibility of concomitant depression in this man, I would place him on an increased observation level to prevent self-harm and/or suicide. I would at this stage ask our team social worker to explore some of the social difficulties that could be addressed during the patient's stay in hospital. In the short term, once this patient was more stable and had finished detoxification, I would continue to prescribe multivitamins and to assess his mood for depression. If indicated, I would prescribe an antidepressant to help his mood and also hypnotics for a few days to aid sleep, if insomnia was a problem. I would ensure that this man had normal LFTs before using antidepressants, particularly SSRIs.

As part of the treatment, the patient would be offered counselling and other psychological treatments in a group setting or individually. We would explore issues surrounding drug and safety awareness, in addition to relapse prevention. In order to consolidate the gains of inpatient admission, I would suggest that we plan a long-term rehabilitation programme for his addiction and that he stay in a halfway house initially while we arranged long-term residential rehabilitation. The aim would be to forestall the chance of him going back to live in an environment that would encourage his drug-seeking behaviour and excessive alcohol consumption. It is possible that after undergoing successful rehabilitation, this man might refuse an offer of residential rehabilitation. I would attempt to continue to engage him and encourage him to attend a day rehabilitation programme, where he could be seen by an alcohol support worker. Attendance at the local Alcoholics Anonymous and Narcotics Anonymous groups would also be recommended.

I would explore this man's social situation to assist the team in focusing our problem-solving strategies. This would include looking into his accommodation situation and addressing his training needs for social and vocational skills. Part of the treatment strategy would be to increase his social networks, particularly encouraging contact with others who are not dependent on alcohol or drugs. In the long term, this might help to boost his self-esteem, reduce boredom and give him opportunities to explore his potential. This might be achieved by attendance at a day hospital or by him taking up a voluntary or part-time job in the first instance. I would hope that, with these strategies in mind, our team would be well placed to meet this gentleman's needs.

(Do not waste time in this vignette establishing whether this man has alcohol and drug dependence. With the use of intravenous drugs and 312 units of alcohol per week, you can safely assume that he has serious alcohol and drug problems.)

ANSWERS TO SUGGESTED PROBES

1. The purposes of a pre-admission assessment in this case are:
   - to clarify whether this man is suitable for admission for detoxification and other treatments at the time of referral
   - to assess motivation for treatment
   - to assess for any medical or psychological risks that could complicate treatment
   - to assess for the risk of suicide and give appropriate suggestions
   - to find out whether he would accept the treatment plan/programme offered on the unit
   - to assess whether the unit is sufficiently well staffed and resourced to meet his complex needs
   - to advise the referrer on alternatives if patient is unsuitable for treatment.
2. My decision to manage him as an outpatient or inpatient would be guided by:
   - severity of illness
   - risk of medical complications such as delirium tremens, and of severe neglect, suicide or harm to others
   - availability of a non-professional support system in the community
   - availability of structures and staff to facilitate treatment as an outpatient
   - ease of monitoring of medical and psychiatric complications
   - logistic issues (is the patient living out of the area?).

3. If I found that this man was depressed but there was a waiting list on my unit, I would:
   - recommend admission to another service, including those in the private sector (while carefully considering the financial implications)
   - suggest admission elsewhere (including an acute psychiatry ward), where his detoxification could be managed with assistance from the addiction services
   - suggest outpatient treatment as an alternative if medically safe, and if intensive treatment could be resourced in terms of staffing and logistics.

BUZZ WORDS AND USEFUL TERMINOLOGY

Harm minimization, physical dependence, neuroadaptation, engagement, relapse prevention, motivational interviewing, opiate substitution, reduced tolerance.

REFERENCES AND SUGGESTED READING

Department of Health 1999 Drug misuse and dependence. Guidelines on Clinical Management. HMSO, London

Schuckit M A, Daepen J B, Tipp J E et al 1998 The clinical course of alcohol-related problems in alcohol dependent and non-alcohol dependent drinking women and men. Journal of Alcohol Studies 59:81

5
Child and adolescent psychiatry

5.1 5-YEAR-OLD BOY WHO IS VERY GOOD AT ART BUT UNABLE TO SETTLE AT SCHOOL

A 5-year-old boy has been referred to you by the family doctor. The boy has not settled down at school since he started 4 months ago. He keeps to himself and is seemingly uninterested during story sessions, but has been noted to be particularly good with his artwork. He behaves similarly at home.

How would you go about assessing this boy with a view to arriving at a diagnosis and management plan?

SUGGESTED PROBES

1. What are your differential diagnoses?
2. What are the core symptoms of childhood autism?
3. What are the salient features of your various differential diagnoses?

PMP PLAN

TASKS TO DO

The following five areas are relevant to this vignette but are not necessarily all-inclusive. The list is also not exhaustive:

a) Show an awareness of the most likely diagnosis and differentials.
b) Demonstrate knowledge of the defining features of each of the differentials and of the core features of childhood autism.
c) Make a comprehensive assessment and take a multidisciplinary approach.
d) Demonstrate an understanding of the processes involved in child psychiatric referral, assessment and multi-agency involvement.
e) Show sensitivity and take an empathic approach to the different forms of management.

ISSUES

- Diagnosis
- Management approaches.

CLARIFY

- Are there other reasons for referring at the present time?
- Does the family have other concerns?
- What help have they sought so far? What have been the benefits of such interventions?
- Is there a history of a neurological problem, hearing difficulties or other neuropsychiatric syndromes?

SEEK MORE INFORMATION

GP

- Investigations and treatment to date
- Family background and dynamics, if known.

FAMILY

- What is meant by 'not settled at school'; history of the problem
- Parents' permission to speak to the school
- Features of autism and other pervasive developmental disorders (PDD); rule out other differentials
- Communication problems, such as delays with language development, repetition of other people's words (echolalia) and using 'he' instead of 'she' (pronomial reversal)
- Set ways or stereotypical behaviour: temper tantrums or hyperactivity if routines are disturbed or changed, evidence of rocking to and fro, tiptoeing or remarkable abilities for age, e.g. art
- Problems with sensory perception
- Change of picture in settings other than school
- Family history of similar problems. Is another child affected?

CHILD

- View of parents on present concern, life at school and problems encountered
- Bullying or intimidation
- Physical causes of the problem
- Depression

- Physical examination to look for soft neurological signs, including neurocutaneous disorders and syndromes associated with particular phenotypes
- Non-specific medical problems: mental retardation (occurs in 80% of classic autism), epilepsy (30% of all children with Kanner syndrome), hearing impairment (20% of classic autism), retinopathy of prematurity (over-represented in autism)
- Specific medical problems: deafness, tuberous sclerosis, fragile X syndrome, Angelman syndrome, Möbius syndrome (congenital bilateral facial nerve palsies usually due to abnormalities in the brainstem).

INVESTIGATIONS

- Hearing tests, EEG and chromosomal investigations (done routinely by some clinics)
- Neuropsychological assessment, especially that of cognitive ability
- IQ test (not favoured by most psychologists).

SCHOOL

- Details of the problem
- School visit to observe behaviour may be useful.

DIFFERENTIAL DIAGNOSIS/DIFFICULTIES

- *Organic.* Autism, another PDD such as childhood disintegrative psychosis, Asperger syndrome, atypical autism, mental retardation not associated with PDD, specific language difficulty, selective mutism. Rett syndrome is another possibility in girls but, being an X-linked disorder, is highly unlikely in boys
- *Functional.* Social anxiety and severe neglect.

APPROACH TO TREATMENT

- Be guided by the diagnosis, the presence of coexisting medical problems and the result of further investigations, including school collaboration and psychometric assessment.
- Ensure that intervention is broad-range, is targeted to the symptoms, and includes biological, psychological and social forms of therapy (including family work and school liaison).

- Make the aim of your intervention the formulation of a strategy for decreasing unwanted behaviours and facilitating learning.

WHAT TREATMENT/ADVICE

SOCIAL

- Teach the child how to tolerate adult guidance and intrusion.
- Teach him how to follow routines.
- Help him develop communicative abilities and move from associational to more conceptual learning models.

BEHAVIOURAL

- Make a functional analysis of the child's behaviour, with the emphasis on antecedent, behaviour and consequence.
- Formulate a management plan based on this analysis to promote desired behaviour and reduce unwanted behaviour.
- Arrange social assistance for the parents; give practical advice on how to manage day-to-day issues; arrange childcare to give the parents space to do other things.

EDUCATIONAL

- Devise a structured educational programme with intensive support.
- Examine the need for special education and appropriate school placement.

PHARMACOTHERAPY

- Show awareness that no medication has proven efficacy in treating the social and relationship problems in autism. Various pharmacotherapeutic approaches have been disappointing. Moreover, most are not licensed by manufacturers for use in children.
- Discuss the need to use anticonvulsant medication, if epilepsy becomes a problem in the future.
- Consider the use of atypical antipsychotics like risperidone (in older children), which may be useful in controlling hyperactivity, impulsivity, obsessional preoccupation and aggressive behaviour.
- Consider the use of antidepressants such as selective serotinin re-uptake inhibitors (SSRIs), which may also be beneficial but should be avoided as far as possible in light of the link with

suicide and paroxetine, in particular. (Due to recent developments in the UK, the Department of Health and the Committee on Safety of Medicines (CSM, 2003) have advised against the prescription of all SSRIs except fluoxetine for depression in people under the age of 18 years.)

FULL ANSWER

The presentation of this 5-year-old boy is very suggestive of a pervasive developmental disorder (PDD). My immediate concern would therefore be to assess him, confirm the diagnosis, devise a management plan in collaboration with other professionals, refer to the appropriate agencies and disciplines for assistance, and return the child to educational learning.

I would first like to clarify with the GP whether there are any other reasons why the patient has been referred at this particular time. I would explain to the parents the need to obtain collateral information and seek their permission to do so. I would find out whether this child's medical record or paediatrician's report suggests developmental delays. In addition, I would reassure myself that there is no history of a neurological problem, hearing or speech difficulties, or syndromes such as Landau–Kleffner. I would find out if the family has any other concerns, and would ask if there has ever been involvement of a social worker or child development staff. I would ask whether any other member of the family is known to the local child development centre or social services department.

The next step would be to arrange an outpatient appointment, inviting members of the family and any other people who have been involved in this child's care. I would do this only with parental permission. The purpose of the appointment would be to seek more information that would be relevant in arriving at a diagnosis. During the assessment, which might take several meetings, I would bear in mind the need to be sensitive and empathic in my approach, given the potential impact the present problem has on the family. I would take a full history from the parents, asking about their concerns, exactly when the problem was first noticed, and what they have done about it to date. I would want to know whether the pregnancy was planned and if there were any problems during the pregnancy or postnatal period. I would ask how the child's very early years were and about previous childhood illnesses or any sensory or hearing impairment. I would also find out whether the child has ever been separated from his parents. I would try to establish how his presentation at school differs from or is similar to the problems encountered at home.

I would ask whether the child is emotionally responsive and if he interacts well with the rest of the family and friends at home (not school). I would ask how he reacts when dad or mum comes home from work. I would find out whether he avoids eye contact when approached or engaged. It would be necessary to investigate any communication problems such as delays with language development, talking to people, repetition of other people's words (echolalia), and using the word 'he' instead of 'she' (pronomial reversal). I would find out if the child is set in his ways and how he reacts to attempts to change his routine. I would also ask if he has temper tantrums or becomes hyperactive when his routines are disturbed or changed. I would enquire about the presence of any repetitive or stereotypical behaviours, such as rocking back and forth or tiptoeing, any unusual abilities for his age (for example, skill in drawing pictures), and problems with sensory perception, such as painful sensitivity to certain sounds or lack of sensation to pain (which might result in a tendency to hurt himself without crying). I would ask the parents if they have any reason to believe the child is depressed or just finding it difficult to settle into school. I would enquire about his appetite and sleep pattern, and whether he has been able to maintain the same level of interest. I would also be interested in knowing about how the family has been coping and how family members have reacted to the present problem.

Bearing in mind the presentation, my working diagnosis would be that of childhood autism, but I would bear in mind other differential diagnoses: for example, another PDD such as childhood disintegrative psychosis, Asperger syndrome, mental retardation not associated with PDD, specific language difficulty, selective mutism, deafness, social anxiety and severe neglect. Furthermore, I would like to exclude the presence of comorbid medical problems or a medical diagnosis that could present with symptoms suggestive of autism, including deafness, tuberous sclerosis, epilepsy, fragile X and Angelman syndrome. It might take more than one visit and liaison with a paediatrician for this diagnostic assessment to be completed. It might be helpful to consider a standardized assessment for PDD, such as the Autism Diagnostic Interview Schedule (ADIS) or Autism Diagnostic Observation Schedule (ADOS). I would ask our clinical psychologist to carry out a psychometric assessment, which might shed more light on the child's cognitive ability, the possibility of mental impairment and the presence of learning difficulties. I would seek parental permission to talk to his nursery teachers in order to hear their views, and would carry out a functional analysis with a view to formulating a strategy for decreasing unwanted behaviours and facilitating learning.

Once I was clear about the diagnosis, my immediate management plan would be to educate the parents about diagnosis, prognosis and treatment options. I would deliver this information in a sensitive manner, giving adequate time for questions and support. Supplying the parents with details of autism support groups might also help. My treatment approach would be guided by a comprehensive review of this boy and his areas of strength and weakness. I would consider a broad range of biopsychosocial interventions, including educational, behavioural and social approaches. Although not curative, medical and pharmacological approaches might be useful in addressing specific problems. There might be a need to use anticonvulsant medication, if epilepsy is a major problem. I would do this with the advice and support of a paediatric neurologist or an epileptologist. Atypical antipsychotics such as risperidone (in older children) might be useful in controlling hyperactivity, impulsivity, obsessional preoccupation and aggressive behaviour. Antidepressants such as SSRIs might also be beneficial, but I would be careful to use them only if necessary in light of the link with suicide in people under the age of 18 years (relating to paroxetine in particular).

I would advise that the child's education be structured in such a way as to take account of his impairments and special skills. I would suggest that we seek the advice of a specialist teacher or psychologist in this regard. Every effort would be made to educate this boy in a mainstream school setting with intensive support. However, if his functioning were very low, special education might be the only viable option and an appropriate school placement would be sought. He would be taught how to tolerate adult guidance and intrusion, to follow routines, to develop communicative abilities and to move from associational to more conceptual learning models.

Concerning psychological treatment, a behavioural approach would involve a functional analysis of target behaviour. A plan would then be formulated to promote desired behaviours and reduce unwanted ones. I would ensure that both his parents and teachers were involved to ensure consistency and also to help them provide an organized, predictable environment at home and school respectively.

As far as social support is concerned, I would provide the parents with practical advice on how to manage day-to-day issues. I would suggest some input from the social services department (in the UK), following a comprehensive assessment of the social care needs of the boy and his family. The parents might need help themselves and would benefit from childcare assistance to give them space to do other things. Should I have reason to believe that the parents are not coping emotionally or that one of them is depressed, I would advise them to seek further help from the GP. I would hope that, if these measures could be carried out effectively in a coordinated fashion, with minimal disruption to the family's life, we would have helped this young boy considerably.

ANSWERS TO SUGGESTED PROBES

1. I have given my differential diagnoses in my full answer.
2. The core symptoms of childhood autism are:
    *   difficulty with communication
    *   social skills impairment
    *   repetitive or stereotypical behaviour.
All of these present before the age of 36 months.
3. The salient features of the differential diagnoses I have mentioned are as follows:
    *   *Childhood autism.* Onset is invariably in the first year of life. The child exhibits problems with communication, social interaction and behaviour, which are often restricted.
    *   *Childhood disintegrative psychosis.* There is normal early development, followed by regression between the ages of 3 and 8 years, the presence of autistic features and mental retardation.
    *   *Rett syndrome.* This occurs only in girls. There is developmental regression after 12 months, with head deceleration, marked mental retardation and a characteristic hand-washing stereotype.
    *   *Asperger syndrome.* This is a mild form of autism with normal early cognitive and language development.
    *   *PDD not otherwise specified/atypical autism.* Some features are indicative of autism but other diagnostic criteria are absent.
    *   *Mental retardation not associated with PDD.* There are social and communication difficulties on a par with the child's IQ level.
    *   *Specific language difficulty.* Social and non-verbal communicative abilities are preserved.
    *   *Selective mutism.* Mutism only occurs in certain situations and towards particular people.
    *   *Social anxiety.* Anxiety arising from social interaction and exposure.
    *   *Severe neglect.* This may arise from inadequacy of learning of social behaviour (experiential learning).

BUZZ WORDS AND USEFUL TERMINOLOGY

Pervasive developmental disorders (PDD), pronomial reversal, developmental milestones, Landau–Kleffner syndrome, fragile X and Angelman syndromes, rituals.

REFERENCES AND SUGGESTED READING

Committee on Safety of Medicine 2003 Selective Serotonin Reuptake Inhibitors (SSRIs) – use in children and adolescents with major depressive disorder. Committee on Safety of Medicines, London

Gillberg C, Billstedt E 2000 Autism and Asperger syndrome: coexistence with other clinical disorders. Acta Psychiatrica Scandinavica 102(5):321–330

Sverd J 2003 Psychiatric disorders in individuals with pervasive developmental disorders. Journal of Psychiatric Practices 9(2):111–127

Tanguay P 2000 Autism. Journal of American Academy of Child and Adolescent Psychiatry 39(9):1079–1095

Volkmar F R, Klin A 2002 Autism and pervasive developmental disorders. In: Gelder M G, López-Ibor Jr J J, Andreasen N C (eds) New Oxford Textbook of Psychiatry, vol. 2. Oxford University Press, Oxford, pp 1723–1732

5.2 8-YEAR-OLD THREATENED WITH EXCLUSION FROM SCHOOL DUE TO DISRUPTIVE BEHAVIOUR

An 8-year-old boy has been referred to you by the family GP. His father left the family home recently following his partner's discovery that he has been having an extramarital affair. Two days ago the boy's mother attended the doctor's practice, bursting into tears because her son has been threatened with exclusion for repeated disruptive behaviour in class. He has apparently been suspended on five previous occasions for similar behaviour.

What would be your line of management?

SUGGESTED PROBES

1. What is the most likely diagnosis and what are the other diagnostic possibilities?
2. What side-effects would you advise the mother to watch for if you prescribe a stimulant such as methylphenidate?
3. What are the key elements of parenting skills training?

PMP PLAN

TASKS TO DO

The following five areas are relevant to this vignette but are not necessarily all-inclusive. The list is also not exhaustive:

a) Show an awareness of the processes involved in child psychiatric assessment.
b) Discuss the need to engage the family in your assessment and in supplying relevant information.
c) Demonstrate awareness of the various diagnostic possibilities.
d) Take a multidisciplinary and multimodal approach to management.
e) Show knowledge of the specific therapeutic options and demonstrate awareness of the medical, psychological and social approaches.

ISSUES

• Determining whether the boy's behavioural difficulties are due to a mental health problem or a reaction to the unfavourable family situation

- Swift assistance to ensure that the boy's education is not disrupted due to exclusion from school.

CLARIFY

- How close is this boy to being excluded?
- Is there a history of aggression towards himself and others?
- Would other children and staff be put at risk if the boy continued to attend school?

SEEK MORE INFORMATION

All the following need parental consent.

GP

- Personal and medical history of the boy and his family.

MOTHER (AND FATHER, IF POSSIBLE)

- Her views; what she has been told by the school, i.e. details of antecedent, behaviour and consequences
- Presence of impulsive, attentional and motor symptoms
- Presence of defiant behaviour, aggression and antisocial behaviour, poor social relationships; social disinhibitions, over-familiarity, cheekiness, disregard for rules and turn-taking
- Information to enable you to rule in or out conditions such as adjustment disorder, mood disorder, attention deficit hyperactivity disorder (ADHD) and autistic spectrum disorder
- History of similar problems in siblings, family history of violence, physical or sexual abuse (need to be sensitive)
- Completion of a Strength and Difficulty Questionnaire (SDQ Parent)
- Parent's relationship. Ask sensitively about the boy's father's views and whether the parents are married
- Parental permission to talk to the school authorities
- Child's referral for special educational needs assessment and support. Does he have a statement?

TEACHER

- Details of the boy's behaviour, what form the disruption takes, management to date, impact on his education and that of other children

- Educational progress and the presence of learning difficulties
- Relationship to peers
- Completion of a Strength and Difficulty Questionnaire (SDQ-Teacher) and Connor's Teacher Rating Scale (CTRS).

CHILD

- Views on his current difficulties
- Bullying
- Assessment of attentional deficit and psychomotor hyperactivity during the interview
- Possible referral for psychometric assessment to exclude learning difficulties and establish cognitive ability. IQ measurement is usually below 75
- Specific learning problems, e.g. reading difficulties (dyslexia) and clumsiness.

DIFFERENTIAL DIAGNOSIS/DIFFICULTIES

- *Functional.* ADHD and conduct disorders, including adjustment disorder, emotional disorders, severe anxiety, depression and, rarely, hypomania
- *Organic.* Autistic spectrum disorder, PDD, mental retardation, chromosomal abnormalities.

Note: request a psychometric test, ask parents to fill in Home Hyperactivity scale and SDQ–Parents form, and teachers to fill in CTRS and SDQ–Teacher form, in order to effectively rule in or rule out ADHD as much as possible.

APPROACH TO TREATMENT

- Take a multimodal and multidisciplinary approach, looking into the enhancement of parenting skills, if necessary.
- Address abnormal family dynamics via family therapy (including other family members, if appropriate).
- Enhance the child's interpersonal skills.
- Treat any comorbid condition.

WHAT TREATMENT/ADVICE

PARENTAL EDUCATION AND SOCIAL SUPPORT

- Avoid blaming the parents for the child's problem.

PSYCHOLOGICAL TREATMENT

- For adjustment and mood disorder, consider cognitive behavioural therapy, interpersonal psychotherapy and counselling.

MEDICAL

- *Major depressive illness.* Consider pharmacological intervention (with antidepressants). There are suggestions from trials that an SSRI may be beneficial but there is little evidence about efficacy in children. Some authorities have advised against the use of paroxetine under the age of 18 years given its link with suicidal behaviour (see previous vignette).
- *ADHD.* Use stimulant drugs, coupled with a psychological approach to promote academic and social learning, and to improve emotional disturbance, self-esteem and family functioning. Allay the mother's anxiety about the possibility of the child becoming 'hooked' on stimulant drugs.
- *Autistic spectrum disorder.* Psychoeducational approaches and family support need particular attention, and should probably constitute the first line of management. Medication may help reduce the behavioural disturbance and hyperactivity associated with this condition. SSRIs such as fluoxetine may help reduce repetitive and maladaptive behaviour in the short term. Clonidine and antipsychotics may help with hyperactivity as a second line.

FULL ANSWER

The mother of this 8-year-old boy is clearly distressed at the prospect of her son being excluded from school. This is a particularly difficult period for her, given the recent split from her partner. One of the issues that I would like to address is to determine whether the boy's behavioural difficulties are due to a mental health problem or are a reaction to the unfavourable family situation. Another issue is how best to provide swift assistance to ensure that the boy's education is not disrupted due to exclusion from school.

I would clarify how close this child is to being excluded from school again and how the mother thinks this could be avoided. I would find out if he has a history of aggression towards himself or others. I would also clarify whether the school authorities think other children or staff would be put at risk by the boy's behaviour if he continued to attend school.

First, I would ask the GP for any relevant records or information he or she might have about this family and the boy's medical history. I would ask if the boy had any contact with the psychiatric or social services during his early years. I would find out if there are other children in the family and their situation at the present time. I would also liaise with the social services department for any information they had on the family, after obtaining permission from the parents to do so.

Then I would offer to see this boy in the outpatient department, encouraging all family members to attend the appointment. I would ask his mother what she thinks of the referral and her understanding of what is happening. I would establish when the problems started and whether the child had any developmental delays, such as speech and language difficulties or clumsiness. I would also ask for the mother's own explanation of events, and what happened when the boy was excluded in the past. I would find out if she has asked the teachers about the child's behaviour and about their explanation of events. I would enquire about his academic performance, any bullying behaviour, whether he enjoys school and if there are similar behavioural disturbances at home. I would be keen to find out about the presence of restlessness, inattentiveness and impulsiveness. I would ask if the child is ever destructive, has difficulty focusing on tasks or sitting still, or becomes involved in dangerous behaviour that leads to him being hurt or to him hurting others. If this does happen, I would like to know whether the child is remorseful afterwards. I would ask how the mother deals with these problems. I would want to be sure that she is not responding or behaving in a way that reinforces this bad behaviour. I would find out about the child's sleep pattern, his appetite, and his relationship with his peers at school and home. I would ask about other children in the family, whether they have a history of similar problems and how are they responding to the present situation. I would like to establish the impact of the present problem on the whole family and know how they are coping. I would find out whether there is a history of violence or criminality in either of the parents. I would ask about the relationship between his parents and if they are married, and would also sensitively seek the father's views, if he attends any of the sessions. I would ask carefully about any history of physical or sexual abuse. I would question the mother as to whether she thinks that the recent split from her partner has had any impact on what is going on at present, and if so, in what way.

After obtaining parental permission, I would talk to other family members to seek their views about what is happening and what help they think is needed. With the mother's permission,

I would talk to the boy's schoolteachers to get a more detailed report in terms of the antecedent, his behaviour, the incident itself, and how they responded to it. I would ask about the impact of this child's behaviour on other pupils and whether the boy is able to appreciate what effect he is having. I would find out what led to the previous exclusions and at what stage the teachers allowed him back to school. It would also be important to hear their understanding of the problem and what they think would help.

I would then proceed to ask the child himself further questions on his understanding of events. I would find out if he has friends in school and whether they have similar difficulties. I would ascertain whether the child realizes his behaviour has become disruptive to others and how he is trying to deal with that. I would pay attention to the presence of attentional deficit and psychomotor hyperactivity during assessments. I would refer him for assessment of his cognitive ability and for psychometry to exclude learning difficulties. IQ measurement is usually below 75. I would look for clumsiness and specific learning problems such as reading difficulties (dyslexia). I would find out if the child has been referred for special educational needs assessment and support and if he has a statement.

Bearing in mind his presentation, the differential diagnosis would include adjustment reaction to a dysfunctional family environment that finally led to his parents' recent separation, emotional disorders (severe anxiety, depression, mania and other mood disorders) and conduct disorders. I would also consider attention deficit hyperactivity disorder (ADHD), given that the core symptoms—namely, impulsivity, inattention and motor overactivity—could have been getting him into trouble at school. Other possibilities include mood disorders presenting with irritability and oppositional symptoms, autistic spectrum disorder, which could also be associated with hyperactivity and oppositional behaviour, PDD and mental retardation or other chromosomal abnormalities. In order to understand the various contributory factors, I would request a psychometric assessment of this boy's level of intelligence and also ask his parents and teachers to fill in the Home Hyperactivity Scale/SDQ–Parents and Connor's (CTRS) Scale/SDQ–Teacher forms respectively. The intention would be effectively to rule out or in ADHD.

In my approach to treatment, I would engage the family as far as possible, avoid blaming the mother (or both parents), arrange convenient assessments—for example, making clinic appointments for late evening to avoid disrupting the mother's work or other activities, and offer her practical help and advice. I would involve other members of the multidisciplinary team but tailor this to the boy's needs. I would ensure that treatment was offered that included biological, psychological and social support. I would advise psychological treatment for specific adjustment and mood disorders, and would consider cognitive behavioural therapy (CBT), interpersonal psychotherapy and counselling. Treatment programmes focused on enhancing the child's interpersonal and social skills would also be useful, and in addition I would treat any comorbid condition. Further psychological treatment in the form of family therapy and parenting skills training might also be useful, depending on the diagnosis. If necessary and feasible, I would suggest addressing family dynamics via family therapy.

There might be a role for medical intervention with psychotropic drugs. If evidence of it existed, a major depressive illness might need pharmacological (antidepressant) intervention. There are suggestions from trials that an SSRI might be beneficial in cases such as these, but there is little evidence about their efficacy in children. However, in light of the link between SSRIs and suicidal behaviour I would avoid their use, with the exception of fluoxetine. Paroxetine would be my last choice, given the difficulties in withdrawing the medication. If the diagnostic assessment carried out by a child psychologist and/or child psychiatrist were highly suggestive of ADHD, stimulant drugs coupled with a psychological approach would be advised to promote academic and social learning, and to improve emotional disturbance, self-esteem and family functioning. I would carefully explain to the mother about the use of stimulants such as methylphenidate, so as to allay her anxieties about the child becoming addicted. I would also warn her about side-effects and what to expect. I would tell her not to expect medication to solve all the problems and that the child will need continuous support, including interventions from other professionals. Parental education will be necessary on the nature of the disorder, the need for medication and reassurance that the child is not going to become addicted, unnecessarily sedated or 'high'.

For a child with an autistic spectrum disorder, medication might help reduce the behavioural disturbances and hyperactivity associated with this condition. An SSRI such as fluoxetine might help reduce repetitive and maladaptive behaviour in the short term. Clonidine and antipsychotics might also help with hyperactivity as second-line medications. I would also pay particular attention to psychoeducational approaches, and to family and social support. There might be a need to involve an educational psychologist, educational social worker and specialist teacher for advice on how this boy's educational and social learning could be promoted. Extra tuition might be necessary, given the child's limited attention span. Fostering would be an extreme solution if the mother were finding it difficult to cope.

ANSWERS TO SUGGESTED PROBES

1. ADHD is a strong diagnostic possibility. Other differential diagnoses include conduct disorder and other conditions I have mentioned in my full answer.
2. If I prescribed a stimulant such as methylphenidate, I would advise the mother to be on the lookout for:
   - reduced appetite
   - insomnia
   - weight loss
   - dysphoric reactions (including depression and irritability)
   - provocation of repetitive activities by over-medication
   - a slight reduction in adult height with long-term use (controversial).

   Note: stimulants can exacerbate tics and are best avoided in some children with tic disorders. Cautious use may be recommended under the supervision of specialists. Other drugs used are imipramine, clonidine and, rarely, antipsychotics.
3. The key elements of good parenting skill training include:
   - promotion of play and a positive relationship
   - praise and rewards for sociable behaviour
   - setting of clear rules and commands
   - consistent and calm consequences for unwanted behaviour
   - reorganization of the child's day to prevent trouble.

BUZZ WORDS AND USEFUL TERMINOLOGY

Core symptoms, stereotypical activities, social skills, parental education, pervasive developmental disorders (PDDs), family dynamics, diagnostic assessment, engagement.

REFERENCES AND SUGGESTED READING

Scott S 2002 Conduct disorder in childhood and adolescence. In: Gelder M G, López-Ibor Jr J J, Andreasen N C (eds) New Oxford Textbook of Psychiatry, vol. 2. Oxford University Press, Oxford, pp 1750–1761

Taylor E 1994 Physical treatments. In: Rutter M, Taylor E, Hersov L (eds) Child and Adolescent Psychiatry: Modern Approaches, 3rd edn. Blackwell Scientific, Oxford, pp 880–899

Werry J S, Aman M G 1993 Practitioner's Guide to Psychoactive Drugs for Children and Adolescents. Plenum, New York

A 7-year-old girl has been referred to your service by her family doctor, following concerns expressed by her parents that she has started to soil herself with faeces. She achieved continence almost 4 years previously.

How would you assess and manage this patient?

SUGGESTED PROBES

1. What are the differential diagnoses of secondary encopresis at this age?
2. What other condition would you rule out before you conclude that the encopresis is due to emotional or psychiatric disorder?
3. What advice (behavioural) would you give to the mother on managing encopresis?

PMP PLAN

TASKS TO DO

The following five areas are relevant to this vignette but are not necessarily all-inclusive. The list is also not exhaustive:

a) Conduct a good and systematic exploration of the presenting problem.
b) Consider biopsychosocial causative factors.
c) Rule out organic causes before assuming a psychiatric aetiology.
d) Take a biopsychosocial approach to management, including liaison with the appropriate professionals.
e) Take an empathic approach to management.

ISSUES

- Assessment of underlying problem, whether due to an organic (physical) disorder or an emotional problem
- Institution of appropriate management including working closely with parents and her physician.

CLARIFY

- Is this a one-off accident?
- Does the presentation fulfil the criteria for a diagnosis of encopresis, whether there is constipation or not?

SEEK MORE INFORMATION

GP

- If physical problems have been excluded.

PARENTS

Details of encopresis.

- Toileting habits: frequency, intervals, amount, diameter and consistency of bowel movements
- Is the stool deposited in the toilet or in underwear? Does the child hide the soiled underwear?
- Presence of constipation (retentive and non-retentive encopresis)
- Situation in which faecal soiling occurs
- Presence of stool withholding
- Presence of abdominal pain
- Dietary habits
- Presence of enuresis and urinary tract infection.

Possible precipitating and perpetuating factors.

- Help received to date and its benefit
- Stressful life events, recent or during toilet training, presence of emotional disturbance, home circumstances/family discord, and effect of the encopresis on the child and the rest of the family
- Parental response to difficulties: punishment of the child/measures taken to resolve the problem
- Professional help at present or in the past.

CHILD

- Awareness of the encopretic event
- Presence of abdominal pain
- Toilet phobia ('monsters'), stress-induced, loss of control, provocative soiling.

INVESTIGATIONS

- Minimal laboratory work-up
- Not necessary if the GP already carried out extensive tests
- Blood studies, urine microscopy and abdominal radiographs may be useful.

PHYSICAL EXAMINATION

- Measurement of weight and height
- Abdominal palpation
- Anal irritation, fissures and faecal impaction
- Sphincteric tone and perianal sensation
- Stool: impacted/soft
- Presence of anorectal malformations, spinal disorders, cerebral palsy, mental retardation and endocrine, metabolic or neuromuscular disorders
- Paediatric advice.

DIFFERENTIAL DIAGNOSIS/DIFFICULTIES

- *Physical.* Constipation, anal fissure, inadequate diet, laxative abuse
- *Psychosocial.* Emotional disturbance, parental over-concern with bowel habit, stressful life events, family discord.

APPROACH TO TREATMENT

- Consider the nature of the encopresis, and whether there is functional constipation.
- Recognize the need to draw parents and child into a therapeutic relationship; take a no-blame approach.
- Involve a multidisciplinary team and minimize disruption to family life.
- Offer psychoeducation and behavioural intervention.

WHAT TREATMENT/ADVICE

- *Health education and counselling (parents and child).* Discuss realistic expectations of the child's response to treatment, once an organic factor has been ruled out. Prepare a detailed plan. Keep a stool diary.
- *Behavioural interventions.* Draw up a programme to reinforce defaecation in the toilet and encourage regular toilet use. Prevent the reaccumulation of stools through reconditioning to normal bowel habit. Ask the child to sit on the toilet for up to 5 minutes, three to four times a day after meals. Combine these measures with a reward system (token).
- *Medical.* Consider retraining as above and use medical therapy in difficult cases. Remove faecal retention if it is

present, using hypertonic phosphate enemas, polyethylene glycol or high-dose laxatives. Prevent the reaccumulation of stools through the use of laxatives, if necessary. Treat constipation, a common cause of secondary encopresis.
- *Biofeedback training.*
- *Monitoring.* Monitor progress and give further advice, if needed.

FULL ANSWER

I would want to address issues of how to assess whether the problem is organic or has an emotional cause, given that she has been referred to a psychiatrist. I would discuss the need for appropriate management to include working with the parents and family doctor.

This will certainly be a distressing development for the young girl and her family. Prior to inviting them to an outpatient appointment, I would clarify whether the soiling is an occasional 'accident', and whether the presentation fulfils the criteria for the diagnosis of encopresis, whether or not constipation is also present. I would clarify with the GP that physical problems such as constipation, anal fissures, inadequate diet and abuse of laxatives have been ruled out. In addition, I would seek to exclude psychosocial factors such as emotional disturbance, parental overconcern with bowel regularity and cleanliness, stressful life events and family discord.

During the assessment itself, I would seek more information on the encopresis, and ask questions about when the child soils (nocturnal encopresis is rare and is often organic), how often it happens and whether she also wets herself. I would ask how independent the child is as regards toileting and how she copes with the episodes of soiling. I would ask if the child is able to sit on the toilet unaided, whether she can take herself to the toilet, and how frequently she does that. I would ask if she is able to undress herself before going to the toilet and dress herself again afterwards. I would want to know what does she do when her pants are soiled and whether she hides her dirty underwear. I would ask the parents whether they feel that the child sometimes becomes preoccupied with more interesting activities and puts off going to the toilet. I would find out whether they are aware of any problem with constipation and, if so, whether any medication has been used. I would ask about abdominal pain and any experience of pain on defaecation. When I saw the child, I would find out if she is aware of the encopretic event and would look for evidence of toilet phobia, if it appears the child is frightened of going to the toilet ('monsters'). The encopresis might also be a stress-induced condition, be due to loss of control, or constitute a form of provocative soiling. I would enquire about stressful life events, either recent or during toilet training, and the presence of any emotional disturbances in the child. I would establish the family's home circumstances, relationships and any discord, and the effect of the encopresis on the child and the rest of the family. I would find out how the parents are responding to the difficulties and whether they have been adopting a punitive approach. I would ask if they have taken any steps towards resolving the problem and whether they are currently receiving any professional help.

As far as the differential diagnosis is concerned, it is possible that the encopresis, which is secondary, might be due to a physical condition such as constipation, anal fissure, inadequate diet or laxative abuse. I would attempt to rule out physical causes and would seek the advice of a paediatrician, who might be able to discount anal irritation, fissures and impacted faeces. I would also consider referral to a paediatrician for assessment of anal pressure, sphincteric tone and loss of perianal sensation, and would screen for anorectal malformations or a neurological condition. The specialist would also be able to carry out appropriate weight and height measurement, perform abdominal palpation, and examine the child's stools and whether they are impacted or soft. I would also ensure that other possible causes, such as spinal disorders, cerebral palsy, mental retardation, and endocrine, metabolic and neuromuscular disorders, have been excluded. I would carry out minimal laboratory investigations, particularly if the GP had already done extensive tests. Otherwise, I would consider routine blood studies, urine microscopy, abdominal radiographs and/or a CT scan.

Having considered and ruled out a physical cause, I would focus on psychosocial aspects, such as emotional disturbance, parental over-concern with bowel habit, stressful life events and family discord.

My approach to treatment would be to involve the child's family very closely with assessment and treatment. I would reassure the parents that they are not the cause of the problem and that the condition is not necessarily due to bad parenting. The assessment and treatment programme would be coordinated in such a way as to cause minimal disruption to their family life. The treatment that I would offer would depend on the nature of the encopresis, which may occur with or without functional constipation. My strategy would focus on psychoeducation, removal of faecal retention if present, prevention of reaccumulation of stools through reconditioning of normal bowel habits, and withdrawal of treatment at a safe time. I would ensure the inclusion of health education and counselling for parents and child, and discuss realistic expectations of the girl's response to treatment once organic aetiological factors had been ruled out. To ensure consistency and the parents' cooperation, I would prepare a detailed plan and give a copy to them. I would encourage them to keep a stool diary to record the frequency and consistency of bowel motions passed in the toilet or in the pants, and the circumstances surrounding the episodes of incontinence. This would help me to assess and quantify the problem, guide the treatment given and assist with monitoring progress.

Behavioural intervention might be quite useful but there might also be a need for medical intervention. Medical therapy might be in the form of removal of faecal retention, if present, with the use of hypertonic phosphate enemas, polyethylene glycol or high-dose laxatives. I would prevent the reaccumulation of stools, if necessary through the use of laxatives, and also treat other causes of constipation, a common cause of secondary encopresis. Osmotic laxatives such as milk of magnesia, mineral oil, lactulose, sorbitol and polyethylene glycol have been found useful. A stimulant laxative such as senna or bisacodyl (10 mg suppositories) might also be of use if the child retains loose stool with the use of osmotic laxatives.

I would consider behavioural intervention programmes to reinforce defaecation in the toilet and to encourage regular toilet use. I would aim to prevent reaccumulation of stools through reconditioning to normal bowel habits. This might involve asking the child to sit on the toilet for up to 5 minutes, three to four times a day after meals. A combination of the above plan with a reward system (token), perhaps a star chart, might improve outcome. I would advise her parents not to over-stress the importance of her keeping her underwear clean, as this could encourage her to retain faeces and so become constipated. I would also suggest that they encourage her to use the toilet after meals or drinks, as this not only is practical but also facilitates defaecation. She should be encouraged to sit on the toilet for long enough to defaecate but not for so long that it becomes boring or punitive (between 1 and 5 minutes). She should be rewarded for sitting on the toilet and given an extra reward for passing a motion.

I am also aware that successes in the use of biofeedback training, acupuncture and withdrawal of cow's milk protein have been reported in the treatment of encopresis with constipation. These would only be considered in this case if there were specific indications for each one after the measures I have already mentioned had been tried. In addition to the obvious physical problems that might be causing the encopresis, any emotional difficulties that may be underlying a functional, non-retentive faecal soiling would require psychological treatment. If the problem is defaecation in inappropriate places, this would raise the possibility of distress in this girl, or dysfunction or problems within the family. In this case, I would assess the response of her parents to the behaviour, bearing in mind that the act might be manipulative. Consequently, family intervention would be offered, looking into the behaviour itself, removing any reinforcer and encouraging more appropriate ways of communicating. Family counselling and support would also be necessary to help the family deal with issues arising from the distress caused by the encopresis. I would arrange for close monitoring of progress and give further advice as necessary.

ANSWERS TO SUGGESTED PROBES

1. The differential diagnosis of secondary encopresis at this age may be divided into:
   - *Physical causes.* Anal irritation, fissures, impacted faeces, anorectal malformations and other causes such as spinal disorders, cerebral palsy, mental retardation and endocrine, metabolic and neuromuscular disorders
   - *Emotional causes.* Emotional disturbance, parental over-concern with bowel habit, stressful life events and family discord.
2. Before I concluded that the encopresis is due to emotional or psychiatric disorder, I would rule out:
   - impacted faeces
   - anorectal malformations and sphincteric abnormalities (check anal pressure)
   - anal irritation and/or fissures, Hirschsprung's disease
   - spinal disorders
   - cerebral palsy
   - mental retardation
   - endocrine and metabolic disorders
   - neuromuscular disorders (loss of perianal sensation?).
3. I have already covered the behavioural advice I would give to the mother in my full answer.

BUZZ WORDS AND USEFUL TERMINOLOGY

Encopretic episodes, stool diary, negative reinforcer.

REFERENCES AND SUGGESTED READING

Borowitz S M, Cox D J, Sutphen J L et al 2002 Treatment of childhood encopresis: a randomised trial comparing three treatment protocols. Journal of Paediatric Gastroenterology and Nutrition 34(4):378–384

Douglas J 2002 Disorders of sleeping, eating and elimination in childhood. In: Gelder M G, López-Ibor Jr J J, Andreasen N C (eds) New Oxford Textbook of Psychiatry, vol. 2. Oxford, Oxford University Press, pp 1793–1794

Loening-Baucke V 2002 Encopresis. Current Opinion in Paediatrics 14(5):570–575

Mikkesen E J 2001 Enuresis and encopresis: ten years of progress. Journal of American Academy of Child and Adolescent Psychiatry 40(10):1146–1158

5.4 11-YEAR-OLD BOY WHO IS REFUSING TO ATTEND SCHOOL

You have been contacted by an educational social worker about an 11-year-old boy who has refused to attend school for the past 4 months. His father left the family home 8 months ago. His mother, who is single, has been threatened with a possible court order, but this has not helped either.

How would you assess and manage this situation?

SUGGESTED PROBES

1. What are the main issues in this case?
2. What are the distinguishing features of truancy and school refusal?
3. During your assessment, you begin to suspect that the mother is complicit in keeping the child at home. What factors in your history support this view?

PMP PLAN

TASKS TO DO

The following five areas are relevant to this vignette but are not necessarily all-inclusive. The list is also not exhaustive:

a) Demonstrate an ability to think broadly about the possible causes of school refusal.
b) Appreciate the need to return the boy to school as soon as possible.
c) Show a good understanding of the various psychological and social approaches.
d) Adopt multidisciplinary thinking and work with the family and the school.
e) Manage social anxieties and bullying, if these are the causes of school refusal.

ISSUES

- Identification of the reason for this child's school refusal
- Dealing with the causative factors
- Measures aimed at returning him to school as soon as possible
- Support for his mother and teachers.

CLARIFY

- Why is the boy refusing to attend school and what has been the approach to this problem to date?
- Why is there a threat to take the mother to court, and is there any suspicion of collusion?
- Is there a family history of contact with social services?

SEEK MORE INFORMATION

Ask for parental consent always.

GP

- Family and background history; medical/psychiatric illness in parents or siblings.

EDUCATIONAL SOCIAL WORKER

- Social worker involvement in addressing the present problem
- Reason for referral to child and family services in the past
- Involvement of other children with the services

MOTHER

- Onset and history of the problem
- What the child does at home if he refuses school (watches television, plays games or does nothing?)
- Recent change of school?

CHILD

- Outpatient review with family members
- Assessment to identify precipitating and maintaining factors
- Physical, psychosocial and emotional reasons: bullying at school, school change, low IQ, chronic anxiety, family discord, maternal illness, attachment problem.

SCHOOL (TEACHERS, SCHOOL NURSE OR EDUCATIONAL SOCIAL WORKER)

- Help given to the family to date
- School's views on the child's development.

DIFFERENTIAL DIAGNOSIS/DIFFICULTIES

- *Functional and psychological.* Panic disorder, depression, generalized anxiety with or without depression, post-traumatic stress disorder (PTSD), agoraphobia, obsessive-compulsive disorder (OCD), separation anxiety disorder, specific phobia, social phobia, sexual abuse, learning disability, substance misuse disorder, alcohol, cannabinoids, stimulant and/or solvent abuse
- *Organic.* Injuries and handicaps, communication difficulties, dyslexia, learning disabilities
- *Psychosocial.* Emotionally dependent mother, maternal anxiety, child labour, conflict and marital discord, child custody issues, bullying at school.

APPROACH TO TREATMENT

- Tailor management to the needs of the child and include psychosocial interventions.
- Involve a multidisciplinary team.
- Coordinate assessment and treatment, ensuring minimal disruption to family life.
- Avoid blaming either of the parents.

WHAT TREATMENT/ADVICE

MEDICAL

- Treat for specific syndromes such as panic disorder, depression, PTSD.
- Take measures to deal with injuries, handicap, dyslexia or any other form of disability.

PSYCHOLOGICAL

- Carry out a functional analysis of the school refusal behaviour and treatment to date.
- Instigate cognitive psychotherapy (individual) and cognitive behavioural therapy.
- Use exposure-based techniques for anxiety and school refusal.
- Advise relaxation and special breathing exercises for anxiety in and out of the classroom.
- Tackle social/performance anxiety—the child needs empowerment.

- Arrange education support therapy and supportive psychotherapy.
- Arrange family therapy for the parents and family counselling if there is discord.

EDUCATIONAL

- Return the child to school as soon as possible; occasionally, a forced return is required.
- Aim for successful reintegration, monitor the child's progress and avoid relapse.
- Minimize the option of education at home.

SOCIAL AND OTHER

- Address communication difficulties with communication skills training.
- If the child is shy, isolated or misunderstood, arrange for social and communication skills training.
- Give practical support to the family.
- Address performance anxiety with empowerment training.
- If the child is a victim of teasing or bullying, adopt strategies of analysis, school intervention, peer refusal training and assertiveness training, along with specific coping skills. A change of school is rarely necessary.

FULL ANSWER

In managing this case, the main issues I would focus on are identifying the reason for this child's school refusal, dealing with the causative factor as far as possible, carrying out measures aimed at returning him to school as soon as possible, and giving support to the mother and teachers. I would bear in mind that the reason why the child is refusing school might be connected with the child himself, the parent, the family situation or even the school.

I would first like to obtain the social worker's views on why the boy has refused to attend school and what attempts have been made so far to address the situation. I would like to know why the education authority has decided to take the route of a possible court order. I would ask the social worker if he or she has any suspicion of collusion on the part of the mother, and whether previous warnings and ultimatums have been ignored. I would find out if the family is known to social services and, if so, why. I would ask if there are other children in the picture and whether they have similar problems or have had them in the past. Since the mother is single, I would find out when she separated or divorced from her partner, and what impact that separation had on the boy's development and day-to-day living. I would find out if the boy's father is involved in his life or his care in any way since his departure 8 months earlier, and what he has tried to do about the boy refusing school.

While making arrangements to see the boy, his mother and other members of his immediate family, I would seek more information from the GP on the boy's medical and psychiatric history and on his family, particularly the mother. I would ask about any family psychiatric illness, and any developmental or medical problems in this boy. I would pay particular attention to any history of anxiety and depression in him and also in his mother.

In my assessment, I would find out when the problem began, how it manifested itself, and whether the mother has any idea of what might have brought it on. I would ask her if her son has recently changed school. I would ask if he has been complaining of physical problems such as headaches or abdominal pain, or whether he just bluntly refuses to go to school. I would find out how the mother deals with the problem, and how the boy occupies himself at home if he does not go to school. I would ask if his physical problems resolve once he is allowed to stay at home. I would also ask what the mother has done so far to rectify the situation, and what help has been sought or given. I would find out about the family environment and situation before and after the mother separated from her partner and how the problem has impacted on family lifestyle and well-being. If, during the interview, I began to suspect that the mother is complicit in keeping the child at home, I would tactically assess for evidence and factors in the history to support this view. It could be that the boy is the oldest child and is able to assist with domestic chores. He might also be assisting his mother in home-based work. It is possible that the mother is suffering from an anxiety disorder, depression and/or other mental illness, or a disability or handicap, and needs the child's support. There might also be secondary gains in keeping the child at home, such as financial support or her being excused from duties or work. Severe social isolation, lack of a confiding relationship in the mother and total lack of support from the child's father would also make the mother's complicity more likely.

Whilst I would seek the opinion of as many members of the family as possible, it might be necessary to talk to the boy on his own to assess his own perception of events. I would allow him to speak about his concerns and fears, and would seek parental permission to talk to his schoolteachers, school nurse, psychologist and/or educational social worker. I would find out if he has just changed schools and, if so, how he has settled down. I would ask if he has made friends and look for any indication that he has been or is being bullied at school. I would find out about the boy's academic performance from his teachers, and whether they think he is worried about his performance or has anxieties about receiving poor grades. I would ask if they think he avoids going to school because of taking a test or to avoid being perceived as stupid. I would ask if the school is aware of any difficulty in communication or social anxiety, and if the boy has any form of learning disability, handicap or language difficulties.

Since the boy has refused to go to school, rather than leaving home in the morning and then not attending class, the most likely problem is that of school refusal. Since school refusal in itself is not a psychiatric diagnosis, I would look for possible underlying problems. For the differential diagnosis, I would consider physical causes such as injuries and handicaps, communication difficulties and dyslexia, which might make the child refuse school if he thinks he is unable to match the performance of his peers. The child might also have underlying emotional and psychological disorder, such as panic disorder, depression, generalized anxiety with or without depression, post-traumatic stress disorder (PTSD), agoraphobia, obsessive-compulsive disorder (OCD), separation anxiety disorder, specific phobia, social phobia and anxiety, sexual abuse or learning disability. There is also the possibility of a substance misuse disorder such as alcohol, cannabinoids, or stimulant and/or solvent abuse. The child might also be refusing school for psychosocial reasons, such as collusion on the part of an emotionally dependent mother, or a mother who suffers from anxiety or another mental illness. The boy might be involved in child labour, family conflict, marital discord and child custody issues, or be suffering from bullying at school or social anxiety. In a very rare situation, the child might have committed an as yet undisclosed or unidentified offence or crime.

To begin with, I would explain the nature of the problem to the mother and also to the school officials (after seeking parental permission). I would discuss treatment approaches with the mother and the teachers to ensure their cooperation in dealing with the situation. I would avoid blaming either of the parents for causing the problem. As far as possible, treatment would be a coordinated joint effort on the part of a multidisciplinary team working with the child, the family and the school. Management, which would include psychosocial interventions, would be tailored to the needs of the child. I would suggest that assessment and treatment are coordinated to ensure minimal disruption to family life and also to avoid duplication of roles.

Treatment would largely depend on the cause of the problem. Overall, it would be necessary to return this boy to school as soon as possible. I would direct specific medical treatment to syndromes such as panic disorder, depression or PTSD. I would give advice on specific measures to deal with injuries, handicap, dyslexia or any other form of disability that might be preventing the child from going to school. To assist psychological treatment, I would carry out a functional analysis of the school refusal behaviour, along with the team psychologist, and would offer treatment in the form of cognitive psychotherapy (individual), cognitive behavioural therapy, exposure-based techniques for anxiety, school refusal and anxiety-based school refusal. If there were a significant problem with social and performance anxiety, treatment would focus on empowering the child. I would also suggest relaxation and special breathing exercises for anxiety in the classroom or school. If, despite these measures, it were still difficult to persuade the child to go to school, I would try slowly separating the parent from the child once he was in school. One approach would be to have the mother attend school with the child initially, but to sit in another room. Then the parent would gradually withdraw, by accompanying the boy almost as far as the school and then just halfway and so on, until he feels confident enough to go to school independently.

The aim of educational management would be to return the boy to school as soon as possible. This might be facilitated by education support therapy, supportive psychotherapy for the child and family therapy for the parents. To encourage the return to school, I would minimize the option of education at home and, if necessary, force a return to school. Successful reintegration would require the support of all concerned, and close monitoring of the child's progress in order to avoid relapse. If there were concurrent family discord and disputes, family counselling might be useful. I would employ other social measures and treatments to deal with social situations that might be encouraging the child to absent himself from school, and if there is a problem with communicating, he would benefit from training in communication skills. This would also help the child if he is shy, or finds himself isolated or misunderstood most of the time. I would advise strict intervention on the part of the school if the child is a victim of teasing and/or bullying. The boy would also benefit from assertiveness and peer refusal training, if peer pressure is contributing to the problem. All these treatments would be accompanied by practical support for the family. In very rare circumstances—for example, if persistent bullying is a problem —a change of school might be necessary.

ANSWERS TO SUGGESTED PROBES

1. The main issues in this case are:
   - finding out why the child is refusing to attend school
   - dealing effectively with any causative factors
   - getting him back to school as soon as possible
   - giving support to the mother and teachers.

2. Truancy is characterized by its wilful nature and is not usually associated with distress (egosyntonic). The parents are not aware of the child's truancy, and it is associated with other antisocial behaviour.

   In school refusal, the child can be upset about not going to school (egodystonic). The parents are often aware of the non-attendance. There is associated anxiety or somatic symptoms and these may disappear during weekends and school holidays.

   It is important to note, however, that truancy and school refusal can overlap.

3. These are the factors in the history that would support the view that the mother is complicit in keeping the child at home:
   - The child is the oldest and is able to assist with domestic chores.
   - The child is assisting the mother in home-based work.
   - The mother suffers from an anxiety disorder, depression or other mental illness.
   - The mother suffers from a disability and/or handicap and needs the support of the child.
   - There are secondary gains in keeping child at home.
   - There is severe social isolation and lack of a confiding relationship in the mother.
   - The mother has a history of poor school attendance herself.
   - There is a lack of support from the child's father.

BUZZ WORDS AND USEFUL TERMINOLOGY

Parental permission, education support therapy, egosyntonic, egodystonic, performance anxiety, functional analysis of behaviour.

REFERENCES AND SUGGESTED READING

Elliot J G 1999 Practitioner review: school refusal: issues of conceptualization, assessment, and treatment. Journal of Child Psychology and Psychiatry 40:1001–1012

Goodyear I 2002 Emotional disorders with their onset in childhood. In: Gelder M G, López-Ibor Jr J J, Andreasen N C (eds) New Oxford Textbook of Psychiatry, vol. 2, pp 1762–1771

Link E H 2003 School refusal and psychiatric disorder: a community study. Journal of the American Academy of Child and Adolescent Psychiatry 42(7):797–807

5.5 9-YEAR-OLD BOY EXCLUDED FROM SCHOOL FOR DISRUPTIVE BEHAVIOUR

A 9-year-old boy has been referred to your child and adolescent psychiatric service by his family doctor after being excluded from school for disruptive behaviour in class. This has persisted for the past 1 or 2 years. He is unable to keep still in class, cannot concentrate on doing just one thing and seems to lack a sense of danger.

How would you go about assessing and managing this case?

SUGGESTED PROBES

1. What are the cardinal features of attention deficit hyperactivity disorder (ADHD)?
2. What else could be making this boy lose concentration in class?
3. What is the possible impact of this condition, if untreated?

PMP PLAN

TASKS TO DO

The following five areas are relevant to this vignette but are not necessarily all-inclusive. The list is also not exhaustive:

a) Mention ADHD/hyperactivity as a differential diagnosis. Show awareness that other situations could mimic this presentation.
b) Demonstrate knowledge of the core symptoms in hyperactivity states and the necessary medical and non-medical investigations.
c) Show familiarity with protocols in the child psychiatric assessment of hyperactivity, with involvement of a multidisciplinary team.
d) Comment on the impact of the condition at present and that of comorbidity if it remains untreated.
e) Demonstrate a good knowledge of treatment modalities, including drugs and their possible side-effects.

Note: this child has already been excluded from school and the management plan should also address how to return him to school as soon as possible.

ISSUES

• Comprehensive assessment to determine the underlying problem, whether due to physical, functional or environmental factors

- Institution of appropriate management strategies including working with the family, family doctors and teachers.

CHILD AND ADOLESCENT PSYCHIATRY

CLARIFY

- Have physical problems such as seizures and epilepsy been ruled out?
- What exactly led to the exclusion?
- Is there a risk of self-harm?

SEEK MORE INFORMATION

GP

- Medical and psychiatric history
- History of atopia, allergies and epilepsy
- Current medication (?use of bronchodilators and anticonvulsants).

PARENTS

- Characteristic core symptoms of inattention, hyperactivity and impulsivity: carelessness, difficulty in watching a film or cartoon to completion from an early age, failure to finish tasks such as school work and homework, distracted easily by extraneous stimuli, always 'on the go', difficulty in awaiting turn, impulsivity (motor, cognitive or verbal), excessive running and climbing, sustenance of frequent injuries
- Family history of mood disorder, ADHD, antisocial personality disorder
- Family and marital discord
- Questionnaires: interview at clinic and use standardized instrument to rate symptoms, i.e. Home Hyperactivity Scale, Strength and Difficulty Questionnaire (SDQ–Parent) and Connor's Rating Scale.

TEACHERS

- Interrupting, intruding, failure to finish games, fighting in school, being 'picked on', lack of friends, difficulty in remaining seated in class, failure to follow instructions, poor academic performance, disregard for rules

- Use standardized instrument to rate symptoms using interviews and questionnaires: 39-item Connor's Teacher Rating Scale (CTRS) or the Abbreviated Connor's Teacher Rating Scale (ACTeRS).

CHILD

- Awareness of the problem: does he think parents or teachers are always 'yelling at him' for no reason?
- Psychologist
- Psychometric and neuropsychological tests to support the diagnosis
- Assessment of IQ by Wechsler Intelligence Scale for Children – Revised (WISC–R)
- Continuous Performance Test (CPT).

INVESTIGATIONS

- EEG.

DIFFERENTIAL DIAGNOSIS/DIFFICULTIES

- *Functional/psychological.* ADHD, conduct disorder, oppositional defiant disorder, depression (look for cognitive blunting or psychomotor agitation), mania, anxiety disorder (impaired concentration, anxious restlessness, fidgeting), pervasive developmental disorder (PDD), mental retardation (look for low mental ability and inattention)
- *Organic.* Infection and seizures, chronic fear, learning disability, poor home environment, use of bronchodilators and anticonvulsants, substance misuse disorder, food allergies (in some cases).

APPROACH TO TREATMENT

- Employ a multimodal approach, psychoeducation and school liaison (stimulant medication is not the whole solution).
- Perform a clinical examination while assessing the child's strengths and developing a therapeutic relationship.

WHAT TREATMENT/ADVICE

MEDICAL

- Prescribe stimulants, antidepressants, rarely antipsychotics, anticonvulsants, clonidine, imipramine.

- Common side-effects of stimulant medications are reduced appetite, insomnia, weight loss, dysphoric reactions (including depression and irritability), and provocation of repetitive activities by over-medication. Long-term use can cause a slight reduction in adult height (controversial). Stimulants can exacerbate tics and are best avoided in some children with tic disorders. Their use with caution may be recommended under supervision by specialists.

PSYCHOLOGICAL AND BEHAVIOURAL

- Take measures to teach the child self-control.
- Arrange cognitive behavioural therapy for anxiety.

PARENTAL TRAINING

- Teach behaviour modification and social learning: use of tracking behaviour, establishment of a reward system, use of points or star charts when the child is good, issuing of clear commands, establishing of clear house rules, establishing a token economy, time out procedures and implementing a daily report card, usually in conjunction with a teacher.
- Arrange for behavioural intervention.
- Describe the use of stimulant drugs.

EDUCATIONAL

- Educate parents and school on the nature of the illness and on treatment.
- Advise on management of different behaviours.
- Hold a conference with school professionals.

DIETS

- There is no conclusive proof that any dietary programme alleviates symptoms but some believe this works.

FULL ANSWER

The presentation in this boy is very suggestive of inattention, hyperactivity and impulsivity. This makes attention deficit hyperactivity disorder (ADHD) a possible diagnosis. I would carry out further assessments to ensure that his presentation is not due to a physical problem, or to a psychological problem such as chronic fear, learning disability or a poor home environment. I would then suggest an appropriate management strategy in a way that would include the family, the family doctor and the teachers, to deal with the problems and return the boy to educational learning.

To begin with, I would clarify when the problems started, what exactly led the boy to be excluded, and whether he is receiving any form of education at this time. I would also find out how the child and his mother have handled the expulsion and clarify whether there is a risk of self-harm or suicide.

I would seek more information from the GP about the boy's medical and psychiatric history, particularly regarding seizures, allergies or atopia. I would also ask about current use of medication such as bronchodilators and anticonvulsants, which may also cause ADHD symptoms. I would make arrangements to interview the parents, the child, his teachers and any other professionals involved. Ideally, I would invite the boy and his family to the clinic to carry out a multidisciplinary assessment.

Prior to assessment in the clinic and in order to save time, I would send the Home Hyperactivity Scale and Strength and Difficulty Questionnaire to the parents, and also seek their permission to get further information from the school. I would also send the Connor's Rating Scale and Strength and Difficulty Questionnaire to his schoolteacher, and would also make arrangements to talk to him or her, in order to ascertain the extent of the problem and the interventions that have been tried so far. When I met the parents, I would establish the exact nature of the problem, in what situations it occurs, how long it has been going on, how old the child was when the problem first started, and its effects on the boy and his family and friends. I would ask about the characteristic core symptoms of inattention, hyperactivity and impulsivity, which can manifest in carelessness, difficulty in watching a film or cartoon to completion from an early age, failure to finish tasks such as school work and homework, and being easily distracted by extraneous stimuli. I would ask if the child is always 'on the go', has difficulty in waiting his turn, and shows impulsivity in a motor, cognitive or verbal way. I would find out if he indulges in excessive running and climbing, and sustains frequent injuries. I would ascertain whether there is any family history of mood disorder, ADHD, antisocial personality disorder, or family and marital discord, and what impact the current difficulties have had on the family. I would conduct the interview at the clinic and use standardized instruments such as those I have already mentioned to assess symptoms.

I would also ask the boy's teachers pertinent questions about his behaviour in school with regard to inattention, hyperactivity and impulsivity. I would ask about any difficulty in remaining seated in class, failure to follow instructions, failure to finish tasks, failure to obey instructions, interruption of scheduled activities, intrusion, failure to finish games, fighting in school, whether his inattentiveness and hyperactivity disrupt other children's activities or intrude on their space, poor academic performance and disregard for rules. I would ask if the child is being 'picked on' and if his behaviour has caused him to lose friends. To support my diagnosis, I would use standardized instruments such as the 39-item Connor's Teacher Rating Scale (CTRS) or the Abbreviated Connor's Teacher Rating Scale (ACTeRS) to assess symptoms.

I would find out if the child is aware of the problem or if he feels his parents or teacher always yell at him for no apparent reason. I would observe his behaviour at the clinic and examine the returned parent and teacher questionnaires to establish whether the behaviour is consistent across different settings. I would use the opportunity afforded by the clinical examination to assess the child's strengths and to develop a therapeutic relationship with him. I would bear in mind that it might be necessary to arrange to observe this boy in class and there might also be a need for further psychological assessment to rule out learning difficulties, which could lead to defeat in classroom situations because he cannot understand what he is being taught. I would ask the team psychologist to carry out a psychometric and neuropsychological test to support my diagnosis. These might involve an IQ assessment using the Wechsler Intelligence Scale for Children – Revised (WISC–R) and a Continuous Performance Test (CPT).

My overall approach in this case would be to ensure multidisciplinary involvement in assessment and treatment, and to coordinate these in such a way as to minimize disruption to family life. My first task would be to give psychoeducation to the boy's parents and the school about both the condition and the treatment options. This would involve the collection of data on the child's behaviour in a form that is accessible to a lay person. The ABC (antecedent, behaviour and consequences) model proves useful to most parents. I would stress that a medical stimulant is not the solution to the entire problem. I would also need to educate the school on how his behaviour can be controlled and how to get the best out of him in class. The advice of a specialist teacher or psychologist might be necessary in this instance. There would also be a need to provide continuous support for his parents and teacher. I would suggest a conference with the school professionals to review the child's special education needs and how best to work with them. This would ensure that the school is able to establish the best learning environment for the child, give instructions and assignments in a consistent manner, modify unacceptable behaviour and enhance the boy's self-esteem.

In terms of the actual treatment, my first line of management would be to consider a behavioural approach, which would be taught to the teachers and parents. This would initially involve giving praise or a reward each time the boy acts in the desired way. As he begins to appreciate what is happening, other psychological measures such as social skills training might be beneficial. Parental skills training might also be offered, but I would reassure the parents that this would not in any way undermine their capability as parents.

The first step would be to continue to collect data on his behaviour and analyse it. The main strategy would be to reward desired behaviour rather than punish undesirable behaviour. I would advise consistent responses to both acceptable and unacceptable behaviour at all times. Behavioural programmes would focus on physical abuse, damage to property, verbal abuse, non-compliance with house or school rules and dawdling. The family dysfunction would need to be addressed in such a way that the child knows that his parents' decision is final. Once his behaviour is better controlled, the child or adolescent can begin to learn new and better techniques that will enable him to function within the family and also to cope with stress. The same thing would apply to management within the school structure. Finally, cognitive behavioural therapy can prove successful in patients with ADHD who have significant anxiety.

If behavioural intervention did not work, I would consider the use of a stimulant drug such as methylphenidate or dexamfetamine alongside. If we chose this approach, there would be a need to explain the side-effects to both parents and teachers. I would suggest a trial of methylphenidate, starting at a dose of 5 mg three times a day. More recently, a once daily, modified release preparation of methylphenidate (18 mg) has become available and could be given instead of split dosages, usually in the morning. The cooperation of the teachers would be needed as they might need to give the medication at midday during the school session. While he was on this medication, the boy's weight and height would be monitored on a regular basis and consideration would be given to taking him off the drug during school holidays (drug holidays).

Once the medication starts to have the expected effect, I would then revert back to psychological and behavioural treatment approaches to deal with unwanted behaviours as above.

ANSWERS TO SUGGESTED PROBES

1. The cardinal features of ADHD have already been described.

2. The following could also be making this boy lose concentration in class:
   - anxiety and depression
   - learning difficulties
   - abuse
   - bullying.
3. If this condition is left untreated, it could result in:
   - risk of academic failure
   - an increased rate of delinquency in the long term
   - increased rate of substance misuse
   - increased risk of antisocial behaviour (aggression, trouble with the law, admission to juvenile facilities)
   - increased risk of psychiatric disorders (such as depression and anxiety).

BUZZ WORDS AND USEFUL TERMINOLOGY

ABC of behavioural assessments, functional analysis, core symptoms, psychoeducation, special education, drug holidays.

REFERENCES AND SUGGESTED READING

Angold A, Prendergast M, Cox A et al 1995 The child and adolescent psychiatric assessment. Psychological Medicine 25:739–753

Babinski L M, Hartsough C S, Lambert N M 1999 Childhood conduct problems, hyperactivity-impulsivity, and inattention as a predictor of adult criminal activity. Journal of Child Psychology and Psychiatry 40:347–355

Goldman L S, Genel M, Bezman R J, Slanetz P J 1998. Diagnosis and treatment of attention-deficit/hyperactivity disorder in children and adolescents. Council on Scientific Affairs, American Medical Association. Journal of American Medical Association 279:1000–1107

Guevara J 2001 Evidence-based management of attention deficit hyperactivity disorder. British Medical Journal 323(7323):1232–1235

Schachar R, Ickowicz A 2002 Attention deficit hyperkinetic disorders in childhood and adolescence. In: Gelder M G, López-Ibor Jr J J, Andreasen N C (eds) New Oxford Textbook of Psychiatry, vol. 2. Oxford University Press, Oxford, pp 1734–1750

Warner-Rogers J, Taylor A, Taylor E, Sandberg S 2000 Inattentive behaviour in childhood: epidemiology and implication for development. Disabilities 33:520–536

5.6 14-YEAR-OLD BOY WITH CHRONIC FATIGUE

A 14-year-old boy has been referred to you by his paediatrician, who has been investigating him for low energy levels and fatigue for over 6 months. Several tests performed to rule out an organic aetiology were negative. The paediatrician is now of the opinion that there are underlying psychological problems that need attending to.

What is your most likely diagnosis and how would you go about your assessment and management?

SUGGESTED PROBES

1. What are your differential diagnoses and why?
2. The boy's mother is asking for tests for Coxsackie virus and other enterovirals, and for functional brain neuroimaging to be carried out. What is your response?
3. What treatments would you give and what is the rationale behind them?

PMP PLAN

TASKS TO DO

The following five areas are relevant to this vignette but are not necessarily all-inclusive. The list is also not exhaustive:

a) Mention chronic fatigue syndrome (CFS) as a very likely diagnosis.
b) Show an understanding of the psychological and psychodynamic factors perpetuating illness in children.
c) Demonstrate knowledge of the various differential diagnoses.
d) Discuss coordinated multidisciplinary assessments and treatments.
e) Consider biopsychosocial modalities in your management plan. Candidates should be familiar with cognitive concepts underlying illness presentation and treatment.

ISSUES

- Determination of underlying psychiatric (or emotional) problem as physical testing has not yielded any positive result
- Systematic assessment with a view to offering the appropriate treatment.

CLARIFY

- Is the child in any immediate danger of medical complications or self-harm/suicide?
- Is the child physically fit to be assessed?

SEEK MORE INFORMATION

GP

- Investigations (and their results) and treatments carried out to date.

PARENTS

- Detailed history of the onset and progression of the disorder
- Any preceding viral illness, unexplained fatigue, tiredness, sadness, irritability, poor sleep, pain, muscle pain (myalgia), recurrent sore throat, headache, feeling of fever
- Exacerbation of symptoms by physical exertion
- Presence of life events, such as illness of a family member, family discord and/or separation
- Psychological symptoms, such as depression and anxiety.

CHILD

- Severe physical and mental fatigue, sleep problems and somatic symptoms
- Physical and mental state examination: anxiety, depression, thoughts of self-harm; cognitive problems, such as difficulties with calculation, attention and wakefulness, diminished abstract thinking, poor problem-solving and forward planning, and in a severe condition, reactive and expressive dysphasia.

SCHOOL

- Academic decline preceding the full-blown symptoms
- Relationships with other children.

INVESTIGATIONS

- Results of physical assessments and investigations
- New investigations only if previous ones are more than 3 months old.

DIFFERENTIAL DIAGNOSIS/DIFFICULTIES

- *Emotional.* Chronic fatigue syndrome, depression, school phobia, Munchausen's by proxy
- *Organic.* Unsuspected drug abuse (including solvents and aerosols), anaemia, childhood malignancy, viral infection, undiagnosed organic condition and other organic disease.

APPROACH TO TREATMENT

- Engagement of the child is paramount.
- Consider family preference and treatment setting.
- Take a biopsychosocial and multidisciplinary approach. Work jointly with the paediatricians.
- Aim to improve the boy's physical and mental well-being.
- Allow what predominates the illness to inform your treatment strategies.
- Tailor treatment to severity: mild, moderate or severe.
- Avoid making rash promises about prognosis.

WHAT TREATMENT/ADVICE

Trying to find out the exact results of all investigations and tests that have been carried out to date would constitute a poor line of discussion or approach, as would not taking a family history, jumping to the conclusion that CFS is the only cause of the problem and not considering a multimodal approach in your treatment plan.

PSYCHOLOGICAL

- Use cognitive behavioural therapy (CBT) for fatigue, with graded activities and cognitive restructuring; also use CBT for depression and anxiety.
- Suggest small achievable goals, one at a time.
- Keep a regular diary.
- Arrange for family therapy.

MEDICAL

- Prescribe antidepressants and anxiolytics.

PHYSIOTHERAPY

- Avoid excessive rest periods and advise graded exercises.
- Avoid undue pressure, and treatment measures introduced too early or too rapidly.

EDUCATIONAL

- Reduce academic pressure or competition.
- Suggest part-time schooling and/or home-based learning (consider use of computers and other information technology).

SOCIAL

- Maintain contacts with peers through short visits and telephone calls.

HOSPITALIZATION

- Consider in extreme disability: if the child is confined to bed or a wheelchair (> 50% of the time), or if there is comorbid depression with suicidal behaviour.

FULL ANSWER

Given the fact that investigative procedures have not suggested any specific diagnosis, I would give consideration to the possibility of non-physical illness in this boy. My preferred and most likely diagnosis would be chronic fatigue syndrome (CFS). I would bear in mind that the child might also be suffering from depression, school phobia, Munchausen's by proxy or unsuspected drug abuse (including solvents and aerosols). I understand that multiple negative test results do not completely rule out the possibility of organic conditions, and that an undiagnosed condition such as childhood malignancy, viral infection or other organic disease is not excluded.

In the first instance I would like to clarify whether this child is in any immediate danger of medical complications, and of self-harm or suicide. I would also ascertain whether he is physically fit to be assessed before making any further arrangements. I would quickly check what investigations and treatment have been performed to date, and would reassure myself that these included an FBC, glucose, U and Es, TFTs, immunological screening for T-cell subsets, antinuclear antibodies and rheumatoid factor, screening for common and uncommon tumour factors, Epstein–Barr virus (EBV), cytomegalovirus (CMV), toxoplasma, HIV and brucellosis.

Following this, I would seek more information from the parents, such as the onset of the illness, the symptoms the child presented with, and how it progressed. I would ask about any preceding viral illness, recurrent sore throat, headache and feverish feelings, unexplained fatigue, tiredness, sadness, irritability, poor sleep and muscle pain (myalgia). I would enquire whether symptoms are exacerbated by physical exertion. I would ask about the presence of life events, including illness of a family member, look for associated depression and anxiety, and find out how long the symptoms have lasted. I would also ascertain whether there are days when the patient seems better and what the circumstances surrounding the boy and the family are at that time. I would ask about the severity of the illness, the disabilities caused by the fatigue, the impact it has had on the boy's emotional and physical well-being, and its effect on his siblings and the entire family. I would take a detailed family history and examine the relationship between the boy and his siblings. I would find out whether any developments in the family have taken away attention from the child, and whether this has meant a role change for him. I would explore the significance of any childhood illness and see whether there are obvious secondary gains involved in this illness.

I would examine for specific stressors at home, at school and among his peers. I would seek parental permission to ask for information about the child from the school authority. I would ask teachers if they were aware of any academic decline preceding the full-blown symptoms. I would find out from the school whether there have been any specific acts of bullying and also about his performance and the peer group he belongs to. I would arrange to see the child at my clinic after I had spoken to the parents and collected other information. I would invite other significant persons in the child's life. As far as possible, I would try to engage the child and would emphasize that, even though the test results have not revealed any specific findings, I believe he is indeed feeling the way he has been describing. I would reassure him that further questioning is to help me understand better how I can be of help to him. The whole assessment might take place over more than one session. I would ask the boy about physical and mental fatigue, sleep problems and somatic symptoms such as chest pain or headache. I would assess the degree of disability caused by the illness and the presence of cognitive disturbances, such as problems with calculation, attention and wakefulness, problem-solving and forward planning, diminished abstract thinking, and (if he were very ill) reactive and expressive dysphasia. I would examine his mental state for evidence of depression, anxiety and thoughts of self-harm. I would explain to his parents that the reason why a definite cause of the problem has not been found might be that the aetiology is multifactorial.

I would suggest that there is no need for further tests and would carry out limited investigations, only if they were strictly necessary.

I would suggest that we explore other means of treatment and explain that, even if the proposed treatment does not bring an immediate improvement, there is usually better functioning and quality of life. In my approach, I would consider the engagement and interest of the child to be paramount. I would also take into account family preferences and the treatment setting. I would work jointly with paediatricians, psychologist, physiotherapists and other professionals. I would adopt a biopsychosocial and multidisciplinary approach to the child's treatment, which would be focused on medical improvement of his physical and mental well-being, and a quick return to educational learning. As far as possible, I would encourage the child to participate in tasks rather than taking the compulsion route. I would allow the symptoms that dominate the illness to inform my treatment strategies, which would depend on whether the illness is mild, moderate or severe. I would avoid making rash promises about prognosis.

My definitive treatment plan would include medical and non-medical approaches and strategies to return the child to educational learning as soon as feasible. A management plan would be agreed with the family after arriving at a common understanding of the child's illness. I would suggest psychological treatment in the form of cognitive behavioural therapy (CBT), supportive psychotherapy, and family therapy if it were necessary. The focus of the CBT would be to explore symptom and illness attribution, to challenge automatic negative (nihilistic and pessimistic) thinking, and to attempt a cognitive restructuring process. This would require a proper understanding of the vicious circles and the negative social and emotional processes involved in the boy's life. The child would be taught to change his thinking pattern and behaviour. The CBT would also focus on the treatment of depression and anxiety, alongside psychological measures centred on the restoration of self-confidence and self-control.

The above treatment would be carried out along with a structured incremental rehabilitation (STIR). I would suggest the setting of small achievable goals, one at a time, and would tailor the programme to the needs of the child. A diary of activities would be kept regularly and would aim to avoid excessive rests, a large fluctuation in activities, undue pressure, and measures instituted too early or too rapidly. I would encourage the cautious use of graded exercise and consistent activities to combat deconditioning. Part of the treatment would also be to re-establish routines in the areas of learning, sleep and eating habits. As this child has missed school for a considerable length of time, reintegration into the educational system would be considered. Management in this regard would include reduction in academic pressure or competition, part-time schooling and home-based learning (perhaps involving computers and other information technology). Home-based learning would form part of an integral treatment package, with clear goals to return the child to school and avoid isolation from his peers. Social contact with peers through short visits, telephone calls and other safe means would be encouraged.

As there is little evidence for specific medical intervention, I would avoid unnecessary treatment such as the use of antiviral agents, immunoglobulins and other controversial treatments for which there has been no conclusive evidence of reasonable benefit. I would, however, suggest the use of antidepressants and anxiolytics, if the evidence suggested clear and severe depressive symptoms in this boy. I would consider referring him to a specialist CFS service if he failed to respond to these measures, if the illness continued for more than 6 months, if he showed marked avoidance with panic attacks and phobia, and if very strong physical convictions interfered with management. Hospitalization might be necessary, if the boy deteriorated and became extremely disabled, and was confined to a bed or wheelchair for more than half of the time.

ANSWERS TO SUGGESTED PROBES

1. My differential diagnoses would include psychological causes such as chronic fatigue syndrome, depression, school phobia and Munchausen's by proxy. Organic causes include unsuspected drug abuse (including solvents and aerosols), anaemia, childhood malignancy, viral infections, or an undiagnosed organic condition or other disease.
2. If the mother was asking for further investigations, I would explain that enteroviral serology, VP-1 (viral protein 1) and neuroimaging would be unhelpful and would not yield any new information. If VP-1 antibody is present, it would only show antibodies the body has made to recent infection. It does not prove the diagnosis of CFS. Further physical tests would only reinforce the theory of an organic aetiology and a strong conviction about a physical cause.
3. Treatment modalities and the rationale behind them are described in my full answer.

BUZZ WORDS AND USEFUL TERMINOLOGY

Preferred diagnosis, consent, engagement, sick role, secondary gains, negative automatic thoughts/patterns, graded exercise, cognitive restructuring, structured incremental rehabilitation (STIR).

REFERENCES AND SUGGESTED READING

Deale A, Chalder T, Marks I et al 1997 Cognitive behavior therapy for chronic fatigue syndrome: a randomised controlled trial. American Journal of Psychiatry 154:408–414

Franklin A 1998 How I manage chronic fatigue syndrome. Archives of Disease in Childhood 79(4):375–378

Theorell T, Blomkvist V, Lindh G et al 1999 Critical life events, infections, and symptoms during the year preceding chronic fatigue syndrome (CFS): an examination of CFS patients and subjects with a non-specific life crisis. Psychosomatic Medicine 61(3):304–310

Whiting P, Bagnall A, Sowden A J et al 2001 Intervention for the treatment and management of chronic fatigue syndrome: a systematic review. Journal of the American Medical Association 286(11):1360–1368

Wright B, Partridge I, Williams C 2000 Management of chronic fatigue syndrome in children. Advances in Psychiatric Treatment 6:145–152

5.7   10-YEAR-OLD BOY REFUSING TO ATTEND SCHOOL AFTER BREAKING HIS ARM ON HOLIDAY

A 10-year-old boy has been referred to you, who has become agitated, is breathing heavily and is refusing to go to school. He broke his left arm 7 months ago when he slipped at a swimming pool in a popular holiday resort. He complains of headaches and dizziness in the mornings.

What are your differential diagnoses and how would you manage him?

SUGGESTED PROBES

1. How do you distinguish between school phobia and school refusal?
2. What medication will you prescribe, and why?
3. What features would make you suspect a syndrome such as post-traumatic stress disorder (PTSD)?

PMP PLAN

TASKS TO DO

The following five areas are relevant to this vignette but are not necessarily all-inclusive. The list is also not exhaustive:

a) Demonstrate skill in assessing and treating a young school refuser.
b) Show understanding that a school refuser usually has symptoms of an underlying differential diagnosis, including psychosocial problems.
c) Appreciate the need to work with the family in accepting illness behaviour as evidence of psychological distress.
d) Discuss the need to coordinate assessment and involve family doctors, psychologists, school counsellors, and other educational and welfare officers.
e) Discuss the differential diagnosis and different treatment options.

ISSUES

- Determination of diagnosis and assessment of contributory underlying physical and emotional factors
- Institution of appropriate management to return the boy to school.

CLARIFY

- Have there been physical sequelae or disabilities since the injury?
- Is the child at risk of self-harm?

SEEK MORE INFORMATION

GP

- Past medical history, history of epilepsy and/or encephalitis, panic attacks, any other medical and organic condition.

PARENTS

- Onset of illness
- Their opinion of the illness
- Presence of anxiety, panic attacks and fear
- Complaints of stomachache, headache, dizziness and nausea during the school day
- Presence of separation anxiety when the child was younger
- Family history of psychiatric illness, including agoraphobia and panic disorder; emotional needs of the parents.

CHILD

- Onset of problems
- Points of anxiety and fear, depression, PTSD, physical symptoms to suggest panic disorder
- Any handicap, e.g. in sports and leisure, or disability arising out of previous falls
- Bullying
- Thoughts of 'escaping' from the situation, of dying or self-harm
- Substance misuse—solvents or alcohol.

SCHOOL

- Negative relationship with others in school, e.g. bullying or problems with teachers, peers and friends
- Awareness of engagement in other activities while not at school
- Recent changes at school.

DIFFERENTIAL DIAGNOSIS/DIFFICULTIES

- *Functional.* Panic disorder, depression, generalized anxiety with or without depression, PTSD, agoraphobia, obsessive-compulsive disorder (OCD), separation anxiety disorder, specific phobia, social phobia, sexual abuse, learning disability
- *Organic.* Substance misuse disorder—alcohol, cannabinoids, stimulants and/or solvents.

APPROACH TO TREATMENT

- Take a multidisciplinary approach involving the school, and refer to a child psychiatrist or psychologist for detailed diagnostic assessment.
- Form a therapeutic relationship with the child.
- Educate child and parents.
- Avoid blaming the parents.
- Liaise with teachers and school and minimize the option of education at home.

WHAT TREATMENT/ADVICE

MEDICAL

- Treat specific syndromes such as panic disorder, depression, PTSD.

PSYCHOLOGICAL

- Do a functional analysis of the school refusal behaviour.
- Consider cognitive psychotherapy (individual) and cognitive behavioural therapy.
- Use exposure-based techniques for anxiety, school refusal and anxiety-based school refusal.
- Propose relaxation training if the child is anxious.
- Give education support therapy, supportive psychotherapy, family therapy for parents.

EDUCATIONAL

- Return the child to school as soon as possible (rarely, this may be a forced return). Aim for successful reintegration.
- Monitor the child's progress and avoid relapse.
- Minimize the option of education at home.

OTHER

- Give practical support to the family.

FULL ANSWER

In approaching this scenario, I would bear in mind that this boy's behaviour might have a relationship to the injury he suffered, or might be related to an undiagnosed psychiatric illness.

First of all, I would like to clarify whether any physical sequelae, injury, disability or handicap arose from the previous fall. I would enquire whether there have been any issues with self-harm or suicidal thoughts in this boy. I would go on to seek more information from the GP, the parents, the child, the school and any other relevant parties. I would ask the GP about any medical or psychiatric history, particularly of panic and anxiety disorder. I would find out whether organic medical conditions such as epilepsy or brain tumour have been ruled out.

As far as possible I would attempt to form a relationship with the family and avoid blaming them in order to gain their cooperation. I would ask the parents, particularly the mother, about the onset of the illness and the time the child started refusing to go to school. I would ask if there has been a recent change of school or a change at the school he normally attends. I would find out if this behaviour started with vague complaints about school or a reluctance to attend. I would ask if the child needed persuasion, recrimination or pressure from the family and school authority to attend school at any time. I would also find out if the child has inconsistently complained of stomachache, headache, dizziness, nausea and other symptoms for which no organic aetiology has been found during the course of this behaviour. I would enquire of the mother whether the child has any features suggestive of anxiety, panics and fear. I would ask her opinions of the child's difficulty and also whether other children in the family have had or are having similar problems. I would ask about a history of separation anxiety when the boy was younger, and whether she has been informed of any negative relationship that he has with others in school, either teachers or peers, or if there has been any bullying. I would ask if she is aware of any specific anxiety-provoking situation at school. I would want to know exactly what the child does when he is at home and absenting himself from school. Does he watch TV or is he continuously engaged in other activities? I would tactfully ask whether either of the parents has any difficulties or mental illness, and whether they have sought help.

I would arrange to see the child with his parents and also with other colleagues such as psychologists and family counsellor.

I would ask the child why he has been refusing to go to school, and find out whether there are any symptoms suggestive of panic disorder or depression. I would enquire further about the morning headaches and dizziness, and ascertain whether they are ever present in the afternoon, at weekends or during school holidays. I would look for any physical symptoms such as headaches, dizziness, abdominal pain, nausea, feeling of choking, loss of control, hyperventilation, sweating or tachycardia, which might suggest a panic disorder. I would ask about the frequency of these symptoms and whether they get worse at school. I would also try to rule out depression and find out whether this boy has been feeling low in his mood. I would enquire about the injury he suffered 7 months ago and whether there have been any sequelae or disabilities. I would ask specifically about pain and discomfort, and his response to prescribed analgesics. I would look for symptoms of intrusive recollection of the traumatic event, hyper-arousal, nightmares, insomnia and avoidance behaviour in this child. I would also check whether he has any flashbacks relating to the incident during which he was injured and whether he has a specific fear of being in open spaces. I would ask him if being at school brings back an unpleasant memory of the injury he suffered and whether he fears he might come to harm again. All this information would help me rule out PTSD. I would also ask the parents about the boy's emotional needs and the presence of mental illness.

Although time-consuming, I would refer to a child psychiatrist or psychologist for detailed diagnostic assessment. The Diagnostic Interview for Children and Adolescents (Herjannick & Reich 1982) or the Anxiety Disorder Interview Schedule for Children (Silverman & Albano, 1996) can be used as a means of ensuring a complete and more reliable diagnostic assessment picture. Other possible instruments are the Screen for Child Anxiety Related Emotional Disorders (SCARED; Birmaher et al, 1997) and the Multidimensional Anxiety Scale for Children (MASC, March et al, 1997).

In dealing with the treatment issue in this boy I would consider a panic disorder, depression, generalized anxiety with or without depression, PTSD, agoraphobia, obsessive-compulsive disorder, separation anxiety disorder, specific phobia, social phobia, sexual abuse and learning disability as differentials. These would be likely to inform specific treatment. In my approach I would involve other professionals, including psychologists, family and school counsellors, and the educational officer at the school, and would suggest the immediate return of this child if possible, while trying to reassure the parents that efforts to remove him from school would be counterproductive.

I would consider medical, psychological and psychoeducational aspects in treating this boy. Since it is likely that he suffers from a panic disorder, depression or a PTSD with depression, I would consider medical treatment using one of the selective serotonin re-uptake inhibitors (SSRIs) such as citalopram at a dose of 5 mg per day or 0.5 mg per kg body weight. I would also consider treatment with imipramine, or very rarely alprazolam, for panic disorder. In view of recent developments and advice from the Committee on Safety of Medicine (CSM, 2003) in the UK concerning the use of SSRIs and venlafaxine in children, I would avoid these and use imipramine instead. I would treat other specific syndromes in the same manner. Treatment with these medications would also help with depression or affective symptoms arising from a possible PTSD syndrome. It is unlikely that there would be any indication for the mandatory prescription of benzodiazepines, and in view of the risk of dependence, I would avoid them as far as possible.

I would consider cognitive psychotherapy (individual form) and cognitive behaviour psychotherapy, consisting of in vivo exposure and coping self-statement training. I would involve the family in these treatments, as this can be very helpful. The graduated in vivo exposure would focus on the child returning to school in a stepwise or gradual manner. I would also consider other cognitive techniques for anxiety-based school refusal, relaxation training for anxious children and educational support therapy as part of my psychological approach to treatment. This would be coupled with family therapy if the family agrees. The parents would be reassured that there is no physical problem with the child, once that fact was established. I would liaise closely with the educational authorities and seek a school contact who would be able to monitor the boy's behaviour and attendance record, and also liaise with the treatment team on progress. As far as possible, I would form a therapeutic relationship with the child and would educate and involve the parents, avoiding a culture of blame.

Having treated specific syndromes that might be underlying this child's behaviour, and giving support to his family, I would hope that he would be able to go back to school again as usual. The main target would be to return him to school as soon as feasible. I would try to discourage suggestions of hospitalization, pupil referral and home tuition. In very rare situations a forced return to school might be necessary. For the child to continue to do well, a successful reintegration programme would be necessary and this would include monitoring of progress and measures to avoid relapse.

ANSWERS TO SUGGESTED PROBES

1. School phobia exists in a situation where a child exhibits specific fear of attending school due to a particular person or object, such as peers or authority figures, or due to situations at school which are found threatening. School refusal is a situation in which a child of school age refuses to go to school for any reason (including school phobia) other than 'simple truancy'.

2. I would consider giving this boy one of the tricyclic antidepressants, imipramine, which has been found to be effective in those patients refusing school who may also have evidence of panic disorder, anxiety and depression. Rarely, I would use a benzodiazepine such as alprazolam to contain the anxiety. In view of the recent developments and advice from the Committee on Safety of Medicine (CSM, 2003) in the UK concerning the use of SSRIs in children, I would avoid citalopram, although it has been found useful in this group of patients.

3. A combination of the following symptoms would suggest a diagnosis of PTSD in this boy:
    * the previous history of a bad fall and injury to his arm in an open place
    * recurrent and intrusive recollections in the form of thoughts, images or perceptions of the trauma
    * reliving the trauma in the form of illusions, hallucinations or flashbacks, particularly ones associated with physical activities or open places
    * persistent avoidance of physical activities or open places
    * hyper-arousal states, such as anxiety, irritability, loss of sleep, agitation, nightmares, increased startle reaction and hypervigilance
    * symptoms causing distress and impairment in social, occupational and other areas of functioning
    * duration of symptoms over 1 month.

Note: school phobia or school refusal is not a specific psychiatric diagnosis but a description of symptoms that may suggest an underlying psychiatric illness.

BUZZ WORDS AND USEFUL TERMINOLOGY

Engagement, functional analysis of behaviour, reintegration, psychoeducation.

REFERENCES AND SUGGESTED READING

Birmaher B, Khetarpal S, Brent D, Cully M 1997 The screen for child anxiety related emotional disorders (SCARED): scale construction and psychometric characteristics. Journal of the American Academy of Child and Adolescent Psychiatry 36:545–553.

Committee on Safety of Medicine 2003 Selective Serotonin Reuptake Inhibitors (SSRIs) – use in children and adolescents with major depressive disorder. Committee on Safety of Medicine, London

Committee on Safety of Medicine 2003 SSRI and venlafaxine use in children. Current Problems in Pharmacovigilance 29:4

Elliot J G 1999 Practitioner review: School refusal: issues of conceptualization, assessment, and treatment. Journal of Child Psychology and Psychiatry 40:1001–1012

Herjanic B, Reich W 1982 Development of a structured psychiatric interview for children: agreement between child and parent on individual symptoms. Journal of Abnormal Child Psychology 10:307–324

Last C G, Hansen C, Franco N 1998 Cognitive behavioural treatment of school phobia. Journal of the American Academy of Child and Adolescent Psychiatry 37(4):404–411

Lepola U, Leinonen E, Koponen H 1996 Citalopram in the treatment of early-onset panic disorder and school phobia. Pharmacopsychiatry 29:30–32

March J S, Parker J D A, Sullivan K, Stallings P 1997 The multidimensional anxiety scale for children (MASC): factor structure, reliability and validity. Journal of the American Academy of Child and Adolescent Psychiatry 36: 554–565

Silverman W, Albano A M 1996 Anxiety Disorders Interview Schedule for Children (ADIS-C). Graywind Publications, State University of New York, Albany

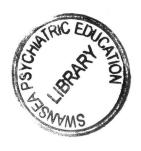

6
Psychiatry in the elderly

A 77-year-old woman has been referred to your clinic following concerns expressed by her daughter and main carer, who works at the local hospital. She has noticed that her mother has become more forgetful recently and is more confused at night. She thinks she may be developing Alzheimer's disease. There is no family history of psychiatric illness. She is very keen for her mother to be prescribed medication to aid her memory and confusion.

How would you go about your assessment and treatment?

SUGGESTED PROBES

1. What are your differential diagnoses?
2. What further information and investigations would help you to arrive at a diagnosis?
3. If she does have Alzheimer's, what treatment would you give, how will you monitor progress and when will you stop treatment?

PMP PLAN

TASKS TO DO

The following five areas are relevant to this vignette but are not necessarily all-inclusive. The list is also not exhaustive:

a) Show an ability to conduct a comprehensive assessment in a patient with cognitive difficulties, including relevant laboratory investigation.
b) Demonstrate an awareness of the various diagnostic possibilities and how to rule out comorbid illness.
c) Consider risk and safety issues.

d) Take a multidisciplinary approach to assessment and management.

e) Demonstrate knowledge of the various settings in which the patient could be managed in the long term, the interventions and the justifications for them.

ISSUES

- Exclusion of a reversible condition that might be responsible for the symptoms
- Ascertaining a firm diagnosis of Alzheimer's disease before making the decision to treat with anticholinesterase.

CLARIFY

- What precipitated the referral and has there been any major incident?
- Where should the assessment take place and would a suitable informant be available?
- Are there any risk issues and what is the patient's current level of support?

SEEK MORE INFORMATION

GP

- Patient's medical history, current medication and investigations done so far.

RELATIVES AND/OR CARERS

- Onset and progression of problem
- Memory problem short-term, long-term or both?
- Associated impairment of language, numerical or visuospatial skills?
- Presence of neglect phenomenon, perceptual disturbance, psychotic symptoms, personality changes
- Comorbid illness such as depression, alcohol misuse or anxiety disorder.

PATIENT

- Full psychiatric history
- Her view of the problem
- Detailed mental state examination, Mini Mental State Examination (MMSE) and physical examination.

INVESTIGATIONS

- Exclusion of treatable causes of dementia, e.g. superimposed delirium
- Dementia screen to include FBC, vitamin B_{12}, folate, serum calcium, TFTs, LFTs, RFTs, Venereal Diseases Research Laboratory (VDRL) test, *Treponema pallidum* haemagglutination assay (TPHA), fasting blood sugar, midstream urine for microscopy, culture and sensitivity, chest X-ray and CT of the brain. MRI may be necessary
- Occupational therapist assessment of needs
- Further neuropsychological tests to assess memory, language and executive functions.

DIFFERENTIAL DIAGNOSIS/DIFFICULTIES

- *Organic.* Common causes: senile dementia of Alzheimer's type, dementia of Lewy body type, vascular dementia. Other degenerative dementia: frontotemporal dementia. Other organic causes: metabolic disorders such as hypothyroidism, hyperparathyroidism, illnesses that cause chronic hypoxia, hepatic disorders, vitamin and folate deficiency, syphilitic infection, medications
- *Functional.* Severe depressive illness leading to pseudodementia.

APPROACH TO TREATMENT

- Carry out a comprehensive assessment, preferably in the patient's home and with an informant present.
- Aim to keep the patient at home for as long as possible with maximum community support (avoid de-skilling).
- Consider a broad range of biopsychosocial interventions.

WHAT TREATMENT/ADVICE

BIOLOGICAL

- Physical assessment and investigations, psychometric assessment with result of MMSE, and assessment of suitability for anticholinesterase treatment. (The MMSE should be used with caution to judge severity as the test may fluctuate very greatly in patients, a high premorbid IQ can hide a dementia behind a score of above 26/30, and pronounced language difficulty can also lead to a spuriously low score.)

- Ensure the patient meets the diagnostic criteria for Alzheimer's disease before commencing anticholinesterase.
- The options for anticholinesterase treatment include donepezil hydrochloride, rivastigmine, galantamine and metrifonate (the latter not routinely used in the UK).
- Educate the daughter about the medication, side-effects and management.
- Increase the dosage gradually and monitor response and side-effects at 2 and 6 weeks, and subsequently every 6 months.
- Administer the MMSE, Instrumental Activity of Daily Living (IADL) and Behavioural Pathology in Alzheimer's Dementia (Behave-AD) again at 6 weeks, 3 months and 12 months to monitor anticholinesterase efficacy.

PSYCHOLOGICAL

- Psychometric assessment: Geriatric Depression Scale to rule out depressive illness.
- Consider the use of the Clifton Assessment Procedure for the Elderly (CAPE) and IADL to assess level of functioning, and Behave-AD to assess behavioural disturbance, Clinical Dementia Rating and Care-giver's Burden questionnaire.
- Bear in mind that the routine use of these questionnaires is often limited to memory clinics, many of which are involved in research.

SOCIAL

- Assess the level of support needed and arrange a care package with the help of social services.
- Involve relatives, as they might have an effective system in place already.
- Arrange community care assessment, if necessary.
- Give advice on Enduring Power of Attorney, if the patient still has the legal capacity to sign.
- Ensure adequate arrangements are in place to manage the patient's day-to-day affairs.

FULL ANSWER

The presentation in this elderly lady arouses the suspicion of possible cognitive impairment. The main issues would be to exclude reversible organic conditions that might be responsible for the patient's symptoms and then to ascertain a firm diagnosis of Alzheimer's disease before making the decision to treat with anticholinesterase. However, in order to make further comments on her presentation, I would need to arrange to see her, preferably with a close relative or carer in attendance for corroborative information. I would clarify as far as possible what precipitated the referral and whether there has been any major incident. I would find out about any risk issues and the current level of support for this lady. I would prefer to see her in her home (in order to look at the home environment and identify obvious risk issues), but if this were not possible, I would see her in the outpatient department. Before that, I would liaise with her GP to seek information on her past medical and psychiatric history, previous alcohol use or habits, and drug history.

When assessing this woman, I would seek more information from her and relatives (after obtaining her permission) on the nature, onset and progression of the memory difficulties. I would find out if the difficulty is short- or long-term, and if there are associated difficulties in the areas of language (word-finding, comprehension and reading), numerical skills (dealing with money, shopping and bills) and visuospatial function (dressing, constructional abilities, spatial orientation and route-finding). I would rule out associated personality changes, and depressive and/or psychotic symptoms. A detailed mental state examination, including mini-mental state, would be conducted. I would take the opportunity afforded by the domiciliary assessment to look at the home environment and see how she is coping.

While carrying out these assessments, I would consider the possible differential diagnoses. I would look at common causes such as senile dementia of Alzheimer's type (SDAT), dementia of Lewy body type and vascular dementia. The other possibilities are frontotemporal dementia and other potentially reversible dementias related to organic causes, such as those due to metabolic disorders like hypothyroidism, hyperparathyroidism, illnesses that cause chronic hypoxia, hepatic disorders, vitamin and folate deficiency, and syphilis. I would rule out any comorbid depressive or psychotic illness that might present as pseudodementia. In order to arrive at a safe diagnosis, I would carry out all the necessary physical investigations including an FBC, renal function tests (RFTs), TFTs, serum calcium, fasting blood sugar, vitamin B_{12} and folate, VDRL, *Treponema pallidum* haemagglutination assay (TPHA), and midstream urine for microscopy, culture and sensitivity. I would also order a chest X-ray, CT scan and/or MRI. All these investigations could be carried out while the patient is in the community, via either the GP or day hospital, where we would have an additional opportunity to assess her mental state and form an idea of her level of functioning. I would suggest that an occupational therapist carried out an assessment of the patient's needs.

As a diagnosis of dementia cannot be taken lightly in view of the implications, I would subject the patient to a battery of different tests to be as sure as possible before making a decision on treatment. I would advise further neuropsychological assessment to ascertain the nature and degree of the cognitive deficit as it affects her memory, language and executive functions. I would use the Geriatric Depression Scale to exclude a depressive illness, the Clifton Assessment Procedure for the Elderly (CAPE) and the Instrumental Activity of Daily Living (IADL) to assess level of functioning, Behavioural Pathology in Alzheimer's Dementia (Behave-AD) to assess behavioural disturbance, the Clinical Dementia Rating to assess severity, and last but not least, the Caregiver's Burden questionnaire. However, I would bear in mind that the use of some of these questionnaires is often limited to memory clinics or other settings, where facilities and staff are available, and that their findings have to be used with caution. I would reassure myself that this lady meets the ICD–10 (or DSM–IV) diagnostic criteria for degenerative dementia.

As far as possible, my approach would be to manage this patient in the community with a multidisciplinary team, unless there was an unacceptable level of risk. Whatever I did, there would be a need to provide education for the family to ensure that they understand what dementia stands for, the likely aetiology and the implications of the diagnosis for the patient. I would explain what they should expect, what services can be given in the community, and the kind and extent of support available for the family or carer. I would make them aware of the risk and safety issues and also encourage them to look out for potential hazards in the house. These might include turning off the gas to minimize the risk of fire, or taking appropriate steps to ensure that doors and windows are not left open at night. All these issues would influence my decision as to treatment type and setting. I would consider admission to hospital, either formally or informally, if the risk of community treatment was far greater than that associated with hospital admission.

Concerning treatment, I would aim to offer a broad range of biopsychosocial interventions. Once a decision had been made on setting, I would rule out or treat any cause of reversible dementia. I would assess and treat any comorbid illness such as depression and anxiety. I would offer anticholinesterase treatment based on the agreed local or national protocol (in the UK, in accordance with the National Institute of Clinical Excellence (NICE) guidelines on the use of donepezil, rivastigmine and galantamine for the treatment of Alzheimer's disease). I would measure baseline cognitive function, activities of daily living and behavioural disturbance using the MMSE, the IADL and Behave-AD instruments respectively. (The

MMSE should be used with caution to judge severity as the test may fluctuate very greatly in patients, a high premorbid IQ can hide a dementia behind a score of above 26/30, and pronounced language difficulty can also lead to a spuriously low score.)

As part of the medical treatment I would offer anticholinesterase medication if the patient was suffering from senile dementia of Alzheimer's type or dementia of Lewy body type. This would also depend on her score on the MMSE. The options for anticholinesterase treatment include donepezil hydrochloride, rivastigmine, galantamine and metrifonate (the latter not routinely used in the UK). I would educate the daughter about the medication and its side-effects, and how these should be managed. I would increase the dose gradually and monitor response and side-effects at 2 and 6 weeks, and subsequently every 6 months. There might be a need for closer monitoring depending on the physical state of the patient, the side-effects and the response to medication. I would also administer the MMSE, the IADL and Behave-AD again at 6 weeks, 3 months and 12 months to monitor the efficacy of the anticholinesterase treatment.

Treatment would also include psychological interventions such as anxiety management, reminiscence therapy or reality orientation therapy. These would be offered to her either individually or in a group at the day hospital. I would enlist the help of our occupational therapist to make a formal assessment of risk issues and activities of daily living (ADL), and seek advice on the necessary adaptations in this patient's environment to minimize risks and make her as independent as possible. Additionally, appropriate arrangements would be made to impose some structure on her day: for example, attendance at a day centre or social club on the days she is not attending day hospital.

I would involve a social worker to facilitate a community care assessment of this woman's needs and, if necessary, to arrange an appropriate care package for her. I would also ask the social worker to look into her finances to ensure these are being attended to, so as to prevent financial abuse. I would advise the patient to make a formal application for an Enduring Power of Attorney if she is still able to make such decisions and has the legal capacity to sign the document, in case it is needed later. Otherwise, it might be necessary to involve the Court of Protection to safeguard the patient's interests. It would also be important to assess the needs of her carer, who might well need treatment in her own right, in order to ascertain whether further help is needed to make the management of this patient in her own home an easier task. If necessary, regular respite care could be arranged to give the carer a break. Should the patient become unmanageable at home, supported accommodation would be considered, including warden-controlled flats, residential homes, or nursing or elderly mentally infirm homes, depending on her level of functioning, psychosocial needs and the outcome of the nursing needs assessment.

ANSWERS TO SUGGESTED PROBES

1. The differential diagnosis has already been described in the full answer.
2. Further information and investigations that would help me to arrive at a diagnosis have already been described in the full answer.
3. Treatment for Alzheimer's and ways of monitoring progress have already been described. I would usually stop treatment when the MMSE falls below 10–12 out of 30 in accordance with NICE guidelines in the UK, although some have disputed the evidence base for this. Stopping treatment would depend not only on the MMSE score, but also on the following factors:
   - presence of intolerable side-effects
   - patient request that treatment be stopped
   - poor compliance with treatment or consistent lack of supervision
   - continued deterioration at the pre-treatment rate after 3–6 months
   - accelerating deterioration
   - if a drug-free period shows the drug is no longer working (rapid deterioration during a drug holiday would indicate efficacy and a need for continuation).

BUZZ WORDS AND USEFUL TERMINOLOGY

Anticholinesterase treatment, carer's assessment, enduring power of attorney, dementia screen.

REFERENCES AND SUGGESTED READING

Bullock R 1998 Drug treatment for early Alzheimer's disease. Journal of Advances in Psychiatric Treatment 4:120–134

Förstl H 2000 Clinical issues in current drug therapy for dementia. Alzheimer Disease and Associated Disorders 14(1):S103–S108

Holden M, Kelly C 2002 Use of cholinesterase inhibitors in dementia. Advances in Psychiatric Treatment 8:89–96

Karlawish J, Clark M 2003 Diagnostic evaluation of elderly patients with mild memory problems. Annals of Internal Medicine 138(5):411–419

Lovestone S, Gauthier S 2001 Management of dementia. Managing the newly diagnosed patient with dementia. Taylor & Francis, London

6.2 42-YEAR-OLD BUSINESS EXECUTIVE SEEKING ADVICE ON HIS RISK OF DEVELOPING ALZHEIMER'S

A 42-year-old business executive has been referred to your clinic as he has become increasingly anxious about his risk of developing Alzheimer's disease. His father died from a dementing illness at the age of 55 years and his own brother has recently started to lose his memory. He is specifically requesting genetic testing as he wants to 'settle it once and for all'.

How would you go about dealing with his request and what action would you take?

SUGGESTED PROBES

1. This patient is confused about gene mutation in Alzheimer's disease, which he read about in one of the national newspapers recently. What simple explanation would you give him about this?
2. He has asked you to advise him on his chances of developing Alzheimer's disease. What advice would you give him?
3. Following neuropsychological assessment, the psychologist thinks he has a mild cognitive impairment (MCI). How would you explain about MCI to this gentleman?

PMP PLAN

TASKS TO DO

The following five areas are relevant to this vignette but are not necessarily all-inclusive. The list is also not exhaustive:

a) Discuss the need for sensitivity in advising on the likelihood of developing early onset dementia.
b) Demonstrate knowledge of the genetic basis of early onset dementia.
c) Show awareness of the local protocol.
d) Discuss the appropriateness of his request and its implications: legal, financial, insurance, family and psychological.
e) Show competence in advising and managing the patient who has a positive result.

ISSUES

- Establishing as far as possible whether this gentleman is presenting with an early onset of dementia
- Need to rule out any treatable organic condition or functional illness associated with this presentation.

CLARIFY

- Why is he making this request now?
- What does he mean by 'settling it once and for all'?
- Are there reasons other than the development of memory problems in his brother?
- What is the medical view of the brother's current problem?

SEEK MORE INFORMATION

GP

Information could also be accessed from hospital records.
- Family history of memory problem
- Results of tests such as CT scan and post-mortem.

PATIENT

- Any memory or cognitive impairment at present?
- Impact on activities of daily living
- Anxiety or depressive symptoms (the presence of these might have exacerbated his present worries)
- Current and past physical/psychiatric problems, including head injury and/or brain infection or abscess
- Drug and alcohol history
- Knowledge of the illness, mode of transmission of Alzheimer's disease, the various genetic tests (apo ε status not conclusive) and the implications of results, whether negative or positive
- Tendency to misinterpret ambiguous health-related stimuli in a threatening way, specific negative beliefs about Alzheimer's dementia and maladaptive behaviour responses to health threats such as test results. (Presence of one or more of these could increase the likelihood of significant distress post-test.)

RELATIVES

- Family pedigree, which includes both unaffected and affected family members with their ages of onset.

INVESTIGATIONS

- Only if indicated (FBC, U and Es, TFTs, LFTs, serum calcium, serum copper, vitamin B_{12} and folate, *Treponema pallidum* haemagglutination assay (TPHA), viral and autoimmune studies, ECG, chest X-ray, EEG, CT scan and/or MRI).

DIFFERENTIAL DIAGNOSIS

- Be aware of the differential diagnoses for early onset dementia but do not discuss them in detail. These are early onset Alzheimer's disease, mild cognitive impairment, cognitive decline secondary to HIV, head trauma, Huntington's disease, Pick's disease, CJD and other infections, brain tumour, chronic cardiopulmonary insufficiency, hypothyroidism, chronic hypovitaminosis and autoimmune disease such as lupus and Wilson's disease.

APPROACH TO TREATMENT

- Give advice based on the patient's history and his knowledge of the subject.
- Know your limitations as a non-geneticist.
- Consider referring to the genetics clinic, if one is available locally, rather than becoming involved without adequate knowledge or services.

WHAT TREATMENT/ADVICE

- Treat any coexisting psychological problem, e.g. depression and/or anxiety.
- Refer to the local genetic centre (advising the patient of what to expect when he attends).
- Give pretest counselling (diagnosis, mode of transmission, prognosis, treatment and implications of test result on legal, financial, career and insurance issues), give genetic counselling if appropriate, and arrange referral to the local genetic centre for testing and follow-up review.
- Arrange for the actual test and disclosure of result.
- Carry out post-test follow-up and counselling: 1 week follow-up by telephone, 1 month follow-up by home visit, 3 month follow-up by telephone and 1 year clinic follow-up. There is always a risk of psychological distress post-test: in the person with a positive test because of the

disease, and in the person with a negative test because of 'survivor guilt'.
- Discharge back to the care of the GP for follow-up.
- Refer to tertiary research centres.

FULL ANSWER

The main issue here would be to establish as far as possible whether this gentleman is presenting with an early onset of a dementing illness. Another issue is the need to rule out any treatable organic condition or functional illness associated with this presentation. It would appear that this man has good reason to be worried about his risk of suffering from a dementing illness like his father, and also like his brother, who has recently been reported as having difficulty with his memory. Although this man is less than 65 years in age, the decision to refer him to our service might be a reasonable one, given the significant family history.

Prior to agreeing to see the patient, possibly on a one-off basis with referral to other more appropriate services, I would clarify with the GP why the man has been referred at this particular time. I would ask whether it is solely because his brother is having problems with his memory or because this man is having a similar difficulty himself. I would find out if the patient knows the age of onset of the memory problem in his brother, and whether his brother has recently been seen by a psychiatrist. If that were so, I would ask him about the working diagnosis for his brother. I would specifically ask him what he meant by 'settling it once and for all'. I would ask whether he has had any thoughts of harming himself or ending his own life if he develops dementia, and find out what plans he has made. I would deal with any acute mental health concern before proceeding further.

My immediate plan would be to seek more information from the GP, patient and relatives. I would ask the GP specifically about the family history of memory problems and dementia and whether he or she has had access to results of any previous investigations, such as a CT scan or hospital record of the patient's father's post-mortem. Next, I would arrange to see the patient at the clinic, where I would enquire about any memory problems, impairment in activities of daily living, anxiety and depressive symptoms. I would also be interested in current and past physical problems, including head injury and/or brain infection or abscess. I would take a detailed drug and alcohol history to make sure that excessive consumption of alcohol or use of drugs has not contributed to the current presentation. With the help of relatives,

I would construct a family pedigree that included both unaffected and affected family members, with their ages at onset of memory and cognitive problems. As part of my assessment, I would examine the patient's knowledge of the illness, the mode of transmission, the test being requested and the implications of the test result. I would assess for the presence of a tendency to misinterpret ambiguous health-related stimuli in a threatening way, specific negative beliefs about Alzheimer's dementia, and potential maladaptive behavioural responses to health threats such as test results. The presence of one or more of these could increase his likelihood of significant distress post-test.

The development of early onset dementia is a realistic possibility in this man but I would bear in mind other conditions that may cause early memory loss and cognitive decline in a 42-year-old man. The differential diagnosis of early memory loss and cognitive decline includes early onset Alzheimer's disease, mild cognitive impairment (MCI), cognitive decline secondary to HIV, head trauma, Huntington's disease, Pick's disease, CJD and other infections, brain tumour, chronic cardiopulmonary insufficiency, hypothyroidism, chronic hypovitaminosis, autoimmune disease such as lupus and Wilson's disease. My approach to management in this case would be first to rule out the conditions that could present as early onset dementia. I would carry out a full dementia screen including an FBC, RFTs, TFTs, LFTs, serum calcium, serum copper, vitamin B_{12} and folate, *Treponema pallidum* haemagglutination assay (TPHA), viral and autoimmune studies, ECG, chest X-ray, EEG, CT scan and/or MRI. One of the possibilities is that this man does not have one of the identifiable physical conditions described above, and this would make the diagnosis of an early onset of Alzheimer's disease more likely. If this were the case, I would then proceed to educate him about dementia as a whole and Alzheimer's in particular, since there would be a probable higher risk in this situation. I would educate him on the genetic basis of the condition and the limitations of the available tests. Since I am not a specialist in genetics, I would feed my findings back to the GP and advise on treatment. For example, if this man had a coexisting anxiety or depressive illness that needed treatment, I would advise the use of an antidepressant, and would suggest referral to appropriate specialists to tackle any treatable cause of dementia. I would advise the GP to refer the patient to the regional genetics centre, where he would be able to access specialist advice. I would describe to the patient what he can expect when he attends the centre. Usually there would be a pretest counselling session, where issues of diagnosis, the risk of developing dementia, mode of transmission, prognosis, treatment, implications of a positive test result and legal, financial, career and life insurance aspects would be explored. If the patient were happy with the explanation, he would be asked to consent to an actual test. The test usually involves taking a small blood sample to analyse for the presence of presenelin 1 (PS1) genes. As it might take days for the test result to become available, I would reassure and support the patient during the waiting time. Whether the test is positive or negative, there is always a risk of psychological distress, either because of the presence of disease in a person with a positive test, or because of 'survivor guilt' in a person with a negative test. This would make post-test follow-up and counselling essential. Usually, this is done 1 week after the test by telephone, 1 month later by home visit, 3 months later by telephone and 1 year later by clinic follow-up. Also bearing in mind the risk of distress in this man post-counselling, whether he has a positive or negative test result, I would advise referral to the local adult psychiatric services, where he would have the opportunity of receiving further psychological support. Of course, this could also be arranged with the man's general practice, or privately for those who prefer and have the financial resources. If a research facility were available, I would consider whether this man might wish to be referred there so that he could be entered into trials in return for continued support, follow-up, and the opportunity to participate in drug trials for MCI.

ANSWERS TO SUGGESTED PROBES

1. I would explain in simple terms that genetic mutation is a permanent change to the genes in our body and can be passed on to children (inherited), even if the manifestation of the effect of the gene is not seen in the person that transferred the abnormal gene (the carrier). I would explain that some genes, called predictive genes (labelled APP, PS1 and PS2), have been associated with an increased risk of developing Alzheimer's. I would also mention a fourth gene, called the apo ε gene (which occurs in different forms: ε2, ε3 and ε4), which is also involved in determining the risk of Alzheimer's. The presence of the ε4 type (or variant) puts people at higher risk of Alzheimer's disease, but does not mean they will necessarily develop the disease. On the contrary, mutation in the APP, PS1 and PS2 genes means the person will most likely develop Alzheimer's disease. I would explain further that, while it is possible to test for all the mutations, clinical genetic testing is only commonly available for PS1.

2. I would suggest that the patient seeks the advice of a clinical geneticist who is experienced in predicting the chances of developing Alzheimer's disease. I would explain that genetic testing for Alzheimer's disease is fraught with uncertainties. I would add that genetic testing for apo ε4 cannot predict who will develop the disease, and that many medical ethicists and geneticists have recommended against such testing in healthy people. Half of those who carry the apo ε4 gene will not develop Alzheimer's, and many people who do not carry apo ε4 will still go on to develop the disease.

3. The diagnostic criteria for MCI include:
   - memory complaints collaborated by a reliable informant
   - normal general cognitive function
   - normal activities of daily living (ADL)
   - absence of dementia and memory impairment in relation to age and education.

   I would explain that this is sometimes referred to as the preclinical phase of Alzheimer's disease. The presence of a diagnosis of MCI increases the person's risk of developing Alzheimer's, which will progress at a rate of 10–15% per year, compared to a typical rate of 1–2% in people who do not have MCI.

BUZZ WORDS AND USEFUL TERMINOLOGY

Pretest and post-test counselling, full dementia screen, 'survivor guilt', genetic mutation, mild cognitive impairment.

REFERENCES AND SUGGESTED READING

Arnaiz E, Almkvist O 2003 Neuropsychological features of mild cognitive impairment and preclinical Alzheimer's disease. Acta Neurologica Scandinavica 179(suppl.):34–41

Friedman J M, McGillivray B 1992 Clinical Genetics. In: Siegfried D (ed) Genetics: the National Medical Series for Independent Study. Williams and Wilkins, Baltimore, pp 149–169

Greicius M D, Geschwind M D, Miller B L 2002 Presenile dementia syndromes: an update on taxonomy and diagnosis. Advances in Neuropsychiatry 72(6):691–700

Grundman M, Petersen R C, Ferris S H et al (Alzheimer's Disease Cooperative Study) 2004 Mild cognitive impairment can be distinguished from Alzheimer disease and normal aging for clinical trials. Archives of Neurology 61(1):59–66

Lovestone S 1999 Clinical genetics of Alzheimer's dementia. In: Howard R (ed) Everything You Need to Know in Old Age Psychiatry. Wrighton Medical Publishing, Philadelphia, pp 31–41

Panegyres P K, Goldblatt J, Walpole I et al 2000 Genetic testing for Alzheimer's Disease. Medical Journal of Australia 172:339–343

6.3   79-YEAR-OLD WOMAN FOUND WANDERING AND CONFUSED IN THE STREET

A 79-year-old female has been brought into the local accident and emergency department after being found by the police, wandering on the street late at night. On assessment, the duty SHO in psychiatry decides to admit her under your care.
How would you manage her?

SUGGESTED PROBES

1. What are your differential diagnoses?
2. What are the safety issues involved in this case?
3. During admission on the ward, you notice the woman has a pulse rate of 153/min and absence of P-waves on the ECG. What is the most likely cause of these abnormal patterns and how would you manage?

PMP PLAN

TASKS TO DO

The following five areas are relevant to this vignette but are not necessarily all-inclusive. The list is also not exhaustive:

a) Take a systematic approach to the assessment and management of acute confusional state.
b) Discuss the possible organic and non-organic differential diagnoses.
c) Show an awareness of safety/risk issues.
d) Demonstrate adequate knowledge of the investigations needed to identify the cause of confusional state and/or dementia.
e) Discuss biopsychosocial interventions in detail.

ISSUES

- Safety, as the patient is wandering
- Need to establish whether she is suffering from an acute confusional state or underlying dementia.

CLARIFY

- Has the necessary information about this lady been sought, e.g. from next of kin?
- What is her psychiatric history, including previous contact with the social services department?

NURSING STAFF

- Mental state since admission; agitation, aggression.

ADMISSION NOTES

- Review, looking especially for any head injury; police report.

GP

- Relevant medical history and medication (digoxin, warfarin, diuretics, benzodiazepines and over-the-counter drugs)
- Recent treatment for systemic infection.

PATIENT

- Subjective view of illness, onset, progression, short-term memory loss, misplacement of items, forgetfulness (appointments, leaving gas on, leaving doors and windows open)
- Getting lost in the neighbourhood
- Worsening of the problem at night
- Activities of daily living
- Family and social support
- Physical factors: history of vascular risk factors, such as hypertension, diabetes mellitus, stroke and hyperlipidaemia
- Frequent falls and head injury
- Medication
- Alcohol and drug history
- Mini Mental State Examination (MMSE): cognitive deficit, depressive features, psychotic features
- Physical state examination: evidence of infection (chest and urinary common), head injury, atrial fibrillation, focal neurological deficit (stroke?).

RELATIVES OR CARERS

- Previous episodes, onset of problem, progression
- Fluctuation in the level of confusion
- Any impairment of memory, language or executive function
- Behavioural abnormality, aggression, impulsivity.

INVESTIGATIONS

- Routine bloods, blood culture, CT scan, urine for microscopy, culture and sensitivity, chest X-ray, random blood glucose, ECG, TFTs, LFTs, RFTs, vitamin B_{12} and folate assay, autoimmune antibodies and calcium to exclude hypercalcaemia
- Further tests: neuropsychology, neurological examination and medical referral.

DIFFERENTIAL DIAGNOSIS

This would include a broad range of causes of cognitive impairment.

- *Organic.* Acute confusional state secondary to dehydration, infection (chest and urinary tract common), alcohol intoxication or withdrawal, medication toxicity, epilepsy, head injury, metabolic problems such as diabetic ketoacidosis (DKA) and uraemia, cerebrovascular event, e.g. transient ischaemic attack (TIA) and cerebral stroke, hypothermia; chronic senile dementia of Alzheimer's type, vascular dementia or dementia of Lewy body type, parkinsonism, normal pressure hydrocephalus (NPH), subdural haematoma
- *Functional.* Severe depression, late paranoid psychosis, acute psychotic episode, delusional disorder.

APPROACH TO TREATMENT

- Be guided by the results of investigations and the underlying diagnosis.
- Take a multidisciplinary and holistic approach.

WHAT TREATMENT/ADVICE

- Treatment should be guided by the diagnosis. It should encompass a wide range of biopsychosocial interventions (see Table 6.1), including advice on the management of the patient's finances and property.

FULL ANSWER

In attending to this lady's case, I would bear in mind safety issues and the need to establish whether she is suffering from an acute confusional state that can be treated, or from an underlying dementia. The presentation suggests the possibility of a

Table 6.1 Treatment strategy in acute confusional state

	Biological/medical	Psychological	Social
Immediate	Treat acute confusional state Rule out life-threatening conditions Low-dose antipsychotics, e.g. haloperidol or risperidone[1] for agitation, aggression and psychotic symptoms Detoxification if alcohol problems	Supportive counselling	Contact family and carers
Short-term	Medical work-up Treat underlying condition Medical referral Dementia screen Treat depression	Neuropsychology Bereavement counselling[2]	Occupational therapist assessment of ADL Social worker assessment of needs Addressing safety issues at home
Long-term	Maintain optimal physical health Anticholinesterase treatment for dementia if indicated Outpatient follow-up Medication monitoring	Reminiscence therapy	Community support package CPN Home care Placements Day care Adaptation to home Alarms

[1] Note that some atypical antipsychotics, such as risperidone and olanzapine, have been associated with increased cerebrovascular stroke and mortality in elderly patients with dementia. This should be considered carefully in patients who have risk factors such as hypertension, diabetes, current smoking and atrial fibrillation. This issue is surrounded by controversy. Risperidone seems to be much safer than haloperidol. There is a risk of parkinsonian side-effects with haloperidol and falls can be much more life-threatening. The Committee on Safety of Medicines (CSM) in the UK has advised that risperidone and olanzapine should not be used for behavioural symptoms of dementia.

[2] Only if necessary.

confusional state, which may be either an acute or an acute-on-chronic condition.

To begin with, I would like to clarify what information the duty doctor and staff have gathered on this patient, particularly about her next of kin, current address, GP details, and psychiatric and medical history. I would find out if there has been any contact with the social services department, which hopefully would be able to shed more light on the patient's current social circumstances, including her support network. I would also like to clarify what investigations have been done to date and whether there are any immediate risk or safety concerns that need prompt attention. I would make sure that any potentially life-threatening organic condition has been ruled out and that this patient is medically fit to be on a psychiatric ward.

I would want to seek more information from the nursing staff on her mental state and cognition since admission to the ward. I would check for evidence of further or fluctuating confusion, memory difficulties, agitation or any symptoms suggestive of a depressive disorder or psychosis. I would review the collaborative information and appraise the results of any investigations. If I were able to speak to her relatives, I would ask whether she has wandered before and enquire further into the onset and progression of the current problems. An acute onset of symptoms would raise the possibility of an acute confusional state. I would look for a history suggestive of short-term memory problems such as repetitive questioning, misplacement of things in the house, leaving the gas on, getting lost in the neighbourhood and leaving doors and windows open inappropriately. I would check for any associated impairment of language function, numerical skills and ability to function independently in the activities of daily living. An additional history of vascular risk factors, such as hypertension, diabetes mellitus, stroke and hyperlipidaemia, would raise the possibility of a vascular type of dementia. I would ask the patient and relatives about any relevant family history, including that of dementia or parkinsonism. The physical status examinations would be reviewed for evidence of an infective process systemic disorder or complications and other organic diseases including parkinsonism. If parkinsonian features were present, other diagnostic possibilities would include dementia of Lewy body type and dementia of Parkinson's disease.

Once I had sourced this initial information, my thoughts on the possible differential diagnosis would include a broad range of causes of cognitive impairment, both organic (acute or chronic) and functional. Acute organic causes include a confusional state secondary to dehydration, infection (especially of chest or urinary tract), endocarditis or heart failure, alcohol intoxication or withdrawal, medication toxicity (especially digoxin, warfarin, diuretics, benzodiazepines and over-the-counter drugs), epilepsy, metabolic problems such as diabetic ketoacidosis, uraemia, hypothermia, or a cerebrovascular event such as transient ischaemic attacks and cerebral stroke. The presentation might also be due to a chronic organic condition, such as senile dementia of Alzheimer's type, vascular dementia, dementia of Lewy body type, parkinsonism, normal pressure hydrocephalus and subdural haematoma. I would also consider functional causes such as severe depression, late paranoid psychosis, acute psychotic episode and delusional disorder. In order to arrive at a safe working diagnosis, I would carry out further investigations, including a comprehensive neuropsychological assessment and a full dementia screen. I would order routine bloods, blood culture, urine for microscopy, culture and sensitivity to specific antibiotics, chest X-ray, random blood glucose, ECG, TFTs, LFTs, RFTs, B$_{12}$ and folate assay, autoimmune antibodies, and calcium to rule out hypercalcaemia. If not already done, I would request a CT scan or MRI of the brain, looking for atrophy, ischaemic changes or any other intracranial abnormality. I would carry out a neurological examination and seek further medical opinion as necessary.

My approach to management would be to confirm the cause of this patient's problem. The overall assessment would involve the multidisciplinary team. I would consider three main possibilities, which are an acute confusional state, an acute-on-chronic state (at which specific treatment can be directed), or an infection. I would treat any infection with the appropriate antibiotics based on sensitivity tests. Treatment would also be directed at any sensory impairment that might be contributing to the confusional state, such as cataract or deafness. I would consider seeking appropriate medical advice in treating other conditions, such as a cerebrovascular event like stroke or acute-on-chronic cardiopulmonary insufficiency, and severe metabolic conditions such as diabetes, chronic renal failure or liver disease. I would carry out detoxification and seek appropriate help if dependence on alcohol were part of the problem. There is also a possibility that the condition is due to one of the reversible dementias, and I would treat any hypothyroidism, hypoparathyroidism, hyperparathyroidism or hypovitaminosis that might be present. Her presentation could also be due to cognitive impairment secondary to a degenerative condition such as Alzheimer's disease or a vascular dementia.

I would consider treatment with an anticholinesterase drug if the diagnoses pointed to Alzheimer's disease or a vascular dementia and if there were no contraindications such as chronic obstructive airways or peptic ulcer disease. In the case of pure vascular dementia, I would consider starting her on aspirin in addition. This medical treatment would be coupled with other psychosocial treatments and support tailored to her needs. I would also consider using a low-dose antipsychotic, which might help with agitation if this is present. In line with recent suggestions from the medicine control agencies, I would avoid the use of atypical antipsychotics if there were any suggestion that this woman has a vascular-based dementia or another risk factor such as stroke or transient ischaemic attack.

While this patient was on the ward, and whatever the cause of her problem, it would be necessary to carry out a comprehensive occupational therapy assessment to look for further safety issues that might impact on her ability to live independently. I would ask the social worker to carry out an assessment of her needs, advise on financial matters, look after her benefit needs, and also make arrangements for carers or support workers to help with certain activities of daily living, should she be discharged back home. There would be a need for a nursing assessment, which would guide my decision on where this patient could be best placed, i.e. in a nursing, residential or elderly mentally infirm (EMI) home. I would ask the social worker to look into the patient's finances to ensure that they are being properly managed. If there were any concerns about this, I would suggest that the need for someone else to manage her money be discussed with the patient while she still has the capacity to make such a decision. This might mean an Enduring Power of Attorney being given to a trusted relative or other person, particularly if her estate were considerable. If she already lacked the capacity to sign an Enduring Power of Attorney, safeguards would have to be put in place by appointeeship or through the Court of Protection, depending on the size of her estate.

ANSWERS TO SUGGESTED PROBES

1. The differential diagnosis has already been discussed.
2. The safety issues involved in this case include:
   - risk of physical harm or death
   - risk of exploitation (sexual, financial, emotional, opportunistic)
   - risk of accidental fire or burglary
   - risk of vulnerability, self-neglect and wandering
   - risk of elder abuse.
3. The most likely cause of a pulse rate of 153/min and absence of P-waves on the ECG is atrial fibrillation. I would make

sure there was no risk of an acute life-threatening event. If there were, I would transfer her to the coronary care unit. I would refer to the medical team for advice on reducing the heart rate, anticoagulation and other appropriate treatment.

BUZZ WORDS AND USEFUL TERMINOLOGY

Reversible dementias, dementia screen, neuropsychological assessment, language deficit, hypovitaminosis, community support package, elderly mental infirm (EMI).

REFERENCES AND SUGGESTED READING

Brown T M, Boyle M F 2002 Delirium. British Medical Journal 325(7365):644–647

Fick D M, Agostini J V, Inouye S K 2002 Delirium superimposed on dementia: a systematic review. Journal of American Geriatrics and Society 50:1723–1732

Karlawish J H T, Clark C M 2003 Diagnostic evaluation of patients with mild memory problems. Annals of Internal Medicine 138(5):411–419

Meagher D J 2001 Delirium: optimizing management. British Medical Journal 322(7279):144–149

6.4   81-YEAR-OLD WHOSE WIFE DIED OF CANCER 3 MONTHS AGO

A bereaved 81-year-old man has been referred to you, whose wife of 55 years died of cancer in a hospice 3 months ago. He has continued to ring the hospice asking to speak to his wife. When told his wife is no longer there, he bursts into tears. The hospice manager has referred him to his GP, who in turn has asked you to see him.

How would you go about assessment and management of this man?

SUGGESTED PROBES

1. You are concerned that a pathological grief reaction may be part of the problem in this man. What would you look for in his history to support this?
2. What would be your approach to treatment and what treatment would you give?
3. Your preliminary investigations have revealed mild cognitive impairment. What would be your line of management?

PMP PLAN

TASKS TO DO

The following five areas are relevant to this vignette but are not necessarily all-inclusive. The list is also not exhaustive:

a) Demonstrate awareness of risk and safety issues and their effect on management.
b) Discuss the issue of bereavement and how pathological grief can complicate the picture, along with the stages of grief and other differential diagnoses.
c) Explore the possibility of an underlying affective, psychotic and personality disorder and cognitive impairment.
d) Appreciate and discuss the role of carers, family and GP in assessment, and the input of a multidisciplinary team.
e) Discuss definitive treatment and aftercare, particularly concerning future placement and/or social support.

ISSUES

- Bereavement
- The possibility of an underlying psychiatric illness
- Safety, self-neglect and risk of suicide.

CLARIFY

- Is there any particular risk, such as suicide, self-neglect, vulnerability and wandering?
- Is the problem bereavement or something else entirely?

SEEK MORE INFORMATION

GP

- Medical history
- Psychiatric illness, such as depression or psychosis
- Memory loss and difficulties
- Ongoing physical problems.

RELATIVES, CARERS, HOSPICE MANAGER

- Nature of wife's illness, patient's role until her death
- Relationship with his wife
- Patient's handling of his wife's death
- Activities of daily living (ADL)
- Support since his wife died (home help, social services)
- Social networks and relationships with his family.

PATIENT

- History as above
- Mental state examination and investigations
- Handling of wife's death, bereavement reaction, stages of grief, opportunity to grieve. Did he have any bereavement counselling?
- Mental health: depression, anxiety, suicidal thoughts, memory difficulties, dementia, psychosis
- Physical health: ADL, presence of physical disability.

INVESTIGATIONS

- To exclude organic conditions, e.g. acute confusional state.

DIFFERENTIAL DIAGNOSIS/DIFFICULTIES

- *Functional.* Grief reaction, pathological grief, depression, mixed depression and anxiety, psychotic illness, adjustment disorder
- *Organic.* Dementing illness.

APPROACH TO TREATMENT

- Arrange to see him with his GP, CPN, social worker and family members, e.g. daughter.
- Carry out a full risk assessment.
- Consider the wishes of the patient and those of family and carers.

WHAT TREATMENT/ADVICE

MEDICAL

- Treat any identified illness (organic and functional).

PSYCHOLOGICAL

- Treat for grief reaction, refer to Cruse for bereavement counselling.

SOCIAL

- Consider support needed for the patient to remain at home, placement issues, if necessary, and day facilities.

FULL ANSWER

In attending to this case, I would look at the issue of bereavement and its possible contribution to this man's presentation on one hand, and the possibility of an underlying psychiatric illness or cognitive impairment on the other. There are also issues concerning safety, self-neglect and risk of suicide in this widower. My focus would be to identify why the man has kept calling the hospice where his wife died, and to examine for factors such as memory difficulties, a dementing illness or pathological grief that might be predisposing to this condition. I would also assess with the aim of arriving at a diagnosis and suggesting an appropriate treatment or management strategy.

First, I would clarify whether there is any particular risk such as suicide, self-neglect, vulnerability and wandering that needs to be taken into consideration. Second, I would seek to establish whether the problem is due to an abnormal grief reaction after his bereavement or to something else entirely. If there are urgent safety issues, I would arrange to see the patient immediately with other colleagues, but if not I would make arrangements to see this man at home.

While I was making these arrangements, I would seek more information from his GP, the local mental health service (if known to them), and his relatives, carers and/or neighbours. I would specifically enquire about any relevant medical history, including ongoing physical problems, psychiatric disorders such as depression, psychosis, memory loss and difficulties, confusional episodes before the bereavement and the treatment received to date. I would ask his relatives, carers and the hospice manager about his relationship with his wife, the nature of her illness, the role he played until her death and how he handled the death. I would find out about his activities of daily living (ADL), the support he received before and after his wife died, and his social networks and relationships with his family.

I would prefer to see the patient with his GP, a member of his family or carer, and/or a member of my multidisciplinary team (CPN, social worker or support worker). I would want to use the opportunity afforded by the interview to examine the condition of his home and check for evidence of self-neglect or whether he is living in squalor. I would ask him why he has continued to ring the hospice and clarify whether he knew his wife had died at the time it happened. I would explore what he knows about the nature of his wife's illness and death, and whether he had an opportunity to say goodbye to her. I would examine factors that might predispose him to develop an abnormal grief reaction (ambivalent relationships, excessively long period of looking after the wife, previous bereavements, unresolved issues, secrets and plans). I would assess for low levels of perceived social support, lack of new opportunities, social isolation, and psychosocial stressors or other life events, such as disabling physical illnesses. If I thought he had an abnormal grief reaction, I would establish the stage he is at (denial, anger, bargaining, sadness and guilt and/or acceptance). This man's repeated phone calls to the hospice might represent a form of denial. I would establish whether this gentleman has had the opportunity to grieve for his wife or whether the process has been disturbed by any concurrent physical illness or impaired by cognitive abnormalities. I would ask if he has ever received formal bereavement counselling. I would check whether there is a preoccupation with thoughts of or yearning for his deceased wife of 55 years, crying and disbelief about her death. I would examine for evidence of memory loss and cognitive deficits.

I would find out from him whether he has a history of depression or another psychiatric illness. I would specifically assess his mood and try to tease out of him whether he has a severe depression or not, given that the repeated crying might point to this. I would ask him if he has felt like dying or not wanting to wake up. I would find out whether he has had any suicidal thoughts or plans. I would look carefully for other abnormal symptoms that might suggest a dementing illness or a psychotic disorder in later life. As part of the differential diagnosis, I would consider grief reaction, pathological grief, bereavement-related depression, recurrent depression, mixed depression and anxiety, comorbid dementing or psychotic illness, and adjustment disorder. Due to the risk involved, my approach to management would be to admit this elderly man to hospital. Admission would also enable the multi-disciplinary team to assess his mental state and physical health, exclude the presence of physical disability, and also carry out investigations to rule out organic conditions that can cause confusional states. We could also arrange an occupational therapy assessment of his ADL, facilitate further assessment of his ADL at home before he is discharged, and suggest and carry out the necessary improvements or adaptations to his home.

Treatment would be along biopsychosocial lines. Medical treatment would be directed at treating any identified organic or functional illness, such as depression and anxiety (with anti-depressants). I would refer him to our unit psychologist for a psychological approach to treatment, and this might include bereavement counselling, other psychological treatments for grief reaction and depression, and activities geared towards reality orientation, such as repeated explanation, showing photographs, and visits to the grave. For the social management, I would consider the support he would need to remain at home, such as home help, social services support and day-care facilities. It might be necessary to discuss placement issues and the multidisciplinary team, including occupational therapy and home assessment worker, would consider the options (respite care, elderly mentally infirm home (EMI), residential home or nursing placement) if we concluded that he would not be able to cope at home on his own. This decision would be informed by a full risk assessment, and the wishes of the patient and his family.

ANSWERS TO SUGGESTED PROBES

1. If I were concerned that a pathological grief reaction might be part of the problem in this man, I would look for the following factors in his history to support my view:
   - *Predisposing factors.* Ambivalent or dependent relationship, previous bereavements, history of depression or other mental illness, low self-esteem.

- *Factors related to the death.* Sudden unexpected death, stigmatised death such as suicide, being an elderly male widower, long-term care for the deceased.
- *Factors after the death.* Level of perceived social support, lack of new opportunities, social isolation, stressors or other life events, e.g. disabling physical illnesses, lack of opportunities to grieve.

2. My approach to treatment would be to:
   - Consider safety.
   - Carry out a full risk assessment.
   - Involve the patient and family/carers.
   - Involve the multidisciplinary team.

   The medical, psychological and social treatment/management options have been described in the full answer.

3. If my preliminary investigations revealed mild cognitive impairment, my specific line of management would be as follows:
   - Assess the nature and level of cognitive impairment.
   - Assess the impact of cognitive impairment on quality of life and activities of daily living.
   - Investigate the cause of the cognitive impairment.
   - Carry out a full dementia screen.
   - Treat reversible dementia.
   - Manage irreversible dementia along biopsychosocial lines.

BUZZ WORDS AND USEFUL TERMINOLOGY

Abnormal grief reaction, bereavement counselling, irreversible dementia, treatable dementia.

REFERENCES AND SUGGESTED READING

Casarett D, Kutner J S, Abrahm J 2001 Life after death: a practical approach to grief and bereavement. Annals of Internal Medicine 134(3):208–215

Parkes C M 1985 Bereavement. British Journal of Psychiatry 146:11–17

Prigerson H G, Frank E, Kasl S V et al 1995 Complicated grief and bereavement-related depression as distinct disorders: preliminary empirical validation in elderly bereaved spouses. American Journal of Psychiatry 152(1):22–30

Raphael B, Minkov C 1999 Abnormal grief. Current Opinion in Psychiatry 12(1):99–102

Sheldon F 1998 ABC of palliative care: bereavement. British Medical Journal 316(7129):456–458

6.5 ELDERLY MAN FOUND SHOUTING AT THE MIRROR

You are currently working with the local old age psychiatry service. A GP has telephoned you about a 79-year-old man who is shouting at the mirror in his bathroom at home. His 78-year-old wife is terrified, as he has smashed one of the mirrors with his fist. He has a history of alcohol misuse, but is not definitely known to be drinking at present.

What would be your approach to assessing and managing the situation?

SUGGESTED PROBES

1. What factors will help you decide whether to admit him to hospital or not?
2. During your physical examination, you discover that this man has moderately severe atrial fibrillation. In what way will this affect your differential diagnosis and management?
3. What findings on physical examination would suggest alcohol-related disorder or alcohol-related dementia?

PMP PLAN

TASKS TO DO

The following five areas are relevant to this vignette but are not necessarily all-inclusive. The list is also not exhaustive:

a) Demonstrate the need to consider safety and risk issues. Consider the risk of violence to the man's wife and others, and also that of suicide.
b) Assess the need for immediate hospitalization or community support.
c) Show awareness of the relevant differential diagnoses and discuss the most likely one.
d) Discuss appropriate investigations to rule out dementia and other organic problems.
e) Discuss relevant management options, including non-pharmacological approaches to treatment, support for carers, and day-care services.

ISSUES

- Understanding of the underlying factors for this presentation, and whether it is due to an organic condition, functional illness or alcohol-related disorder

- Management of the risk that this man poses to himself, his wife and others.

CLARIFY

- How safe are the man and his wife?
- Has he sustained any injury to his hand or fist whilst smashing the mirror?
- Is there a need for immediate treatment for any injury or for immediate hospitalization?
- Has he done anything else, apart from smashing the mirror?

SEEK MORE INFORMATION

GP

- Medical and psychiatric history.

PSYCHIATRIC SERVICES

- Any history of psychiatric illness and treatment in the past.

WIFE

- Onset of the problem, agitation, confusion, wandering and memory loss
- Pervasiveness; do the problems occur in the bathroom when her husband is alone?
- Relieving factors; worsening of the problem at night
- Strange ideas and abnormal beliefs, including ideas of persecution.

PATIENT

- Interview to take place at home in the presence of the patient's wife and with other colleagues such as approved social worker, another mental health worker or his GP
- Mental state examination: visual hallucinations, delusions of misidentification, persecutory ideas and auditory hallucinations; affective symptoms, including mood disorder, anxiety, anger and agitation; cognitive deficit (MMSE)
- History as above
- Physical examination to rule out space-occupying lesion, normal pressure hydrocephalus, visual and hearing impairment.

INVESTIGATIONS

- Routine blood analysis, FBC, white cell count, blood film to look for macrocytosis (increased red cell mean corpuscular volume, or MCV), urine microscopy, culture and sensitivity, CT scan and/or MRI (for possible dementia, widening of sulci, cortical and subcortical infarcts), TFTs, LFTs, gamma-globulin transferase (γ-GT), RFTs, vitamin B_{12} and folates, ECG, viral and autoimmune studies.

DIFFERENTIAL DIAGNOSIS/DIFFICULTIES

- *Functional.* Late-onset paranoid psychotic disorder, acute psychotic episode, delusional disorder, psychotic depression
- *Organic.* Acute confusional state, dementia, medication toxicity, drug and alcohol toxicity and withdrawal, space-occupying lesion, normal pressure hydrocephalus, viral infections, cerebrovascular accident (stroke).

APPROACH TO TREATMENT

- Consider compulsory admission, if necessary.
- Treat organic problems as far as possible.
- Rule out other psychopathology.
- Establish a therapeutic relationship.
- Explore the establishment of regular CPN visits or brief hospital admission. Hospitalization would give the opportunity of further neuropsychological assessment, including the use of the Wechsler Adult Intelligence Scale – Revised (WAIS–R) and the Wisconsin Card Sorting Test.

WHAT TREATMENT/ADVICE

BIOLOGICAL

- Use a pharmacological agent, taking into consideration age, side-effects, tolerability, compliance with medication and memory difficulties.
- Low-dose antipsychotics may be useful.

PSYCHOLOGICAL

- Arrange supportive psychotherapy, cognitive behavioural therapy, support for wife and carer, supportive psychotherapy to allay anxiety.

- Suggest a means of coping with distress.
- Show an understanding of the illness from the patient's point of view.

SOCIAL

- Arrange a place at a day hospital to give the man's wife some respite and to engage him in enjoyable activities.
- Offer respite care.
- Allocate to a CPN for closer monitoring.

FULL ANSWER

I think the main issue in this man is his own safety and that of his wife, who is terrified due to his aggressive behaviour. The other issue is to understand the underlying factors for this presentation, and whether it is due to an organic condition, a functional illness or an alcohol-related disorder. I would also consider the risk this man poses to himself, his wife and others, and would institute appropriate management.

First of all, I would clarify whether there is any emergency situation other than that already highlighted. I would also find out whether this man injured himself when he smashed the mirror. If he were in need of immediate treatment in hospital, I would arrange for this. I would also ensure that his wife was both safe and able to take care of her husband whilst help was being sought. As this man might refuse assessment and further treatment, I would consider using an appropriate legal framework such as the Assessment Order under Section 2 of the Mental Health Act 1983 in England and Wales. (Legal frameworks for compulsory admission differ between jurisdictions.) I would therefore invite our team's social worker to attend the interview.

In order to go about my assessment, I would seek more information from the patient himself, his GP, the psychiatry services (who might already know him) and his wife. I would ask the GP about his relevant medical and psychiatric history, and also seek information on diagnosis and treatment from any other psychiatric services that he might be known to. I would ask his wife about the onset of the problem, and whether this was associated with any agitation or confusion. I would also find out whether this man has a tendency to wander, possibly at night, and whether there have been any problems with memory loss. I would also ask about any history of aggression and strange ideas and beliefs, paranoia and persecutory ideas. I would ask whether the problem is pervasive or only crops up in the bathroom. I would arrange to see this man in the presence of his wife, along with my colleagues, including the GP and social worker, if possible. My aim would be to take a further relevant history, assess his mental state and review the necessary physical examinations. I would be particularly concerned about the presence of auditory and visual hallucinations, delusions of misidentification, persecutory delusions and ideas, paranoia and whether he has any ideas that his life is in danger or feels he should retaliate against perceived aggressors. I would also look for affective symptoms such as mood disorder, anxiety and agitation.

As this man also has a history of alcohol consumption, I would look for features suggestive of falls or head injury, and signs suggestive of alcohol-induced liver disease (jaundice, pallor of anaemia, hepatomegaly, spider naevi, distended abdominal veins). I would look for signs of alcohol intoxication (smelling of alcohol, slurring of speech) or alcohol withdrawal (shakes, sweats) or even delirium tremens (characterized by nystagmus, ophthalmoplegia, ataxia and confusion). I would conduct a cognitive assessment using a Mini Mental State Examination (MMSE) in the first instance. If this man were admitted to hospital, we would have an opportunity to carry out further neuropsychological assessment. During this time, a Wechsler Adult Intelligence Scale – Revised, Wisconsin Card Sorting Test, Wechsler Memory Test, Warrington Recognition Memory Test and also a test of verbal fluency would be carried out. If we decided to admit this gentleman to hospital, we would carry out further investigations including a dementia screen, which will include a FBC, blood film to look for macrocytosis or raised MCV, white cell count, urine microscopy, culture and sensitivity, ECG, CT scan and/or MRI (to rule out possible dementia, widening of sulci, cortical and subcortical infarcts), TFTs, LFTs (including γ-GT), RFTs, vitamin B_{12} and folates and autoimmune studies.

The aim of the overall assessment would be to arrive at a safe diagnosis. I would consider a differential diagnosis such as late onset paranoid psychotic illness (late paraphrenia), delusional disorder, acute psychotic episode, dementia, depressive disorder, alcohol intoxication, alcohol withdrawal, acute or chronic confusional state, cerebrovascular accident, antipsychotic toxicity, cerebral infections, normal pressure hydrocephalus, brain tumour and subdural haematoma. From the details given, the most likely diagnoses are those of late onset paranoid schizophrenia, problems related to alcohol intoxication or withdrawal, and a possible dementing illness.

In my approach to treatment, I would consider the most likely diagnosis, assess the risk of violence and suicide, and assess for immediate hospitalization and support for the wife. I would also rule out other psychopathology and treat any organic condition identified. It would be essential at this stage to establish a therapeutic relationship with the patient and this might mean exploring the possibility of a brief hospital admission or the establishment of regular CPN visits. If dementia were suspected, I would carry out a full dementia screen.

Concerning medical treatment, I would consider the use of low-dose antipsychotics to treat any psychotic symptoms and this might mean the use of low-dose risperidone, olanzapine or, rarely, haloperidol. I would consider the man's age, the possible side-effects, and his ability to consent and comply with medication and other treatment. I would also take into consideration the issue of his memory disorder and the availability of support for him at home. I would look for any sensory deficit including visual or auditory impairment. If compliance were likely to be a problem, I would consider the use of low-dose depot medication such as flupentixol decanoate or fluphenazine decanoate, which have proved successful in some patients. I would consider the use of low-dose long-term injectable risperidone, if the side-effects of these typical medications proved problematic. Due to its low anticholinergic activity and relatively weak blockade of striatal dopamine-D_2 receptors, low-dose clozapine might prove useful in the treatment of this elderly man with psychotic symptoms, who could have individual sensitivity to the extrapyramidal symptoms caused by typical neuroleptics. This would, however, be the last option on my list, given the risk of seizures and also the need for regular blood monitoring, which might prove very difficult in a confused patient.

In addition to this medical treatment, I would offer the patient and his wife supportive psychotherapy sessions to allay his anxiety, suggest further means of coping with their distress, and help with understanding the illness from the point of view of the patient. There is also a place for psychological treatment, including cognitive behavioural therapy, in elderly patients with psychotic symptoms. The use of a day hospital would give the wife some respite. I would arrange a carer's assessment for her to determine whether she is able to care for her husband adequately, and also offer them the necessary support to continue to live independently in their house. If I suspected that dementia was the main problem, I would carry out a full dementia screen and then, if necessary, institute the appropriate anticholinesterase treatment. This would have the aim of effecting symptomatic relief, improving cognitive and behavioural functions, slowing down disease progression, and maintaining well-being and safety.

I would liaise with the appropriate professionals to ensure community and social support, with the provision of home care and CPN services. As far as possible, the plan would be to manage this man briefly in hospital and then discharge him home. Following discharge, I would refer him to a day hospital to engage him in enjoyable activities and also to give his wife some respite. Regular respite admission could also be arranged to give her some space to rest and attend to other things in her life. If these options were not feasible or the patient's symptoms did not abate despite treatment, I would plan for alternative living arrangements with possible discharge to a halfway home before eventual discharge, or even discharge to supported and staffed accommodation if his wife continued to find it difficult to care for him in their own home.

ANSWERS TO SUGGESTED PROBES

1. The following factors would help me decide whether to admit this man to hospital:
    *   the wife's safety and her ability to continue to support the man at home
    *   the patient's continuing aggression, risk of harm to himself and others, and his general safety
    *   the need to clarify the causative factors
    *   our ability to treat this man as an outpatient, including the availability of support.
2. If I discovered that this man had moderately severe atrial fibrillation, I would be concerned about a possible cerebrovascular event, which might cause a thromboembolic phenomenon. I would immediately refer the man to the geriatrician, with a view to him receiving appropriate medical treatment in the form of digoxin to reduce the heart rate and control arrhythmias. It would be necessary to give aspirin or dipyridamole afterwards to prevent thromboembolism.
3. The findings on physical examination that would suggest an alcohol-related disorder or alcohol-related dementia are:
    *   alcohol intoxication: smelling of alcohol, slurring of speech, head injury
    *   alcohol withdrawal: smelling of alcohol, shakes, sweats, nystagmus, ophthalmoplegia, ataxia and confusion (the last four signs may suggest delirium tremens)
    *   dementia: memory loss, forgetfulness, confabulation
    *   findings on investigation: CT scan or MRI shows widening of cerebral sulci, infarction and atrophy or

hypoplasia of the cerebellar vermis; blood tests show abnormal LFTs, raised pancreatic amylase, increased MCV and hypochromia

- other: evidence of jaundice, pallor of anaemia, hepatomegaly, spider naevi, distended abdominal veins.

BUZZ WORDS AND USEFUL TERMINOLOGY

Late paraphrenia, Wernicke–Korsakov encephalopathy, space-occupying lesion, therapeutic relationship, neuropsychological assessment, anticholinergic toxicity.

REFERENCES AND SUGGESTED READING

Howard R 2002 Late-onset schizophrenia and very late-onset schizophrenia-like psychosis. In: Jacoby R, Oppenheimer C (eds) Psychiatry in the Elderly (3rd edn). Oxford University Press, Oxford, pp 744–761

Howard R, Rabins P 1997 Late paraphrenia revisited. British Journal of Psychiatry 171:406–408

Howard R, Rabins P V, Seeman M V et al 2000 Late onset paraphrenia and very late onset schizophrenia-like psychosis: an international consensus. American Journal of Psychiatry 157:172–178

6.6 ELDERLY WOMAN WHOSE HUSBAND IS SUSPECTED OF ABUSING HER

You are the registrar in old-age psychiatry for the local community mental health team. One of your community psychiatric nurses has brought to your attention the possibility that an elderly patient, a 78-year-old female you have not met before, is a victim of abuse, the husband being the possible perpetrator. She suffers from mild to moderate dementia of Alzheimer's type and is also being treated with an antidepressant.

How would you manage this case?

SUGGESTED PROBES

1. What further information would you need to assess the situation?
2. What are the risk factors for abuse in the elderly?
3. You have been able to make a case for both physical and emotional abuse in this patient. How would you proceed?

PMP PLAN

TASKS TO DO

The following five areas are relevant to this vignette but are not necessarily all-inclusive. The list is also not exhaustive:

a) Appreciate the need for a thorough and systematic interview, including giving consideration to interviewing the partner separately.
b) Appreciate the need to examine relevant risk issues, and situational and environmental factors that could have precipitated and be maintaining the present problem.
c) Appreciate the need to involve the husband, if necessary, whilst fulfilling your main duty of care to this woman.
d) Look into the current support network, the possibility of stress in the carer, and his physical/mental well-being.
e) If abuse or maltreatment is confirmed, give prominence to the patient's safety and appreciate the need for involvement of a multidisciplinary team.

ISSUES

- Ascertaining whether this lady is being abused or not; if so, the kind of abuse she suffering
- Determining the risks involved and instituting appropriate management.

CLARIFY

- Are there any urgent reasons or indications for removing this lady from the situation of abuse?
- Is she having suicidal thoughts or demonstrating suicidal behaviour?

SEEK MORE INFORMATION

GP

- His/her concerns
- History of repeated, unexplained physical problems.

CPN

- Seek objective facts
- Nature of abuse, duration, when and where it is happening, previous occurrences
- Who else is involved, any other family members and their view of the current situation
- Risk of future occurrence and anticipated risk.

RELATIVES (WITH PATIENT'S CONSENT)

- Awareness of any abuse, concerns and views of the current situation
- Nature of the abuse: longstanding marital abuse that has worsened or that has not changed over many years.

PATIENT

- Assessment of her capacity to give an accurate account of events
- Awareness of the abuse
- History of previous maltreatment: type, frequency and intensity
- Antecedent to current maltreatment situation and likelihood of recurrence
- Current mental state, activities of daily living functions, physical condition, socioeconomic situation, care and treatment needs, adequacy of care provided and living arrangements
- Impact of abuse on patient's mental state, e.g. anxiety and worsening of depressive symptoms.

HUSBAND

- Assessment, in person when possible or via the GP, of his emotional and physical state (including pain), and emotional, physical and financial responsibilities to his wife
- Any cognitive impairment or other organic or functional illness that may affect his judgment
- His understanding of the current concerns and his perceived need for change
- Disparity in the husband's and wife's story
- Use of drugs and/or alcohol.

ENVIRONMENT

- Adequacy of accommodation
- Adequacy of care/acceptance of support from outside agencies
- Financial resources.

DIFFERENTIAL DIAGNOSIS

Not relevant. There is a possibility with this presentation that the CPN has a total misunderstanding of what is going on. It is also possible that the patient really is being abused, and there are many reasons or factors that would increase the likelihood of this happening. These include:

- *Factors in the woman (the abused).* Worsening of cognitive impairment with increased physical and emotional dependency on her husband
- *Factors in the husband (the alleged abuser).* Presence of emotional disturbance, mental illness, alcohol or substance misuse, carer's stress, particularly if he is overwhelmed with the task of caring for his wife
- *Factors in the environment.* History of violence in the marriage, social isolation, inappropriate shared living situation, stressful life events.

APPROACH TO MANAGEMENT

- Decide whether abuse is present or not. Carry out a risk assessment.
- Establish the predisposing, precipitating and perpetuating factors.
- Evaluate whether the maltreated person wants to do something about it. She may dread consequences such as retaliation and abandonment.

- Discuss various ways of bringing an end to the abuse.
- Make your highest priority the safety of the patient, while respecting her autonomy.
- Report to the local social services department or consider reporting to the police, if appropriate.
- Consider admission to bring maltreatment to an immediate end. Bear in mind the patient's wishes; the seriousness of the maltreatment, the history of and nature of the violence; whether the pattern is escalating; the level of the husband's insight into the problem and his motivation to change; treatability of the precipitating and perpetuating factors.

WHAT TREATMENT/ADVICE

This depends on the perceived cause(s) of the problem. Give consideration to a broad range of biopsychosocial interventions and multidisciplinary approaches.

- *Biological.* Review the need for cognitive enhancers and antidepressants in the patient, if she has not already been prescribed one.
- *Psychological.* Arrange family/marital therapy for family/marital problems.
- *Carer support.* Provide help with the burdens the husband suffers from caring for his wife.
- *Social.* Ask for a social worker's assessment of the adequacy of current support: carer's burden and benefits issues. Arrange attendance at a day hospital. Provide regular respite care, and consider residential care if the risk to the patient outweighs the benefit of trying to keep the couple together. Provide information on a carer support association.
- *Occupational therapy.* Ask an occupational therapist to suggest necessary adaptations or aids to enhance independent living.
- *Legal.* If social support and other interventions are unlikely to succeed in stopping the maltreatment, consider advice from a senior colleague and legal advice from the hospital or trust solicitors. This is a worrying development that would need to be attended to promptly.

FULL ANSWER

The main issues would be to ascertain whether this woman is being abused or not, what kind of abuse she is suffering, who is the perpetrator, and what factors in abused and abuser underlie the situation. This would help to determine the risks involved, in order to institute appropriate management.

First, I would clarify from the CPN what he or she has noticed to generate concern. I would find out whether there is any serious risk of harm to the patient or her husband, and if there is a need for her immediate hospitalization or removal from the situation of abuse. I would quickly assess if she is having thoughts of self-harm or suicide or demonstration of any suicidal behaviour in response to frustration about being abused. I would also clarify whether the husband has any urgent issues that need attention. Before arranging to see this lady and her husband, I would clarify whether the CPN has any objective evidence of abuse and whether this has been recorded in the client's notes. I would ask the CPN about the nature of the alleged abuse, how long it has been going on, and when and where the abuse happened or is happening. I would also ask who else is involved, whether any family members know about it, and if so, their view of the current situation. I would find out if abuse has occurred in the past, and whether relatives think there is a risk of it happening again in future. I would ask for evidence of any physical abuse or witnessed evidence of any psychological abuse, or both. I would find out why the maltreatment issue has been raised at this particular time. I would also find out what other family members have done about it to date. I would ask the CPN what he or she thinks needs to be done, given that she knows the patient better than I do. I would clarify whether there is an immediate and urgent risk or concern necessitating the urgent removal of the patient from the abuse situation. I would speak to the GP and ask if he or she has any concerns, and whether there have been repeated presentations to the practice of unexplained physical problems such as bruises, fractures or falls. I would be careful to be specific and to differentiate clearly between factual history and what has been reported by others.

Next, I would arrange via the CPN to meet with the client, preferably with a family member present to provide more information. Given the nature of the problem, I would bear in mind that I might need to interview the patient, her husband and her family separately. During my meeting with the client, I would as far as possible assess her capacity to give an accurate account of events and would document this properly. I would be particularly careful about my line of questioning, to ensure that I did not suggest answers or discourage her from disclosure. I would start with general and then specific questions about the type, frequency and intensity of the maltreatment. I would also enquire about antecedents to the current situation, any previous history of maltreatment and the likelihood of its recurrence. I would assess the patient's current mental state (using the mini-mental state examination), activities of daily living function, physical state, socioeconomic situation, care and treatment needs, adequacy of the care provided and living arrangements.

Next, I would talk to the husband to hear his version of developments. I would avoid confrontation and be non-judgmental in my approach. I would demonstrate empathy and show understanding of the burdens shouldered by care-givers, in order to develop a fairly accurate picture of the problem. I would try to ascertain whether the husband has any cognitive impairment or other organic or functional illness that might affect his judgment. I would try to assess his satisfaction with the support mechanisms in place, adequacy of care, the couple's acceptance of support from outside agencies, and their financial resources.

Lastly, I would seek the views of family members on the current situation. I would find out if the abuse is a longstanding marital problem that has worsened or which has not changed over many years.

Having taken a detailed history, I would hopefully have clarified whether the CPN has misunderstood the situation or whether he or she is right to think that this woman is being abused. While it might be difficult to establish why she might have been abused, I would give consideration to issues in this woman, her husband and their environment that would make abuse more likely. In the woman, these factors include worsening of cognitive impairment with increased physical and emotional dependency on her husband, a history of violence in their marriage and social isolation. The presence of emotional disturbance and/or mental illness, including misuse of substances in the husband, an unfavourable environment and shared living situations, and stressful life events would also increase the likelihood of abuse.

As regards my approach to management, I would first decide whether abuse is present or not. I would evaluate whether the maltreated person wants to do something about it or not, bearing in mind that she might be dreading the possible consequences, such as retaliation or abandonment. I would assess her capacity to make decisions on the issue at hand, and also discuss with my colleagues the various ways of bringing an end to the abuse. My highest priority would be to ensure the safety of the patient while respecting her autonomy and family life. I would report the identified abuse to the local social services department, who would be able to implement the agreed local Adult Protection Procedures. I would also consider reporting the case to the police, if appropriate, particularly if a crime had been committed. I would carry out a risk assessment and assess the impact of the abuse on the patient's mental state: for example, increasing anxiety and worsening of any depressive symptoms. I would definitely consider admission to hospital to bring the maltreatment to an end, immediately if necessary. I would bear several issues in mind, including the patient's wishes, the seriousness of the maltreatment, any history of violence and its nature, an escalating pattern of abuse or violence, the level of the husband's insight into the problem, his motivation to change, and the treatability of the precipitating and perpetuating factors. It might also be necessary to remove the abuser through legal means rather than removing the abused.

The treatment and management that I would offer would depend on the perceived cause of the problem, and would include a broad range of biopsychosocial interventions and multidisciplinary approaches. Treatment would be directed to the patient and the husband both as individuals and as a couple. As depression and cognitive deficits might be important problems in this lady, medical treatment in the form of antidepressants and cognitive enhancers would be attempted, if it had not already been tried. Psychological treatment, such as family and marital therapy, would be offered to deal with marital and family problems. A social worker would carry out an assessment of the adequacy of current support, housing and living arrangements, carer's burden, and support needed for the husband in his capacity as carer. I would ask an occupational therapist to suggest adaptations or aids to enhance independent and more pleasant living, and to improve the couple's environmental situation. Other social assistance measures would include looking into money and benefit issues, the provision of home helps and the funding of regular respite care. We would also look into attendance at a day hospital for the patient and referral of her husband to the local carer's support association. Consideration would be given to residential care or an alternative placement, if the risk to the patient outweighed the benefits of keeping the couple together.

If social support and other interventions were unlikely to succeed in stopping the maltreatment, separating the couple might be the last resort. I would seek opinions and advice from my senior colleagues, and legal advice from the trust or hospital solicitor. I would refer to the adult protection team at the local social services department, if appropriate. I would suggest placement with family members who were willing and who had been assessed as having the will, ability, time and resources to look after either the wife or husband. I would recommend that the social services department should continue to offer assistance and support to the abused woman.

ANSWERS TO SUGGESTED PROBES

1. The further information necessary for assessing the situation is described in the full answer.

2. The risk factors for abuse in the elderly are as follows:
   - in the abused: worsening of cognitive impairment with increased physical and emotional dependency on the abuser, history of marital violence, social isolation, and presence of learning difficulties or dementia
   - in the abuser: presence of emotional disturbance/mental illness, including misuse of alcohol and other substances
   - in the environment: shared living situation and stressful life events, which provide opportunity for tension.
3. If I were able to make a case for both physical and emotional abuse in this patient, I would carry out the following measures:
   - Follow the local protocol for abuse of the elderly and vulnerable adults, as far as possible.
   - Remove the abused or the abuser from the situation of abuse.
   - Treat any physical illness.
   - Ask the duty social worker to assess the woman and her living situation.
   - Inform the police if a crime had been committed.
   - Organize an early Older Adult Protection conference.
   - Offer assistance to the family.
   - Offer help to the abuser himself, if necessary: e.g. with mental or physical illness, alcohol or substance misuse, and carer's stress.
   - Carry out a carer's assessment if the abuser remained as the main carer.

BUZZ WORDS AND USEFUL TERMINOLOGY

Non-judgmental, empathy, care-giver's burden, autonomy, adult protection team, vulnerable adult, adult protection conference.

REFERENCES AND USEFUL READING

Hirsch R D, Vollhardt B R 2002 Elder maltreatment. In: Jacoby R, Oppenheimer C (eds) Psychiatry in the Elderly, 3rd edn. Oxford University Press, Oxford, pp 896–918

Kahan F S, Paris B E 2003 Why elder abuse continues to elude the health care system. Mount Sinai Journal of Medicine 70(1):62–68

Kruger R M, Moon C H 1999 Can you spot the signs of elder mistreatment? Postgraduate Medicine 106(2):169–173, 177–178, 183

Lachs M S, Pillemer K 1995 Abuse and neglect of elderly persons. New England Journal of Medicine 332(7):437–443

6.7 DEPRESSION IN A 78-YEAR-OLD WOMAN

A 78-year-old female has been referred to your team by her GP because of a 'worsening depression' that has failed to respond to citalopram 40 mg daily. She suffers from many physical problems, which include severe arthritis, diabetes mellitus and hypertension. She has lost two of her sons and her only daughter was recently diagnosed with what appears to be Creutzfeldt–Jakob disease (CJD).
How would you assess and manage her?

SUGGESTED PROBES

1. What further information would you like to have?
2. On cognitive assessment, the patient scores low on the Mini Mental State Examination (MMSE). How would you manage this situation?
3. What psychosocial treatment would you offer her?

PMP PLAN

TASKS TO DO

The following areas are relevant to this vignette but are not necessarily all-inclusive. The list is also not exhaustive:

a) Make a comprehensive and systematic assessment of the patient's current symptoms to ascertain what role physical problems and bereavement play in this presentation.
b) Demonstrate awareness that depression can present with atypical symptoms in the elderly.
c) Appreciate the need to look into the various psychosocial issues in both the assessment and management of the patient.
d) Demonstrate the need to assess risk and possible impairment of activities of daily living (ADL).
e) Include a range of biopsychosocial interventions in your management plan.

ISSUES

- Need to determine whether this lady has a functional depressive disorder or whether depression is related to her various physical and psychosocial problems
- Comprehensive risk assessment to inform an appropriate management plan.

CLARIFY

- Why is she being referred now and are there any immediate safety concerns?
- Is any informant available, does she live on her own and how recent are the various losses in her life?
- Is there any risk of self-harm or suicide? Is there a need for immediate hospitalization?

SEEK MORE INFORMATION

GP

- The patient's current symptoms and their impact on her ADL
- Control of her various physical problems, in particular pain
- Current medication; some antihypertensive might be depressogenic
- Psychiatric history, including self-harm.

CARERS/RELATIVES

- Current support network.

PATIENT

- Current depressive symptoms, especially atypical ones (elderly patients may not admit to feeling depressed)
- History of affective disorder and medication that she has found helpful in the past
- Her view of her physical problems and hopes of getting better
- Her various losses: help such as bereavement counselling? Did she grieve normally or has she never been able to do so? Factors that would make abnormal bereavement reaction more likely. Daughter's physical state and prognosis
- Any misuse of substances such as alcohol and her coping strategies
- Any financial worries
- Social interests and current level of involvement in social activities
- Impact on her day-to-day functioning
- Detailed mental state and physical examination, looking for evidence of depressive illness, depressive cognition, psychosis, cognitive impairment and disabling physical conditions.

INVESTIGATIONS

- Review of results of investigations into physical illnesses.

DIFFERENTIAL DIAGNOSIS/DIFFICULTIES

- *Functional.* Grief/bereavement reaction, depressive illness, possibly exacerbated by physical problems.

APPROACH TO TREATMENT

- Give strong consideration to domiciliary assessment, as it would be very informative in this case.
- Assess risks and consider inpatient treatment. Otherwise offer a comprehensive package of community care, which should ideally include day hospital attendance.
- Liaise with other professionals, e.g. medical specialists, psychologists and occupational therapist. Reassess the diagnosis.
- Assess whether the patient is compliant with medication.
- Assess the impact of her current physical and psychosocial problems.
- Offer a broad range of biopsychosocial interventions.

WHAT TREATMENT/ADVICE

- *Medical/biological.* Treat physical, emotional and/or psychiatric problems. Change the antidepressant. Arrange augmentation therapy and ECT. Treat physical conditions adequately. Arrange physiotherapy for the arthritis.
- *Psychological.* Consider bereavement counselling, CBT and psychodynamic psychotherapy.
- *Social.* Improve community support, including a comprehensive care package, if necessary.

FULL ANSWER

The GP referral raises the possibility that this patient has some degree of resistance to treatment of her depression. One of the issues would be to determine whether she has a functional depressive disorder or whether her depression is related to her various physical and psychosocial problems. I would also want to assess the role that physical problems, psychosocial problems and bereavement play in this lady's presentation. I would need to carry out a comprehensive risk assessment to inform an appropriate management plan.

To begin with, I would clarify why she has been referred at this particular time, how soon the GP thinks she should be seen, whether there are any immediate risks or concerns, and if so, what they are. I would find out if there is any risk of self-harm or suicide and any need for immediate hospitalization.

While making arrangements to see this lady, I would also seek more information from the GP on her current physical and emotional symptoms, the impact of these on her activities of daily living, and details of any antidepressant or other treatment she has received to date. I would be interested in how well the GP has been able to control her physical illness and the medication she is taking for it at present, especially if that included antihypertensive drugs, some of which might be depressogenic. I would also enquire about her psychiatric history, including treatment for depression, duration of treatment, extent of compliance and progress to date. I would ask the GP if there have been any concerns about deliberate self-harm or suicidal behaviour. I would enquire about her various losses, how recent they are, and if she received appropriate help and support, including bereavement counselling. I would also speak to any identified carers or relatives to obtain their views about her current problems and to ascertain the level of support they provide. I would find out whether the GP and carers think an outpatient appointment or domiciliary visit would be more appropriate. I would ring the patient in advance of any appointment to make sure an informant was available.

When I saw this elderly lady, I would look for evidence of depression, psychosis and cognitive impairment. I would ask her about the impact of the current difficulties on her activities of daily living and how she thinks things can be improved. I would also enquire about any history of affective disorder and the treatments she found beneficial in the past. I would seek her views about her physical problems, the treatment she is taking, what she has been told about the progress of the different physical conditions she is suffering from, and her hopes of getting better. Next, I would tactfully ask about the various losses in her life and how she coped with them. I would look for various risk factors that might predispose her to an abnormal grief reaction, such as ambivalent relationships with the deceased sons, excessively long periods of looking after them, unresolved issues, secrets and plans. I would assess for a low level of perceived social support, lack of new opportunities, social isolation, psychosocial stressors or other life events such as her physical illnesses. If I thought she had an abnormal grief reaction, I would establish what stage she has reached (denial, anger, bargaining, sadness, guilt and acceptance). I would also ask whether she received formal counselling after her bereavements, if she had the opportunity to grieve for her sons, or whether the grieving process was disturbed by hospitalization for her physical illness or impaired by cognitive abnormalities. I would find out about her daughter's state of health and also about her prognosis. I would ask if the patient has been drinking more alcohol or simply keeping to herself.

Given her presentation, my thoughts on differential diagnosis would be that this woman is suffering either from a treatment-resistant depression, a poorly treated recurrent depressive disorder, a grief- or bereavement-related depressive reaction or a depressive illness secondary to multiple or disabling physical or organic conditions. It is also possible that her depressive state is being exacerbated by her physical and psychosocial problems or her current medication. The other alternative is that all these problems play a part, in one form or the other.

My approach to management in this case would be first to appraise all the available information, review the diagnosis and the various investigations, ensure good medication compliance, assess the impact of the current physical and psychosocial problems, make an assessment of risk, and then decide on treatment type and setting. I would be inclined to manage this woman as an inpatient if there were significant risk issues, if she had a moderate to severe depressive illness with the risk of self-harm or suicide, or if there were complicating physical problems and a lack of social support. Should I decide to manage her in the community, however, I would ensure that she received a comprehensive package of care, including attendance at the psychiatric day hospital for closer monitoring.

Whatever the treatment setting, I would offer a broad range of biopsychosocial interventions including a change of antidepressant, augmentation therapy, electroconvulsive treatment, bereavement counselling, cognitive behavioural therapy, psychodynamic psychotherapy (psychological) and social interventions. As far as medical treatment is concerned, the aim would be to treat her physical problems in order to stabilize them and minimize distress. I would refer to the appropriate specialist to oversee these treatments. Adequate treatment of her physical conditions might also include physiotherapy for her arthritis, with input from the local pain clinic if the pain became unmanageable. For her depression, I would consider a change of antidepressant, or try augmentation therapy and ECT as a last resort if her physical condition allowed.

There would be roles for psychological treatments in the form of bereavement counselling, CBT for depression and/or a psychodynamic psychotherapy approach to treatment. This lady would also be referred for social and community support, if necessary, with the aim of arranging a comprehensive care package. This would include identifying and funding the appropriate day services, and arranging for a home help, health visitor or district nurse, community psychiatric nurse and a befriending service. The care package would be organized and coordinated in such a way as to ensure that functions were not duplicated, time was saved, and the lady was not overwhelmed by the presence of multiple professionals. The treatment would ensure that she did not become de-skilled and remained able to perform basic tasks for herself without relying on other people.

ANSWERS TO SUGGESTED PROBES

1. The information needed for diagnosis and management is covered in the full answer.
2. Cognitive impairment is not uncommon in depressive illness due to poor attention and concentration, but memory impairment more often than not improves on recovery from depression. I would therefore not be worried about this patient's low score on MMSE at this present time. However, because the presence of cognitive impairment during a depressive episode is said to be a risk factor for future memory problems, I would make sure that her condition was monitored on a regular basis in order to assess the need for anticholinesterase treatment.
3. Psychosocial treatment is covered in the full answer.

BUZZ WORDS AND USEFUL TERMINOLOGY

Bereavement counselling, package of care, de-skilling.

REFERENCES AND SUGGESTED READING

Baldwin R 1999 Approaches to treatment-resistant depression in the elderly. In: Howard R (ed) Everything You Need to Know about Old Age Psychiatry. Wrighton Biomedical Publications, Petersfield, pp 187–197

Baldwin R 2002 Mood disorders in the elderly. In: Gelder M G, López-Ibor Jr J J, Andreasen N C (eds) New Oxford Textbook of Psychiatry, vol. 2. Oxford University Press, Oxford, pp 1644–1651

7

Eating disorders

A GP has referred to you a 14-year-old girl who has been losing weight in the last 4 months. She is described as 'very fussy' about her food, measures the calories she consumes, and is 'obsessed with watching her weight'. Her stepfather started working abroad about 6 months ago and her mother is now very concerned she will come to harm if she does not receive help soon.

How do you go about assessing and managing her?

SUGGESTED PROBES

1. Are there any obvious psychodynamic inferences in this case?
2. What in her premorbid history makes a diagnosis of an eating disorder or anorexia more likely?
3. What factors will guide your suggestion and/or acceptance of an outpatient treatment?

PMP PLAN

TASKS TO DO

The following five areas are relevant to this vignette but are not necessarily all-inclusive. The list is also not exhaustive:

a) Demonstrate an ability to decide on safety and risk issues, including ruling out organic conditions and suicidality.
b) Discuss the assessment and physical investigation of eating disorders, focusing particularly on anorexia nervosa.
c) Explore psychological factors, e.g. parental separation and divorce, stepfather working abroad, feelings of rejection and self-blame.
d) Show an understanding of the role of other professionals in the assessment and management of eating disorders.
e) Consider medical management, and psychological and social treatment in this girl. Cover the need to engage the child and work with the parents.

ISSUES

- Establishing whether the girl has an eating disorder and understanding the psychological factors underlying the abnormal eating pattern
- Instituting treatment for anorexia nervosa.

CLARIFY

- What is the girl's physical status? Are there any life-threatening complications or suicidality?
- Is there an urgent need to hospitalize her?

SEEK MORE INFORMATION

GP

- Extent of physical investigations and results
- Ruling out an organic condition.

PARENTS

- Onset of illness
- Any history of getting rid of food surreptitiously.

CHILD

- Body mass index (BMI)
- Preoccupation with food, fear of gaining weight, effort to lose weight and methods used, disorder of body image, amenorrhoea, clarify type of eating behaviour (restricting or binge eating)
- Impulsive behaviour, obsession with cleanliness and studying, delayed psychosexual development
- Ruling out depression, suicidality, obsessive-compulsive disorder (OCD).

INVESTIGATIONS

- BMI
- FBC, U and Es, LFTs, RFTs, TFTs, hormonal assay, serum amylase and ECG
- Bone scan for osteoporosis, if the history dates from more than 6 months ago.

PHYSICAL EXAMINATION

- Evidence of weight loss, lanugo hair, cachexia, low blood pressure, anaemia, distension of abdomen.

DIFFERENTIAL DIAGNOSIS/DIFFICULTIES

- *Functional.* Anorexia, bulimia, depressive disorder, somatization disorder, OCD
- *Organic.* Crohn's disease, hyperthyroidism, Addison's disease, diabetes mellitus.

APPROACH TO TREATMENT

- Work with the family and other professionals.
- Base assessment and treatment on the needs of the individual.
- Take a multifaceted treatment approach, which includes medical management, nutritional counselling, psychoeducation and other psychological treatment including individual therapy.
- Put discharge planning in perspective.

WHAT TREATMENT/ADVICE

MEDICAL

- Hospitalize, and restore and monitor weight. Instigate nutritional rehabilitation, rehydration and correction of serum electrolytes. If the patient's weight is not too low, i.e. BMI >14 kg/m^2, refeeding could take place in an outpatient or day patient setting.
- Prescribe an antidepressant and cyproheptadine, if necessary.

NURSING

- Monitor for suicidality, impulsive behaviour and self-harm.
- Give support at meal times.

PSYCHOLOGICAL

- Start cognitive behavioural therapy, problem-solving and motivation enhancement therapy.
- Educate while on the ward.
- Start the discharge planning process.

RELATIVES/CARERS

- Offer family therapy and parental counselling.
- Provide support.

The main issues I would want to address would be to determine whether this 14-year-old girl has an eating disorder, to understand the psychological factors underlying the abnormal eating pattern, and then to institute the appropriate treatment.

My initial approach would be to clarify whether there is any physical and life-threatening condition that requires prompt attention. Prompt intervention would be necessary if there were a BMI of less than 13.5 kg/m², a higher BMI but rapid weight loss, severe electrolyte imbalance or multiple abnormal physical tests. I would also decide whether there is a need for immediate hospitalization and would want to rule out any parasuicidal behaviour plan or intent to self-harm. I would find out what exactly is worrying the mother about her daughter's health. Once I was satisfied that the girl was stable and not at immediate risk of medical complications, I would make proper arrangements to see her.

Prior to the appointment, I would seek more information from the GP and her parents to enable me to carry out a proper assessment. I would find out from the GP what physical investigations had been done to date, and would want to see the results of investigations to rule out organic conditions such as Crohn's disease, hyperthyroidism, Addison's disease and diabetes mellitus. When I saw her parents, I would ask about the girl's history, focusing on the onset of the problem and the family's psychosocial situation. I would ask if the girl had ever been caught getting rid of food surreptitiously and/or making an effort to lose weight. I would ask the parents how the family has been coping with the girl's condition and what other help they have sought. I would ask about other children in the family to make sure they do not have similar problems. As far as possible I would try to engage the patient. I would concentrate on the relevant history and onset, and explore the girl's view of the present problem. I would carry out a mental state examination and relevant physical examination, and then review the relevant investigations. I would try to establish the extent of her preoccupation with food and find out whether she has a preference for particular types of food. I would also ask whether she is very concerned about getting fat or has a fear of being a normal body weight. I would find out about the onset of the illness and when her concern about gaining weight started, and whether she is preoccupied with the calorific value of food every time she eats. I would find out about any attempts the patient has made to lose weight and whether these include jogging, ritualistic cycling and exercise, self-induced vomiting, and misuse of laxatives or diuretics. I would check whether her eating behaviour is of a restricting or binge eating type (when she regularly binges and later vomits). I would find out whether she has feelings of rejection due to her parents' separation and to her stepfather leaving home to work abroad. I would ask if she associates any feelings of rejection with increasing weight.

I would also look for evidence of a disorder of body image or over-concern with her body weight or shape. Her assessment would also give me the opportunity to look for evidence of inflexibility, rigidity, and perfectionist, obsessive and rule-bound traits, all which would make the diagnosis of anorexia nervosa more likely. I would also seek evidence of impulsive behaviour such as stealing, drug abuse, misuse of alcohol and parasuicidal behaviour. I would look for symptoms of depression and ask her about thoughts, plans and intentions to harm herself. I would look for signs of obsessional behaviour, such as excessive cleanliness and studying, and find out more about her psychosexual development. I would find out if she acknowledges that she is now dangerously underweight or whether she sees loss of weight as an improvement. I would carry out a physical examination and measure her body mass index (BMI), which I would expect to be between 20 and 25 kg/m^2. I would document clearly any evidence of starvation, including weight loss, cachexia, presence of lanugo hairs, low blood pressure, anaemia and distension of the abdomen. I would assess this girl's sexual development and document it appropriately. I would also carry out further investigations if none had been done recently, and order an FBC, U and Es, LFTs, RFTs, TFTs, serum amylase, bone scan, ECG and other tests as suggested by the differential diagnosis. If the girl had amenorrhoea, I would consider checking the serum level of luteinizing hormone (LH), follicle-stimulating hormone (FSH) and oestradiol, and also carrying out a pelvic ultrasound.

From the description given, it would seem to me that this girl is suffering from anorexia nervosa. I would consider other differential diagnoses including bulimia nervosa, depressive disorder, somatization disorder, obsessive-compulsive disorder, and organic conditions such as Crohn's disease, hyperthyroidism, Addison's disease and diabetes mellitus.

In my approach to treatment I would seek to work with the family and other professionals, and to engage the girl as much as possible. I would base my treatment strategy on her individual needs and consider a multifaceted treatment approach. This would include medical management, nursing management and monitoring, nutritional counselling, psychoeducation, psychological treatment, discharge planning and support for the family and carers.

In light of the information that this girl may be severely underweight and at risk of harm, I would consider hospitalization for weight restoration and monitoring as part of the medical management. Depending upon the severity of the weight loss and the girl's motivation to get better, I would decide whether to manage her as an outpatient or inpatient. If this particular young girl were not severely underweight, I would consider outpatient management with regular weekly family therapy, dietetic input, medical review and possibly individual therapy. If the weight loss were severe, I would consider admitting her to hospital, but would involve the parents at a very early stage so that they can learn how to refeed their child. After brief psychoeducation, we would need to agree on a reasonable target weight gain of about 0.5–1.0 kg per week initially, to approach a target BMI of 19 (about 85%–100% of weight for height). If this girl were severely malnourished on admission to hospital, I would stabilize her weight before attempting to increase it. I would rehydrate her, and if necessary, I would give intravenous fluids and correct any serum electrolyte imbalance. I would also monitor elecrolytes, phosphates and magnesium carefully for evidence of refeeding syndrome, which can be fatal. I would liaise with the dietician to advise on the calorie contents needed for refeeding, and would generally aim to start at around 1500 kcal a day, ensuring that she is eating three meals or so a day. The total calorie intake could be divided into moderately sized meals and snacks.

I would monitor the patient's progress using a Cole's Slide Rule or BMI chart. I would ask nursing staff to offer support at meal times, monitor her food intake, and watch for any attempt to hide food or activities that might promote further weight loss. As her weight increased, the girl might become distressed, and I would ask staff to monitor her for any suicidal or self-harm behaviour. Once she had reached a healthy weight, efforts would be made to stabilize that weight. In the long term, I would monitor whether she was menstruating or not.

As far as psychological treatment is concerned, I would consider cognitive behavioural therapy, whereby feelings and emotions about her food intake would be monitored, analysed and treated. The psychologist in the team would attempt cognitive restructuring to identify automatic negative thoughts and to challenge core beliefs. I would also consider family therapy and parental counselling at the appropriate time. I would arrange for educational support while the girl was on the ward, particularly if the admission was likely to be a long one. Further psychoeducation would focus on the health hazards of weight loss and starvation, abuse of medications (laxatives, diuretics, emetics and/or illicit drugs), appearance and body image, the components of long-term treatment, the process of recovery, what constitutes a relapse, its indices and how to deal with it. It would also be useful to give support to her mother, the main carer, and also refer her to any carer or support group that might be available locally.

ANSWERS TO SUGGESTED PROBES

1. The obvious psychodynamic influences in this case are issues of loss, self-blame and low self-worth. The illness may serve as a strong positive function in this girl's life by allowing her to escape uncomfortable interpersonal problems or feelings. These include developmental issues involved in becoming an adult, parental divorce, her upbringing, her relationship with her mother and stepfather, and the absence of a paternal figure following the stepfather's departure to work abroad. These life events are things the girl does not have control over, and she may see her weight as the only thing she can control.
2. The factors in her premorbid history that would make the diagnosis of anorexia more likely are inflexibility, rigidity, and perfectionist, obsessive and rule-bound traits.
3. The factors that would guide me towards outpatient treatment are:
   - illness of moderate degree dating from less than 6 months ago
   - absence of an acute or imminent life-threatening condition
   - absence of suicidal thoughts and behaviour
   - absence of binge eating and excessive vomiting
   - presence of parents who are likely to cooperate and participate in outpatient treatment
   - availability of staff who can carry out outpatient treatment and monitoring.

BUZZ WORDS AND USEFUL TERMINOLOGY

Engagement, body mass index, psychoeducation, multifaceted treatment, refeeding, refeeding syndrome, automatic negative thoughts, cognitive distortions, cognitive restructuring, multifactorial problems, multidisciplinary team, family therapy.

REFERENCES AND SUGGESTED READING

Fairburn C, Harrison P J 2003 Eating disorders. Lancet 361:407–416
Lask B, Bryant-Waugh R 2000 Anorexia Nervosa and Related Eating Disorders in Childhood and Adolescence, 2nd edn. Psychology Press, Hove
Szmukler G, Dare C, Treasure J 1995 Handbook of Eating Disorders: Theory, Treatment and Research. John Wiley, Chichester
Treasure J 1997 Anorexia Nervosa: A Survival Guide for Families, Friends and Sufferers. Psychology Press, Hove

7.2 21-YEAR-OLD WOMAN WITH DENTAL CARIES WHO BINGES ON CHOCOLATES

You have been asked to see a 21-year-old single woman who has been dieting for the last 3 years. She has presented to her dentist with severe dental caries. On further questioning she discloses that she has been eating large amounts of chocolates in binges, at the same time as she has been attempting to lose weight. She feels low in her mood, has low self-esteem and thinks her boyfriend is about to leave her. Her BMI is 21.3 kg per m^2.

How would you go about your assessment and management of this lady?

SUGGESTED PROBES

1. What features enable you to distinguish between this presentation and anorexia nervosa?
2. After attending clinics for a couple of months, the patient admits she has started to binge, vomit and use laxatives again. What complications must you watch for?
3. The patient is more stable. What factors will help you choose between individual and group therapy?

PMP PLAN

TASKS TO DO

The following five areas are relevant to this vignette but are not necessarily all-inclusive. The list is also not exhaustive:

a) Demonstrate an ability to decide on severity and risk issues and awareness of the need to rule out organic conditions.
b) Utilize the relevant information to arrive at the most likely differential diagnosis.
c) Examine the patient's relevant history and mental state, and carry out a physical examination and investigations to support your diagnosis of an eating disorder, particularly bulimia nervosa.
d) Explore psychological factors and other interpersonal problems that may be responsible.
e) Include medical, psychological and social treatment and support in your management plan.

ISSUES

- Establishing whether the patient has an eating disorder and understanding the psychological factors underlying her abnormal eating
- Instituting treatment for bulimia nervosa.

CLARIFY

- What is the main issue at hand?
- What is the patient's physical status?
- Is there a life-threatening situation, suicidality or an urgent need to bring her into hospital?

SEEK MORE INFORMATION

GP

- Relevant medical history, results of referrals and investigations to date.

PATIENT

- History of onset, recurrent bingeing, purging or non-purging type of eating disorder
- Compulsive behaviour of eating yet trying to lose weight, timing and frequency of bingeing, negative cognitions and preoccupation with body weight and shape
- Menstrual periods
- Preoccupation with thoughts of binge eating, feelings of guilt, depression, self-disparagement, high level of anxiety
- Evidence of impulsivity, poor self-concept, substance misuse and a chaotic lifestyle.

PHYSICAL EXAMINATION

- Previous history of being overweight, current weight, body mass index (BMI)
- Menstrual periods
- Abrasions and scars on the back of hands.

INVESTIGATIONS

- FBC, U and Es, LFTs, TFTs, RFTs (plus ECG, chest X-ray, abdominal X-ray and serum amylase, only if indicated, particularly in cases of hypokalaemia or intestinal obstruction)

- Other measures—Bulimic Investigatory Test, Edinburgh (BITE) (Henderson & Freeman 1987) for the assessment of symptoms and severity of bulimia.

DIFFERENTIAL DIAGNOSIS/DIFFICULTIES

- *Functional*. Bulimia nervosa, anorexia nervosa, binge eating disorder, eating disorder not otherwise specified (EDNOS)
- *Organic*. Klein–Leventhal syndrome.

APPROACH TO TREATMENT

- Work with other professionals.
- Be gentle but firm.
- Consider other factors that might undermine treatment, such as chaotic lifestyle and substance misuse.

WHAT TREATMENT/ADVICE

MEDICAL

- Prescribe an antidepressant to reduce binge eating and depression.

PSYCHOLOGICAL/PSYCHOTHERAPY

- CBT, interpersonal therapy, individual therapy, group therapy, motivation enhancement therapy.

FAMILY THERAPY

- This is mainly appropriate for younger patients.

OTHER TREATMENTS

- Look at problem-solving for chaotic lifestyle, and treatment for substance misuse and alcohol disorder.
- Reduce boredom, loneliness, isolation, stress, tension and depression.

FULL ANSWER

The issue of diagnosis would be paramount in my mind in considering this scenario. As far as possible, I would try to establish whether this woman has an eating disorder, and to understand the psychological factors underlying her abnormal eating behaviour. I would exclude the presence of an organic condition and institute the appropriate treatment depending on my findings.

I would quickly clarify the patient's current physical status and condition to ensure that there is no life-threatening situation that would warrant immediate medical attention. I would also find out about the plan for her dental treatment from the dentist who referred her, and would take this into consideration while planning her assessment and treatment for a possible mental disorder. I would also establish whether there was any suicidal behaviour or suicidality in this lady. I would consider admission to hospital only if there was a severe electrolyte imbalance such as hypokalaemia, or if the patient was considered to be at risk of significant self-harm or suicide.

Prior to seeing her, I would ask her GP about any relevant medical and psychiatric history. I would concentrate on any history of contact with the psychiatric services, and assessment and treatment by psychologists and/or psychiatrists for depression. I would arrange to see the patient in the outpatient clinic with one of my colleagues (preferably female), if there were no emergency situation. I would be particularly interested in finding out about the onset and escalation of her symptoms. I would attempt to establish how she has been dieting, and also the pattern and frequency of her bingeing. I would also find out whether there is a sense of lack of control over the amount she eats and when to stop, and whether this behaviour serves to relieve tension or anxiety. I would also assess her fear of gaining excess weight and her preoccupation with body weight and shape.

I would also check what methods this woman is using to lose weight and whether she has engaged in self-induced vomiting, misuse of laxatives, diuretics and enemas, ritualistic exercise and fasting. I would also ask if she has used amphetamines on any occasion to reduce her appetite or even taken ipecac to induce vomiting. I would decide whether her eating disorder is of a purging or non-purging type, and find out if there have been episodes of bingeing and vomiting up to twice a week. I would ask her about her menstrual periods, whether these are still present and how regular they are. Bulimia nervosa may be the main problem in this lady, whether there is amenorrhoea or not, given that she has other symptoms to suggest this diagnosis. My history would also include exploration of any impulsive behaviour, such as substance and alcohol misuse or a chaotic lifestyle. In the mental state examination I would focus particularly on her preoccupation with binge eating, feelings of guilt, depression and self-disparagement, high level of anxiety, impulsivity, poor self-concept and morbid over-valued ideas about her body. I would also assess her for thoughts, plans and intentions to harm herself. Since up to 70% of patients with bulimia have comorbid depression, I would carry out a full depression screen.

I would carry out a physical examination and measure the patient's weight and height, in order to determine the body mass index and to ensure this is the same or close to the BMI value stated by the referrer. As part of the physical examination, I would carefully check the back of her hands and fingers for abrasions and scars, which might be due to repeated self-induced vomiting achieved by putting her hands down her throat. I would carry out basic laboratory investigations and these would include an FBC, U and Es, LFTs, TFTs and RFTs. An ECG, chest and abdominal X-rays, and serum amylase would be ordered if there were hypokalaemia, intestinal obstruction or parotid gland enlargement respectively. I would carry out an objective rating of symptoms and severity of the bulimic eating disorder, using validated instruments such as the Edinburgh Bulimic Investigatory Test (Freeman 1987).

Given the patient's BMI of 21.3, the presence of bingeing and vomiting, and prominent and severe dental caries, I would concentrate on the diagnosis of bulimic nervosa. I would consider other differential diagnoses and bear in mind that this lady might be suffering from another eating disorder, such as binge eating or an eating disorder not otherwise specified (EDNOS). The diagnosis of Klüver–Bucy syndrome, although rare, and that of Kleine–Levin syndrome, both of which include hyperphagia, would also be at the back of my mind. (Klüver–Bucy syndrome is a disorder involving bilateral temporal lobe damage associated with indiscriminate sexual behaviour, hyperphagia and pica. Kleine–Levin syndrome consists of inordinate eating or bulimia (some texts describe hyperphagia or compulsive eating), hypersomnia and hypersexuality. It occurs mainly in males.) In order to fulfil a diagnosis of bulimia nervosa, the patient must have a normal BMI or even be overweight, and the vomiting and binge eating must occur at least twice a week for a minimum of 3 months. Psychologically, I would carefully establish that this woman's self-esteem is based largely on her shape and weight. If she clearly has disordered eating but is not binge eating and vomiting as frequently as twice a week, she might have binge eating disorder or EDNOS.

In my approach to her treatment I would work with other professionals, particularly those who would be involved in the psychological treatment of her condition. I would be gentle but firm, and try to deal with any chaotic lifestyle or substance misuse that might undermine treatment.

Essentially, my treatment strategy would consist of psychological treatment, pharmacotherapy and psychosocial management to deal with other problems such as social isolation, substance misuse, alcohol abuse, impulsivity, chaotic lifestyle and suicidal behaviour. In my psychological treatment I would consider cognitive behavioural therapy to be the first line, as this has been shown to bring about an improvement in binge eating, dieting and vomiting in up to about 70% of bulimia patients. CBT may involve the use of rigorous detailed manner, which the patient will work, and its effect in decreasing depression in this group of patients. The essence of individual CBT is to interrupt the behavioural cycle that tends to perpetuate or maintain her bingeing and dieting, and also to alter her abnormal thinking pattern (dysfunctional cognition) and her abnormal beliefs about food, body image and herself. While receiving this treatment, this lady needs to normalize her eating habits and develop a structured meal plan. Following the stabilization of eating patterns, CBT can also take the form of group therapy with the aim of improving interpersonal skills, but I am aware that some patients might find sessions difficult to attend due to shame. I would also consider motivation enhancement therapy in this lady, if such treatment were available locally. Interpersonal therapy (IPT) might also be useful to help her focus on interpersonal functioning, although it might take longer to have an effect. The outcome of IPT after 1 year is broadly comparable to that of CBT.

The other line of management would be the use of antidepressants to reduce binge eating and depression. Fluoxetine at a high dose of up to 60 mg a day has been shown to be effective. I would consider other selective serotonin re-uptake inhibitors (SSRIs), such as fluvoxamine, which has been found useful in bulimia. Comorbid problems such as alcohol misuse, self-harm and previous anorexia nervosa predict a poorer outcome, and these might require inpatient assessment and treatment. I would attend to other problems which need practical problem-solving and also deal with chaotic lifestyle, misuse of drugs, boredom, loneliness, isolation, stress and tension. I would hope with this treatment plan to alleviate symptoms in this woman, so that she can return to a normal life.

ANSWERS TO SUGGESTED PROBES

1. The features that distinguish this presentation from anorexia nervosa are:
   - BMI, which is less than 17.5 kg/m² in anorexia nervosa but equal to or greater than 19 kg/m² in bulimia nervosa

- phobia of normal body weight in anorexia, as opposed to fear of fatness in bulimia.
2. If the patient started to binge, vomit and use laxatives again, the most likely complication would be severe hypokalaemia, which might lead to cardiac arrhythmia or cardiac arrest. Other complications, which are less common but do occur, are aspiration pneumonia, acute dilatation of the stomach from persistent vomiting and binge eating, cardiac failure or cardiac myopathy from chronic ingestion of ipecac used to induce vomiting, other electrolyte imbalance and death from all other complications.
3. Once the patient was more stable, I would consider individual therapy:
   - in order to tailor treatment to the specific needs of the individual
   - if the patient could not cope with a group program
   - if there was evidence of a chaotic lifestyle and/or severe interpersonal problems that need a specific individual treatment plan.

   I would consider group therapy in patients:
   - who often keep their disorder (bulimia nervosa) secret
   - who feel isolated and ashamed about their symptoms
   - who have difficulty in asking for help from others
   - who also have interpersonal problems.

   Sharing their problems in a group setting might relieve their sense of isolation and also offer the opportunity to gain from the practical experience of other people.

BUZZ WORDS AND USEFUL TERMINOLOGY

Poor self-concept, body image, dysfunctional cognition, BMI, motivational enhancement therapy.

REFERENCES AND SUGGESTED READING

Fairburn C G, Cooper Z, Doll H A et al 2000 The natural course of bulimia nervosa and binge eating disorder in young women. Archives of General Psychiatry 57(7):659–665

Fairburn C, Harrison P J 2003 Eating disorders. Lancet 361:407–416

Henderson M, Freeman C P 1987 a self-rating scale for bulimia. The 'BITE'. British Journal of Psychiatry 150:18–24

Keller M B, Herzog D B, Lavori P W et al 1992 The natural history of bulimia nervosa: extraordinarily high rates of chronicity, relapse, recurrence, and psychosocial morbidity. International Journal of Eating Disorders 12:1–9

Russell G F M 1979 Bulimia nervosa: an ominous variant of anorexia nervosa. Psychological Medicine 9:429–448

8
Forensic psychiatry

As specialist registrar with a forensic psychiatric team, you have been asked to see a 24-year-old male at a local police station, who handed himself in for arrest shortly after he became violent and attacked people with a machete. A local shopkeeper later died in hospital and another person was seriously injured. Whilst in the police cell, he was noticed to be talking to himself and behaving strangely, as if fending off attack from unseen objects.

How would you go about assessing and managing him?

SUGGESTED PROBES

1. How would you assess this patient's fitness to be interviewed?
2. How would you assess his fitness to plead in court?
3. How would you assess the risk of reoffending in this man?

PMP PLAN

TASKS TO DO

The following areas are relevant to this vignette but are not necessarily all-inclusive. The list is also not exhaustive:

a) Gather details of the offence and the witness statement.
b) Mention information-gathering regarding the patient's psychiatric history. Attempt to contact the GP, relatives, and probation and social services.
c) Demonstrate systematic information-gathering from the offender regarding his own account of the incident, psychiatric history, forensic history and current mental state, including assessment of suicidality.
d) Discuss the possible causes of this presentation.
e) Appreciate the need for risk assessment and give consideration to safe disposal/management setting.

ISSUES

- Immediate management options for a man who may be acutely disturbed
- Safety considerations: should this man remain in custody or be in hospital?
- Level of security if this man has to be transferred to hospital.

CLARIFY

- In what capacity am I being asked to see him?
- Is it safe to interview the patient at this time?
- Is this man fit to be interviewed?
- Have the police interviewed him and were any charges brought against him?
- Who else is involved: for example, GP, forensic medical examiner, social worker and/or probation officer? Are they available for a joint assessment?
- Has there been previous psychiatric contact? What is his forensic history and what are the details of his next of kin?

SEEK MORE INFORMATION

OFFICER IN CHARGE OF CASE

- Details of the offence, witness statement, details of the police interview, if already held, and charges brought against the patient.

CUSTODY OFFICER OR SERGEANT

- Unusual, strange, bizarre, aggressive or self-mutilating behaviour
- His interactions, communication and responses to officers.

CUSTODY RECORD

- Interaction, appetite and sleep since remand in custody.

FORENSIC MEDICAL EXAMINER

- Under the influence of drugs or alcohol? Breathalyser or drug screen, and results
- Findings on physical examination
- Patient's recollection of events and how reliable it is

- Perceived level of intelligence
- Any indication of mental subnormality or mental illness; if present, was an appropriate adult asked to attend prior to the police interview?

SOCIAL WORKER/PROBATION OFFICER

- Detailed family background, history of offending and past convictions.

RELATIVES

- Observed changes in mental state in the days leading up to the incident
- Any life events or changes in social circumstances.

GP

- Medical and psychiatric history, including that of epilepsy, head injury, paranoid psychotic illness or depression
- Last appointment with the patient
- Current medications.

PSYCHIATRIC SERVICES

- Details of psychiatric history, including history of violence
- Any relationship between the attack and aspects of the patient's mental state when unwell
- Current medications
- Key worker or care coordinator.

PATIENT

- Sensitive and empathic questioning on details of the incident
- Mental illness: suggested by control override phenomenon/symptoms, paranoid and persecutory delusions and the link to the alleged attack. Poor compliance, engagement with the services and the presence of a poorly controlled mental disorder
- Learning difficulties: special schooling, reading or writing difficulties, and extra tuition
- Substance and alcohol misuse: alcohol and drug history, use of alcohol or drugs before or around the time of the incident

- Presence of life events, pre-existing vulnerabilities such as disorganized or abusive childhood, irritability, impulsivity, and social and other personal factors (poor social network, lack of education and work skills, recent life events, poverty and homelessness)
- Mental state at present and at the time of the alleged incident; thoughts of self-harm or suicide
- Victim awareness: did he know the victims or are they complete strangers?
- Fitness to plead: legal criteria ('Pritchard criteria') that apply at the time of trial.

DIFFERENTIAL DIAGNOSIS/DIFFICULTIES

- *Functional.* Paranoid psychotic illness such as schizophrenia or schizoaffective disorder, severe depression with psychotic symptoms, mania and acute stress reaction; also culture-bound syndromes like Amok, found in South-east Asia and characterized by a depressive withdrawal state followed by indiscriminate murderous frenzy (not top of the list for candidates in Europe)
- *Organic.* Alcohol and drug intoxication or withdrawal state; organic brain disease, temporal lobe epilepsy, head trauma, brain infections (viral encephalitis, AIDS, tuberculosis, fungal meningitis), cerebrovascular disease, tumours and post-hypoglycaemic state with brain damage; learning disability; other medical diseases that may cause a severe acute confusional state, such as hepatic and renal diseases, electrolyte imbalance, hypoxia, vitamin deficiency (B_{12}, folate, thiamine), systemic infections, systemic lupus erythematosus, Cushing's disease, hyperthyroidism
- *Personality difficulties.* Antisocial personality disorder
- *Malingering.* Person feigning illness (ICD–10, Z 76.5)
- *Intermittent explosive disorder (classified under DSM–IV).* An impulse control disorder manifested by several discrete episodes of loss of control over aggressive impulses, resulting in serious assaultative acts or destruction of property. Not everybody accepts the existence of this 'disorder', which was previously called 'episodic dyscontrol syndrome'.

APPROACH TO TREATMENT

- Liaise with the forensic medical officer to ensure there are no obvious medical problems that need immediate attention.

- Decide on the man's fitness to be interviewed, if not already interviewed by the police.
- Decide whether he is mentally ill or not, the need for treatment and the setting for such treatment.

WHAT TREATMENT/ADVICE

See Table 8.1.
- Carry out a comprehensive risk assessment.
- Consider the need for immediate or rapid tranquillization.
- Advise on the need to implement hospital diversion if necessary.
- Carry out detailed biological, psychological and social investigations following admission to hospital.
- Consider the need for a detailed psychometric assessment if there are concerns about the possibility of a learning disability.

Table 8.1 Management of violent patients

	Biological	Psychological	Social
Immediate	Comprehensive review of available information Physical investigations: bloods, urine for drugs CT scan, EEG Consider medium secure unit	IQ assessment Nursing assessment	Social investigation
Short-term	Psychotropic medication	CBT	
Long-term	Relapse prevention	Hare's Psychopathic Checklist – Revised (PCL–R) or Historical/ Clinical/Risk Management 20-Item Scale (HCR-20) violence risk assessment scheme	

- Carry out an assessment of the man's personality. Any indication of submissiveness, compliance with authority figures and dependence on others may point towards suggestibility. This would raise the possibility of someone who might be unreliable.
- Include a broad range of biopsychosocial interventions in your treatment plan, including psychotropic medications and psychotherapy as deemed necessary.
- Decide whether the man is fit to plead, bearing in mind his understanding of the nature of the charges brought or about to be brought against him, whether he can instruct counsel, whether he will be able to follow the proceedings in court and whether he will be able to challenge a juror.

FULL ANSWER

This is clearly an emergency in several respects, as someone has been killed and another person seriously injured by a man who appears to be suffering from a psychiatric disorder, given that he is talking to himself and behaving strangely. I would clarify in what capacity I am being asked to see the patient and also ask the forensic medical examiner (FME) if it is safe to interview him at this time. The main issues in this case would be, first, to carry out a detailed psychiatric assessment with a view to ascertaining whether this man has an underlying mental disorder that has contributed to his dangerous and very aggressive behaviour. The second issue is to gain an understanding of his mental state at the time of the incident and decide on the immediate management options if he is acutely disturbed, aroused or aggressive. The other issue is to determine if it is safe for this man to remain in custody or whether he should be transferred to hospital with the appropriate level of security. This would be followed by a detailed assessment to clarify the diagnosis so as to offer appropriate treatment and advice. If the police have not formally interviewed him, there might be a need to assess whether he is fit to be interviewed. It is possible that he is suffering from a form of learning disability, in which case it would be necessary for an appropriate adult to be summoned. Acute psychosis and intoxication with alcohol or drugs at the time of offence and the aftereffects during interview could mean he is unable to appreciate the significance of the questions put to him and the presence of mania might affect his fitness to be interviewed. I would ask if the police have interviewed him or brought any charges against him, and would find out if the GP, FME, social workers and probation officers are going to be involved in the assessment. I would also notify the duty consultant psychiatrist or the duty responsible medical officer.

I would clarify from the arresting officer whether he or she is aware of any previous psychiatric or forensic history and the details of the man's next of kin. I would seek more information about him, if possible before seeing him at the police station. I would ask the arresting officer for details of his offence, the witness statement, details of the police interview and the charges brought against him. I would look into the record of his behaviour since he has been in police custody and also talk to the FME about what he or she found on initial assessment. I would ask the custody officer if there has been any unusual, strange, bizarre, aggressive or self-mutilating behaviour. His interactions, communication and responses since he has been in custody would also be important. I would ask if there is any evidence of drug or alcohol misuse, or any significant findings on the physical examination to suggest medical problems like epilepsy or diabetes. I would ask about the results of alcohol and drug testing, if they have been carried out. Also prior to seeing this man, I would make an effort to speak to his social worker or probation officer (if he is known to these services) about details of his contact, offending history and past convictions. I would talk to his relatives to find out if they saw any changes in his mental state in the days leading to the above incident. When I talked to his GP, I would ask about this man's medical history, especially that of epilepsy or head injury, and would ask if he is currently on any medication. I would also enquire about any history of psychiatric illness, such as paranoid psychotic illness or depression. If he has a history of contact with the local mental health services, I would speak to the key workers and ask about any history of violence and symptoms suggestive of paranoia, persecutory delusions, delusion of control, passivity phenomena and hallucinations (command hallucinations would be very important).

I would arrange to see this man, with the key worker if time permitted or preferably with a forensic psychiatric nurse or another member of the multidisciplinary team. I would bear in mind the need to develop a comprehensive picture of what actually happened, with attention paid to antecedent, behaviour and consequences. I would ask him if he is aware of the fatality and the injuries he has caused and if he thought the victims deserved it. I would find out if he knew the victims or whether they are complete strangers. I would assess whether there is any element of psychosis and would pay particular attention to the presence of a poorly controlled mental disorder with active symptoms, especially delusions of control, passivity phenomena, and paranoid or persecutory delusions.

I would also ask if there is a history of poor compliance with treatment, poor engagement with services, or substance misuse. I would also look for evidence of a depressive illness and thoughts, ideas, plans and intention of self-harm or suicide. I would enquire about pre-existing vulnerabilities such as a disorganized or abusive childhood, irritability, impulsivity and poor anger control, disordered personality, and social and interpersonal factors such as poor social network, lack of education and work skills, poverty, homelessness and past life events. I would want to exclude the possibility of learning difficulties and ask about special schooling, reading or writing difficulties, extra tuition and general under-achievement. I would take a detailed account of his family and personal history, and of significant recent life events and circumstances such as separation, divorce, bereavement and unemployment.

Having taken the above history, I would bear in mind that his presentation could be due to an organic or a functional psychiatric illness. The important differential diagnoses are a paranoid psychotic illness, schizophrenic illness, severe depression with psychotic symptoms, manic state and acute intoxication, malingering and dissocial or antisocial personality disorder. Other differential diagnoses are rare in this context but not irrelevant. They include severe acute stress reaction, learning disability, intermittent explosive disorder, and culture-bound syndromes like Amok. The possible organic causes include organic brain disorders such as temporal lobe epilepsy, brain tumour, head trauma, brain infections (viral encephalitis, AIDS, tuberculosis, fungal meningitis), cerebrovascular disease and post-hypoglycaemic state. Other medical problems that may cause a severe acute confusional state, such as hepatic and renal diseases, electrolyte imbalance, hypoxia and vitamin deficiency (B_{12}, folate and thiamine), systemic infections, systemic lupus erythematosus, Cushing's disease and hyperthyroidism would be excluded. *(Note: it is not necessary to mention all these during a PMP session.)*

The outcome of my interview with this man would inform my decision on whether he is mentally ill or not, and the need to divert from custody for further assessment and treatment in an appropriate setting. If necessary, I would suggest urgent treatment to calm him down at the police station. My approach following this would be to carry out a comprehensive risk assessment. If this man is suffering from a psychiatric illness, I would advise a psychiatric disposal to hospital to enable us to carry out further assessment and to arrange any relevant investigations such as EEG, CT scan or MRI and blood tests if there were indications of an organic problem. I would consider the need for a detailed psychometric assessment if there were a possibility of learning disability. The admission would also give us the opportunity to assess his personality to look for any longstanding tendencies to be aggressive to others. As this man could have been charged for the offences, there might be a need to assess his fitness to plead, bearing in mind the relevant legal criteria. I would examine whether this man understands the nature of the charge(s) brought or about to be brought against him, if he understands the difference between a plea of guilty and a plea of not guilty, and if he could instruct counsel. I would also assess whether the man can follow and understand evidence in court and if he is able to challenge a juror whom he might object to.

His treatment would include a broad range of biopsychosocial interventions, including psychotropic medication (antipsychotics and antidepressants) and psychotherapy. Once he had been treated and prior to discharge from the hospital, I would carry out a comprehensive risk assessment, and I would consider using instruments such as the Violence Risk Assessment Tool, which aims to assess the risk of further violence after discharge from the hospital. There would also be a need to do relapse prevention work and victim awareness before discharging him to the community.

ANSWERS TO SUGGESTED PROBES

1. Fitness to be interviewed is based on clinical and not legal criteria and can usually be determined by a sound clinical judgment. This has already been covered in the PMP plan.
2. Fitness to plead involves legal criteria (which are covered in the PMP plan). The defendant must be able to:
   - understand the charge
   - understand the difference between a plea of guilty and a plea of not guilty
   - instruct counsel
   - follow the evidence in court ('understand the evidence')
   - challenge a juror to whom he might object.
3. In assessing the risk of reoffending in this man, I would give consideration to three major factors based on the HCR–20 scheme.
   - *Historical factors.* These include a history of violence (of the escalating pattern, in particular), young age at first violent incident, relationship instability, employment problems, comorbid substance misuse, early maladjustment, personality disorder and psychopathy. These factors, i.e. characteristics, traits and tendencies, reflect the kind of person he is, and psychopathy is closely related to violence. The cluster of traits from the

Hare's Psychopathy Checklist includes lack of anger, guilt and empathy; impulsivity; forcefulness; tendency to violate social norms; sensation-seeking; and dominance. There may be a history of a major mental illness.

- *Clinical factors.* These include active symptoms of major mental illness, such as the presence of irritable mood or disinhibition in the context of a mood disorder, delusions and hallucinations, control override symptoms and impulsivity. Records show negative attitudes, including poor compliance with treatment, both medication and attendance at clinics or day centres. The patient shows a poor response to treatment and lack of insight.
- *Risk management and contextual factors.* These include a plan that lacks feasibility, lack of personal support, exposure to destabilizers, increased stress levels and non-compliance with remediation attempts.

BUZZ WORDS AND USEFUL TERMINOLOGY

Witness statement, forensic medical examiner, probation service, fitness to plead or to be interviewed, diversion scheme, diminished responsibility, comprehensive risk assessment.

REFERENCES AND SUGGESTED READING

Gray N S, Hill C, McGleish A et al 2003 Prediction of violence and self-harm in mentally disordered offenders: a prospective study of the efficacy of HCR—20, PCL—R, and psychiatric symptomatology. Journal of Consulting and Clinical Psychology 71(3):443–451

Rix K J B 1998 Fit to be interviewed by the police. In: Lee A (ed) Recent Topics from Advances in Psychiatric Treatment, vol. 1. Gaskell, London, pp 123–129

Bluglass R 1998 Preparing medico-legal reports. In: Lee A (ed) Recent Topics from Advances in Psychiatric Treatment. vol. 1. Gaskell, London, pp 130–135

Stone J H, Roberts M, O'Grady J, Taylor A V, O'Shea K 2000 Dangerousness, risk assessment and risk management. In: Stone J H, Roberts M, O'Grady J, Taylor A V, O'Shea K (eds) Faulk's Basic Forensic Psychiatry, 3rd edn. Blackwell Scientific Publications, London, pp 257–271

8.2 MAN REMANDED IN CUSTODY FOLLOWING VIOLENT ATTACK ON WIFE'S NEW PARTNER

A solicitor has asked you to see a 38-year-old man, who is currently remanded in custody. Six months ago he separated from his wife, who could no longer cope with his constant accusations of infidelity and alleged violence against her. He came back to his former home one afternoon in an intoxicated state and met his wife's new partner. A struggle ensued, during which his wife's partner was severely injured, but his wife escaped without injury. When the police came, he was found crying outside the door.

How would you go about your assessment and recommendation to the court?

SUGGESTED PROBES

1. What are your differential diagnoses?
2. What further information do you need and how would you go about collecting it?
3. What would be your recommendation for treatment, supposing this man is admitted to hospital?

PMP PLAN

TASKS TO DO

The following five areas are relevant to this vignette but are not necessarily all-inclusive. The list is also not exhaustive:

a) Show familiarity with the assessment of a remanded offender in a prison setting.
b) Discuss the need to gather relevant information from a wide variety of sources.
c) Demonstrate knowledge of the differential diagnoses. Mention delusional disorder (alcoholic jealousy, ICD–10, F10.5).
d) Assess fitness to plead.
e) Give specific advice on the various disposal options.

ISSUES

- Determination of relevant underlying factors for the man's behaviour with a view to reaching a working diagnosis
- Assessment of fitness to plead and suggestion of appropriate disposal options.

- Where exactly is the prison located?

SOLICITOR

- Specific written instructions
- Depositions and indictments. What has the offender been charged with?

GP

- History of depression, psychosis, head injury and treatments
- Current treatment.

PSYCHIATRIC OR DRUG AND ALCOHOL TEAM

- History of and treatment for depression and/or psychosis
- History of paranoid and persecutory delusions, command hallucinations and aggression
- History of violence against person and/or property
- Forensic history
- Drug and alcohol history, alcohol dependence, compliance with treatment plans.

PRISON HEALTH WING STAFF

- Observations since client was remanded in prison
- Evidence of distractibility, response to abnormal perceptions, delusions, thought disorder, violence and self-harm
- Inmate medical record (IMR).

PATIENT

- Informing the client of the reason for your visit; warning about confidentiality issues
- History of index offence; alcohol history in light of the possibility of alcoholic jealousy, history of morbid jealousy and use of substances at the time of the index offence
- Relationship between offender and wife; history of domestic violence, anger and rage
- Previous visit(s) to his former home before the time of incident; why he returned there on previous occasions and at the time of incident

- Mental state at the time of the index offence and careful assessment of current mental state: depression, mania, suicidality and/or homicidal thoughts; overvalued ideas, ruminations and anxious preoccupations about his wife having affairs; presence of auditory hallucinations (in particular, command hallucinations), persecutory and referential delusions; personality type—antisocial, asocial or schizoid personality disorder
- Forensic history: reason(s) for attacking his wife's new partner, thoughts after the assault, intention to repeat the action
- Any underage children living at home
- Fitness to plead: understanding of the charge and its implications, understanding and appreciating the importance of entering a plea, ability to instruct counsel, ability to challenge a juror he might object to, ability to follow the course of the trial and understanding the evidence.

DIFFERENTIAL DIAGNOSIS/DIFFICULTIES

- *Functional.* Depression, paranoid schizophrenia, delusional disorder, mania, substance misuse disorder, learning difficulties and/or dual diagnosis with psychiatric illness and morbid jealousy. Morbid jealousy may be due to all of these conditions *(Note: the delusion that an individual partner is unfaithful is categorized under Paragraph 297.1 (Delusional Disorder) of the DSM–IV)*
- *Organic.* Learning disabilities, organic brain damage secondary to alcohol misuse.

APPROACH TO TREATMENT

- Arrange to see the client with a colleague if necessary.
- Determine if he has a mental illness or not.
- Carry out a risk assessment.
- Determine if there is an immediate need to transfer this man to hospital for treatment.
- Advise on the level of risk and observation in prison.
- Identify a bed, if necessary, to divert this man to hospital for treatment.

WHAT TREATMENT/ADVICE

- The court report may carry the recommendation that the patient is fit to plead, fit to stand trial or unfit to plead or stand trial.

- The insanity defence (M'Naghten Rules) could be used, but this is practically confined to murder cases and is rarely used nowadays.
- Choose between hospital disposal, under the relevant mental health law (Sections 35–38 of the Mental Health Act 1983 in England and Wales, with restriction under Section 41 of the MHA 1983), or non-hospital disposal, such as a Community Rehabilitation Order with attached conditions of treatment.

FULL ANSWER

In attending to the solicitor's request that I see this 38-year-old man, I would first ask for a specific letter of instruction. I would ask the solicitor to supply me with a copy of the deposition, indictments and a summary of convictions. I would clarify whether the solicitor only wanted me to specify a diagnosis of mental illness in this man, to comment on his mental state at the time of the offence, or to assess his fitness to plead, with a view to producing a full psychiatric report for the court. The solicitor could also be requesting my opinion on the appropriate disposal options to be suggested to the court. I would ask the solicitor what offence the man has been charged with, how long he was remanded in custody, and how far the court case has proceeded. I would ask the local probation office, if the man was known to the service, for reports of past convictions, probation orders and the extent of his cooperation with probation services.

Before going on to assess this man, I would seek relevant information to help me form an opinion as to what is wrong with him so that I could advise on the appropriate disposal options and/or assist the court in its proceedings. I would ask this man's GP about his or her knowledge of any past psychiatric history, treatment for depression or psychosis, head injury, epilepsy and learning difficulties. I would find out why any current medication had been prescribed, and the patient's compliance with treatment. If this man was known to the local psychiatric or drug and alcohol team, I would ask them about their knowledge of him, his history of admissions and treatment for depression and/or psychosis. I would find out if his previous presentations were characterized by paranoia, persecutory delusions, command hallucinations and aggression. I would enquire about any history of interpersonal violence, especially marital violence, violence in previous relationships (including domestic violence) and destruction of property. I would ask if any previous episodes of violence have led to criminal charges or convictions in the past. I would ask about his forensic history and if there were any pending court cases before the present incident. I would ask those who know him about his drug and alcohol history, the possibility of alcohol dependence, previous and current treatment, and his compliance with treatment plans.

Once I had this background information, I would then proceed to assess the man. I would ask the prison's health wing staff if they have observed any abnormal movements or behaviour, such as evidence of distractibility, responses to abnormal perceptions, delusions, thought disorder, unusual preoccupations, severe agitation, restlessness and aggressive behaviour since the man was remanded in custody. I would then request his inmate medical record. When I saw the man, I would inform him of the reason for the visit, who has sent me to see him and why it is important for me to ask him several questions, some of which he may already have been asked in the past. I would warn him that I would not be able to guarantee confidentiality concerning the information he disclosed to me, as the content of the interview might form part of the report that his solicitor might ask me to produce for the court. I would carefully ask him about the relationship between him and his wife before and after they separated. I would ask about his previous and current thoughts about infidelity. I would ask if the couple have underage children living at home. I would elicit any history of domestic violence, and feelings of anger and rage before his wife left him. If I strongly suspected morbid jealousy, I would ask about any history of controlling and checking behaviour, such as checking his wife's underwear for stains, following her for the purpose of observation, opening letters and checking electronic mail or mobile telephone numbers.

I would ask him relevant questions to try to determine as far as possible his mental state at the time of the index offence. I would ask him to give a chronological account of the events preceding the index offence, take a history of the index offence, and examine how much of the incident the inmate can actually recollect. I would ask him if he had visited his former home before the time of incident, the reasons he visited on those occasions, the reason for his visit at the time of incident, and whether he knew his wife's new partner would be there. I would ask him why he attacked this man, if he planned the attack beforehand and if he carried weapons with him on that day. All these questions would help me to assess the degree of pre-planning and premeditation. I would take a drug and alcohol history in light of the possibility of morbid jealousy, and ask him if he used illicit drugs or alcohol on the day of the incident. I would conduct an assessment of his current mental state, focusing particularly on his mood for depression, mania, and suicidal or homicidal thoughts. I would assess for the presence of auditory hallucinations, command hallucinations, persecutory and referential delusions. I would make a brief assessment of his personality type and determine whether he has an antisocial or asocial personality trait. I would examine his insight into the consequences of his actions, whether he thinks the victim deserved what happened to him, or if he feels any remorse. I would assess whether he is fit to plead or stand trial. I would find out whether he understands the nature of the charges against him, the implications of pleading guilty or not guilty, and the consequences of being found guilty. I would also assess whether he is able to instruct a solicitor, follow the course of the trial and understand the evidence, along with his ability to challenge a juror he might object to.

Having asked for other relevant information and taken an extensive history, I would consider a range of functional and organic problems as the cause of this incident. High on my list of differential diagnoses would be paranoid schizophrenia, psychotic depression, mania, delusional disorder leading to a morbid or alcoholic jealousy, drug abuse or dependence, organic brain damage secondary to alcohol misuse, a learning difficulty and antisocial personality, including psychopathic traits.

My approach to treatment in this case would be first to determine whether this man has a mental illness or not, and if there is an immediate need to transfer him to hospital for treatment. I would then carry out a detailed risk assessment, determine the appropriate level of security that would be necessary to treat the man in a hospital setting and give advice on the level of observation, should he remain in prison.

My recommendation to the court would depend on the findings of my assessment of his current mental state and fitness to plead, and might be that the patient is fit to plead, fit to stand trial, or unfit to plead or stand trial. If he has a mental illness and is moderately or severely psychotic and unable to plead, I would recommend a hospital disposal for further assessment and treatment with restrictions under the relevant mental health laws. A hospital disposal, under Sections 35–38 of the Mental Health Act 1983 in England and Wales, with restriction under Section 41 of the Mental Health Act 1983 would apply in this case. A non-hospital disposal, such as a Community Rehabilitation Order with attached conditions of treatment, is also a possibility. These disposal options would be necessary for this man's health, for his safety and for the protection of others. I would therefore refer him to his local medium secure (regional) or high-security (special) hospital for assessment with a view to an admission, if these institutions agreed that an admission to hospital would be appropriate. Admission to hospital would give the treatment team more opportunity to carry out a comprehensive risk assessment, institute appropriate management, identify clear relapse indicators and arrange adequate follow-up and support on discharge.

In the event that the man continued to be remanded in custody or sentenced to serve a prison term, I would advise the prison healthcare department on the need for closer monitoring of his mental state, for treatment with psychotropic medication, and management of the risk of suicide and harm to others.

ANSWERS TO SUGGESTED PROBES

1. Differential diagnoses are covered in the full answer.
2. The further information required and how to collect it is described in the full answer.
3. If this man were admitted to hospital, I would recommend the following treatment:
   - *Nursing and medical.* Nursing observation and monitoring, treatment with antipsychotics and/or antidepressants, treatment of addictive behaviour
   - *Psychological.* Relapse prevention programme, family work, psychosexual issues, victim awareness work, anger management
   - *Psychosocial support.* Identification of appropriate community support, closer monitoring, with the condition that he does not enter his wife's area of residence as part of his treatment plan. This would best be enforced by a restriction order under Section 41 of the Mental Health Act 1983 in England and Wales
   - *Vocational treatments.* To include day care
   - *Post-discharge.* Geographical separation from his wife.

BUZZ WORDS AND USEFUL TERMINOLOGY

Index offence, morbid jealousy, command hallucinations, solicitor's letter of instruction, bundle of indictment, depositions, confidentiality, fitness to plead, defences, diminished responsibility, insanity.

REFERENCES AND SUGGESTED READING

James D 1999 Court diversion at 10 years: can it work, does it work and has it a future? Journal of Forensic Psychiatry 10(3):507–524

Michael A, Mirza S, Mirza K A et al 1995 Morbid jealousy in alcoholism. British Journal of Psychiatry 167(5):668–672

8.3 39-YEAR-OLD FEMALE TRANSFERRED FROM A MEDIUM SECURE (REGIONAL) UNIT

A 39-year-old female patient, whose index offences were arson, has been transferred from the local medium secure unit (MSU, sometimes called regional secure unit (RSU) in the UK) to your rehabilitation unit. Prior to her transfer, she had been attending a catering course at the local college as part of the programme for her rehabilitation. During one of your team discussions, you become aware that the MSU has not disclosed her previous child abduction offence to the college. Team members are concerned about whether to disclose this or not and are seeking your opinion.

What information would assist you in arriving at a decision and what would be your approach to her future care?

SUGGESTED PROBES

1. After discussions with the patient, she objects to disclosure. What would you do?
2. In what situation would you consider breaching confidentiality in regard to this patient?
3. Six months after her admission to your service, you are planning discharge. What factors would you take into consideration?

PMP PLAN

TASKS TO DO

The following five areas are relevant to this vignette but are not necessarily all-inclusive. The list is also not exhaustive:

a) Discuss the main issues of confidentiality, risk and safety.
b) Demonstrate awareness of the need to weigh the disclosure of confidential patient information against the risk of harm to the public.
c) Show an understanding of the systematic evaluation of the patient's current problems, whether they have anything to do with the child abduction offence, and the risk involved.
d) Involve the patient and the multidisciplinary team, seeking appropriate legal advice if necessary.
e) Discuss management of the patient in the event of disclosure.

ISSUES

- Necessity to disclose versus breach of patient confidentiality
- Risk of harm to others, particularly children, if the offences are not disclosed
- Risk of liability if the offence is not disclosed and others are harmed.

CLARIFY

- Are there any immediate risk/safety concerns and does the patient have access to children?
- Is there any relationship between her current difficulties and previous child abduction offence?

SEEK MORE INFORMATION

TRANSFER DOCUMENTS

- Details of index offences and outcomes
- Psychiatric history, treatment history and management plans, pre-admission assessment, care plan and Care Programme Approach (CPA) documents.

REFERRING TEAM

- Reason for non-disclosure of the previous child abduction offence
- Issues of concern, including those relating to employment, that need closer monitoring
- Relapse indicators.

REHABILITATION STAFF

- Activity on the ward, attendance at other programmes
- Mental state of the patient, use of alcohol and drugs
- Any perceived risk to children or others. Do they think the disclosure of child abduction is necessary and would disclosure threaten her continuation on the course?

PATIENT

- Arson offences and the context in which they happened; what she has learnt about the index offences to date
- Previous offences: reasons for abducting the child and location of the incident, any physical harm involved.

Motivation for abducting the child: anger, revenge, feelings of abandonment, sexual fantasies or secondary to abnormal psychotic experiences, such as paranoid delusions or beliefs that she was the mother or that the child needed to be cared for by her

- Reason why she is doing the present catering course, her plans for work in the future, including the possibility of finding catering jobs in schools
- Has she told the college or others (personal tutor, classmates) in the college about the index offences and previous child abduction offence? Reasons for objecting to disclosure; her concerns.

COLLEGE

- Patient's presentation at the college, interaction with others
- Any concern of tutors and other students.

DIFFERENTIAL DIAGNOSIS/DIFFICULTIES

Note: the arson and previous offence might be due to one of many possible causes, but candidates should be aware of the differential diagnoses. You do not necessarily have to mention them in your response to the PMP but they may come up during probing by examiners.

- *Functional illness and personality disorder.* Paranoid schizophrenia, schizoaffective disorder, delusional disorder, mania, bipolar affective disorder, depression, antisocial and borderline personality disorder
- *Organic.* Learning disability, organic brain damage.

APPROACH TO TREATMENT

- Seek the opinion of other colleagues; seek legal advice (from the Caldicott Guardian in the UK: a medical doctor, usually very senior and experienced, who is appointed by a hospital or health trust and given the responsibility of overseeing the protection and use of patient information. This clinician, who is in charge of information governance, advises individuals working in the organization, the ethics committee and departments on issues relating to patient confidentiality and disclosure of patient information).
- Seek the advice of the local medical defence organization and licensing body.
- Seek the consent of the patient.
- Carry out a full risk assessment.

Tailor your advice to the nature and level of risk posed by the patient.

DISCLOSE

- If the pertinent risk outweighs patient confidentiality
- If the patient agrees to the disclosure
- If the risk of danger to the public is imminent
- If the risk of harm to others is sufficiently specified
- If disclosure would be an exceptional means of averting danger.

DO NOT DISCLOSE

- If there is no pertinent risk
- If the patient disagrees with disclosure.

RISK MANAGEMENT

- Consider access to children.
- Ensure adequate treatment and supervised employment.

FULL ANSWER

I would consider several main issues before I gave my opinion on this scenario. There is, on the one hand, the issue of whether it is necessary at this time to disclose information about this woman's previous child abduction offence, and on the other, the issue of patient confidentiality. There is also the issue of risk to the public, particularly children. I would bear in mind the need to approach this case with extreme caution and sensitivity, and would seek more information and appropriate advice before giving a definite opinion.

To begin with, I would like to clarify with staff whether they have any concerns about immediate risk and/or safety issues. I would ask whether they anticipate any particular problems and if this patient has access to children at the present time. I would clarify whether they know why the local medium secure unit failed to disclose the child abduction offence to the college and if they thought that it was unnecessary. I would also ask about the patient's diagnosis, current mental state, and current compliance with medication and other treatment plans.

I would seek more information on this patient by looking through the pre-admission assessment records, discharge risk assessment documents, transfer and discharge documents, care plans and the Care Programme Approach (CPA, in England and Wales) documents. I would also speak to relevant members of the referring team, her probation officer and social worker, our rehabilitation staff, the patient herself and the college authority, if that became necessary at any point. I would also be interested in the details of the child abduction offence, the relation of the offence to her mental state at the time, and whether the abduction occurred while the patient was psychotically ill or depressed. I would clarify whether the abductee was a stranger to her or not. I would investigate her compliance to medication and other treatments at the time of the child abduction. I would ask the referring team why the offence was not disclosed to the college. I would ask them about this lady's relapse indicators and if they have any particular concerns relating to employment that need closer monitoring. I would ask staff about her participation in activities on the ward, attendance at other programmes, use of alcohol and drugs and her current mental state. I would speak to other staff (such as the team psychologist and social worker) presently involved in her care about her progress since being admitted to our unit. I would review her previous and current treatment and monitor her response so far.

I would interview this patient to hear her account of the offences and to ascertain her level of insight, in particular in relation to the victims, and to empathy and remorse. I would examine the arson offences that led to the present admission and check whether there is any relationship with a psychotic illness, severe depression, boredom or a personality disorder. I would find out why she abducted the child (victim), where the offence took place and if any of the factors I have already mentioned could have been involved. I would carefully assess her motivation for abducting the child and whether this was connected with anger, revenge, feelings of abandonment or sexual fantasies, or was purely secondary to abnormal psychotic experiences such as paranoid delusions or command hallucinations. I would also ask whether the patient believed that she was the child's mother or that the child needed to be cared for by her, and would find out if the child came to any physical harm during the abduction. I would ask about the outcome and whether she was convicted of the offence, served a prison sentence or was diverted and sentenced to hospital under the relevant mental health legislation (Mental Health Act 1983 in England and Wales). I would find out why she chose the present catering course, her plans for work in the future, and if she has plans to work with children on completing her course: for example, as a caterer or school dinner lady where she would have access to children. I would ask if she has told the college or others (personal tutor or classmates) in the college about the index offences or the child abduction offence. I would ask if she thinks a disclosure would threaten her continuation on the course. I would ask her if she has unsupervised access to children at the moment and if so, the context of that contact and whether she thinks she is a risk to children. I would find out if she is in any relationship at present and if she has plans to have children in the future.

Armed with this information, I would call a meeting to seek the opinions of members of the multidisciplinary team. I would carry out a formal risk assessment, bearing in mind the possibility of an underlying mental illness. The possible differential diagnoses would include functional illnesses such as paranoid schizophrenia, schizoaffective disorder, delusional disorder, mania, bipolar affective disorder and psychotic depression, organic problems such as learning disability and organic brain damage, and antisocial and borderline personality disorders. I would focus on the risks that this woman poses to others, at present and in the future, particularly to children and other vulnerable people. Her current mental state, and factors such as compliance with treatment plans, illicit drug use, circumstantial stressors, opportunities for vocational activities and the availability of support, would play a crucial part in determining the level of current and future risk. In giving an opinion, my approach would be to consider all the relevant information and, because of the complexity of the case, to seek further advice from senior colleagues, and legal advice from the hospital legal department and the local medical defence organization. The advice of the local medical registration or licensing body (General Medical Council or GMC in the UK, Irish Council in Ireland) and the hospital's 'Caldicott Guardian' (in the UK) would also be invaluable.

If this woman were stable and compliant with medication, my advice would be not to disclose the child abduction offence to the college at present, particularly if her current presentation had little or nothing to do with the previous offence. If, however, she had potential access to children and there was any suggestion that she had been behaving in a way that might put children or others at risk, I would make her aware of our concerns and the reasons why we might want to disclose her previous offence to the college. As far as possible I would seek the consent of the patient and make her aware of what information needed to be disclosed, to whom that information would be disclosed, and how it might possibly be used. In a situation where she was mentally unwell or not complying fully with treatment plans, and already had access to children or had plans to have such access, there would be a strong argument for breaching confidentiality and disclosing the offence to the college. I would apply the GMC test, which suggests that breach of confidentiality may be justified if there is a 'grave risk of death or serious harm to others'. The decision to breach confidentiality would only be taken if the risk were imminent and sufficiently specified, and if it were exceptionally appropriate to avert danger. If a decision were made to breach confidentiality, this would be strictly on a need-to-know basis.

I would give advice on how to manage the risk this patient poses, particularly if there were any suggestion that she was becoming unwell again. While the patient might find it difficult to accept, I would advise her to postpone attending college until she was well and the risks were considered to be low and manageable. I would then institute the appropriate medical and psychological treatment, including treatment for substance misuse. I would advise that she be discharged from hospital under an enhanced CPA to enable much closer monitoring and support. If she had her own children, I would find out who normally takes care of them, what kind of access she has, and the kind of support she would receive to help her care for them when she left the unit. I would also refer her to the appropriate local social services to give support and care after discharge. I would consider referring her to the local Multi-Agency Public Protection team (MAPP in England and Wales) if I considered that she posed a danger to members of the public, given her previous and index offences.

ANSWERS TO SUGGESTED PROBES

1. If, after discussion with the patient, she objected to disclosure, I would:
   - Inform her that further information would be sought, along with professional and legal opinions.
   - Warn her that confidentiality would be breached if there were overriding safety issues.
   - Review the risk assessment to make sure all aspects of risk had been covered.
   - Seek a forensic opinion.
   - Seek legal advice as above.
   - Make a decision to breach confidentiality or not, guided by the risk assessment and legal opinion.
   - Accept the patient's wishes if there were no overriding risk to members of the public.

2. I would consider breaching confidentiality:
   - if the risk of danger to the public were imminent
   - if the risk of harm to others were sufficiently specified
   - if disclosure would be an exceptional means of averting danger
   - if the patient gave her consent.
3. I would consider the following factors in my discharge planning:
   - *Progress of the disorder.* The degree of control and stability in the patient's mental state; her response to other modalities of treatment apart from medication; whether she has insight into her illness and treatment; the presence of other conditions that might affect progress, e.g. substance and alcohol misuse disorder, learning disabilities, organic brain disorder, personality disorder and/or sexual disorder; and whether everybody involved in her care is aware of the relapse indicators and contingency plans
   - *After-discharge arrangements.* Specific accommodation arrangements; follow-up under a restriction order or absolute discharge; the patient's ability to cooperate with the various staff who would be involved in her after-care, e.g. community responsible medical officer, social workers, support workers, housing officers and landlords; availability of staff and facilities to ensure safe monitoring and follow-up
   - *Issues with victims.* Severity of the offence and/or violence; whether the patient understands the impact of previous violence on her victim; the present location of the victim; the views and feelings of the previous victim, relatives or neighbours
   - *Social skills and factors.* Whether the patient would be able to live with others independently or in a supported environment; availability of vocational activities.

BUZZ WORDS AND USEFUL TERMINOLOGY

Pre-admission assessment, index offence, relapse indicators, 'Caldicott Guardian', Tarasoff's rule, breach of confidentiality, 'need-to-know basis', Human Rights Act 1998, right to privacy.

REFERENCES AND SUGGESTED READING

Applebaum P S 1985 Tarasoff and the clinician: problems in fulfilling the duty to protect. American Journal of Psychiatry 142:425–429

Gates J J, Arons B S 1999 Privacy and Confidentiality in Mental Health Care. Paul H. Brookes, Baltimore

General Medical Council 2000 Confidentiality: Protecting and Providing Information. General Medical Council, London

Roch-Berry C 2003 What is a Caldicott guardian? Postgraduate Medical Journal 79:516–518

Shaw J 2000 Assessing the risk of violence in patients. British Medical Journal 320:1088–1089

8.4 MENTALLY DISORDERED OFFENDER WHO INDECENTLY ASSAULTED SCHOOLGIRLS

You have been asked to see a 42-year-old man in a local prison. He is awaiting sentencing for a series of indecent assaults and a rape incident against schoolchildren, which took place over the past year. He has been noticed to be talking to himself and behaving strangely whilst in prison. You have been asked to review him so as to advise on his short-term and long-term management and to prepare a report for the court.

How would you proceed with the above request?

SUGGESTED PROBES

1. What do you know about the sexual offenders treatment programme?
2. What factors would increase the risk of recidivism in this patient?
3. What do you understand by 'cycle of offending' and the essential components of cognitive behavioural therapy in the treatment of sexual offending?

PMP PLAN

TASKS TO DO

The following five areas are relevant to this vignette but are not necessarily all-inclusive. The list is also not exhaustive:

a) Appreciate the need to exclude an underlying mental illness, to determine the motivation for this man's behaviour and to understand that this man might be feigning mental illness in light of the impending conviction.
b) Appreciate the need to gather as much information as possible and to demonstrate an understanding of the criminal justice system as it relates to offenders.
c) Discuss the multidisciplinary assessment and management of this sexual offender patient.
d) Demonstrate an understanding of one type of treatment method for a sexual offender.
e) Demonstrate knowledge of other biopsychosocial interventions in the management of this patient.

ISSUES

- Risk of sexual assault against schoolchildren and issues of public safety and protection at large
- Diagnosis of mental illness and suggestion of treatment strategies
- Advising the court on the appropriate psychiatric disposal, treatability and future risk.

CLARIFY

- In what capacity have I been asked to see him?
- Are there specific questions to be asked?
- What was the onset and duration of the observed behaviour? Was it before or after the court appearance?
- Is there any previous psychiatric history and is the man on any medication at present?
- Is he in the main prison, the hospital wing or a Vulnerable Prisoner's Unit?
- Are there any concerns over self-harm behaviour and risk of harm to others?
- What is the name of his probation officer or local consultant, if he is known to the probation or mental health services?

SEEK MORE INFORMATION

PRISON MEDICAL OFFICER

- Observed behaviour, other evidence of psychosis, such as hallucinations and delusions
- Current treatment and response.

PROBATION OFFICER

- History of repeated sexual offences, which suggests the possibility of similar behaviour in the past. Information from the probation officer would shed light on past sexual and related offences.

GP

- Previous psychiatric and medical history, including treatment details
- Family and other background history.

PSYCHIATRIC SERVICES

- Psychiatric diagnosis, treatment and follow-up plan
- Community key worker and when the man last saw him/her.

PATIENT

- Details of index offence, onset of offending behaviour, relationship to any of the victims. Involvement of others. Acting alone or part of an organized paedophile ring? Duration of behaviour, degree of force, violence or coercion used. Past history of sexually abusive/assaultative behaviour. Presence of inappropriate sexual fantasy and the use of pornography including the Internet (whether adult or children). Evidence of learning difficulties. Grooming of victims, level of planning and preparation. Previous violent or sexual offences, such as exhibitionism
- Personal history of sexual, physical and emotional abuse. Detailed psychosexual and developmental history. Sexual orientation: homo-/hetero-/bisexual, level of adult sexual functioning, capacity for intimacy, capacity to engage and maintain appropriate inter-adult relationships, psychosexual knowledge, view of his sexual orientation and offences; egosyntonic or egodystonic, level of fulfilment from adult relationships, and presence of sadomasochistic tendencies
- Assessment of premorbid personality (preferably by talking to a reliable relative), social skills and ability to express anger appropriately. Presence of antisocial personality trait. Forensic history and other non-sexual related offences and convictions. Use of illicit drugs and alcohol. Presence of psychiatric symptoms, either now or in the past, in particular schizophrenia and affective psychosis. Distorted cognition about child sexuality and consent to sexual activities. Exclusion of cerebral organic diseases, such as epilepsy and frontal lobe disorder due to various causes.

The above assessment will help to develop a picture of the internal world of this man, identify possible motivating factors for his behaviour, and develop a behavioural analysis of antecedents, behaviour and consequences, and also possibly the cycle of his offending. The latter is well represented in Wolf's cycle of offending, as depicted in Figure 8.1. There is a need to bear in mind that this man may not volunteer all the above information in one session. It may take two or more sessions, along with collaborative work with other agencies and professionals such as the psychologist, forensic social workers, probation officers and

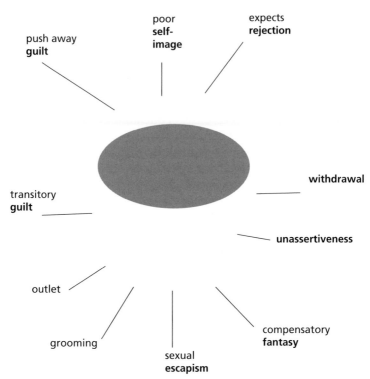

Fig. 8.1 Wolf's cycle of sexual offending.

forensic community psychiatric nurses, if he has had past involvement with the mental health services.

RISK ASSESSMENT

- Assessment of risk of reoffending, focusing on variables in this man and victims. The presence of these variables would increase the risk of reoffending (see Box 8.1).

DIFFERENTIAL DIAGNOSIS/DIFFICULTIES

- Paedophilia of unknown aetiology
- Paedophilia secondary to pathology such as schizophrenia, affective psychosis and organic cerebral disease
- Substance misuse also a potential contributory factor
- Adjustment disorder ('prison reaction') might account for his acute behaviour in prison.

Box 8.1 Assessment of the risk of reoffending

Offender variable	Victim variable
History of two or more sexual offences	Offending against both sexes
History of serious sexual offence	Offending against pre- and post-pubertal girls or boys
Unstable early attachment	Intra- and extra-familial abuse
Lack of intimate adult relationship	
Substance misuse problem	
Sexual deviancy	
Personality disorder	
Denial of problem	
Abnormal emotional attachment	
Cognitive distortion	
Factors identified by the Sexual Offenders Treatment Programme (SOTP) as indicative of high risk:	
Higher level of social inadequacy	
A greater lack of empathy for the victims	
Distorted thinking	
Higher level of sexual obsession	
Abnormal emotional congruence	

APPROACH TO TREATMENT

- Review the available information.
- Liaise with the multidisciplinary team as far as possible.
- Carry out a detailed risk assessment.
- Arrange necessary investigations, such as psychometric testing and a CT scan if there is any evidence of an organic cerebral condition.
- Consider penile plethysmography to measure the man's level of sexual arousal when subjected to visual and/or auditory depictions of sexual and violent acts. (One of the drawbacks of this investigative technique is that it has been criticized for displaying pornographic materials to sex offenders.)
- Give advice, depending on whether the behaviour is due to mental illness, the treatability of such illness, the availability of an appropriate treatment setting and also the risk of reoffending.

WHAT TREATMENT/ADVICE

ADVICE TO THE COURT

- Advise on sentencing and the setting of any treatment at the discretion of the court.
- Bear in mind that the safety of the public is paramount.
- Advise the court of the need to reconcile public safety with the need to treat this man.

ADVICE ON THE TREATMENT SETTING

- Treatment can either be in the prison, in hospital as an inpatient, or in the community.
- Be guided by the presence or absence of psychiatric illness such as schizophrenia or affective psychosis.
- Gain an impression of the level of risk presented by this man.
- Ascertain the perceived risk of him reoffending, as documented above.
- The presence of severe mental illness and/or these risk issues would suggest the need to manage in a secure environment, such as a psychiatric medium secure unit with expertise in the treatment of sex offenders.
- Arrange treatment under the Sex Offenders Treatment Programme (SOTP) in prison, if there is no evidence of mental illness.

TREATMENT

- Give consideration to a range of biopsychosocial interventions, including cognitive behavioural therapy (CBT) and psychosocial support.
- The essential components of CBT include: understanding the offence cycle, challenging distorted thinking, understanding the harm done to victims, fantasy modification, social skills and anger control, relapse prevention work.
- Consider chemical castration as a last resort.

FULL ANSWER

One of the main issues in this case is the risk that this man poses concerning sexual assault against schoolchildren, public safety and public protection. The other issue is to establish the presence of mental illness, with a view to suggesting appropriate treatment strategies and advising the court on the appropriate psychiatric disposal, treatability and future risk.

To deal with this request, I would want to be sure what capacity I have been asked to see this man in. I would clarify the onset and duration of the observed behaviour. I would ask if he started talking to himself and behaving strangely before or after his court appearance, whether he has a past psychiatric history, and whether he is on any medication at present. I would also like to clarify his present location in the prison: whether he is in the healthcare department, the main prison wing or the Vulnerable Prisoner's Unit. I would find out if there is any specific concern about self-harm, risk of harm to others or risk of harm from others. Before any visit it would also be useful to obtain more background information from his probation officer, GP, local psychiatric consultant or community psychiatric nurse, if he is known to the probation or local psychiatric services respectively. I would speak to the probation officer to obtain further details of past sexual and non-sexual offences. The local psychiatric service would be able to give useful information on his diagnosis, treatment plans, compliance with treatment and the follow-up arrangements. If he has a community key worker, I would ask when he was last seen, and his presentation and mental state at the time.

Next, I would make arrangements to see this man at the prison, with one of my colleagues if possible. Prior to assessing him, I would seek more information from the prison medical officer and the prison's hospital wing staff about any observed behaviour, including evidence of psychosis such as distractibility, response to hallucinations, delusion or thought disorder. I would inform the patient of my proposed visit and ask staff to make available the inmate medical record (IMR). When I saw him, I would ensure that he understood my role and also make him aware of the information I have had access to. I would explain clearly to him that whatever we discuss might be included in the report that has been requested of me by the court, and that I could not guarantee the confidentiality of anything he tells me, as the court might decide to use it as it deemed fit. Next, I would establish the details of his index offences, the onset of his offending behaviour, which he might not see as a problem, any close relationship to any of the victims, and how long this behaviour has been going on. I would try to find out if he is acting alone or is part of an organized paedophile ring, and if he has ever used violence at any time. I would also seek more information on his past sexual offences, the presence of inappropriate sexual fantasies and the use of pornography including the Internet (whether involving adults or children). I would look for distorted cognition about child sexuality and children's consent to sexual activities. I would assess whether he groomed his victims, and the level of planning and preparation of his offences.

I would ask him about any personal history of sexual, physical and emotional abuse and if there is a family history of similar behaviour. I would also enquire about his psychosexual and developmental history. I would ask about his sexual orientation to find out if he is homosexual, heterosexual or bisexual. I would ask about his level of adult sexual functioning, his capacity for intimacy, his capacity to engage and maintain appropriate inter-adult relationships, his psychosexual knowledge, his view of his sexual orientation and offences, whether egosyntonic or egodystonic, his level of fulfilment from adult relationships and the presence of sadomasochistic tendencies. I would assess his level of social skills and his ability to manage anger appropriately. I would look for evidence of premorbid substance abuse and antisocial personality traits, and also exclude the possibility of a learning difficulty.

I would carry out collaborative work and assessments with other professionals, particularly probation officers who have been involved with this man in the past. I would also speak to relevant staff such as the psychologist or forensic social worker, if the local psychiatric team knows this man. This assessment and further information would enable us to develop a picture of his internal world, identify possible motivating factors for his behaviour, and develop a behavioural analysis of antecedents, behaviour and consequences. This information would also help us to build up a picture of the cycle of his offending (as in Wolf's cycle of offending). I would specifically assess the risk of reoffending in this man, focusing on variables in both him and his victims. The presence of a history of two or more sexual offences, a history of a serious sexual offence, an unstable early attachment, abnormal emotional attachment and lack of intimate adult relationships would increase the risk of him reoffending. The presence of substance misuse problems, sexual deviancy, personality disorder, cognitive distortion and denial of the problem would also be a danger. Risk would also be increased if the offending was against both sexes or pre- and post-pubertal girls or boys, and if the abuse was intra- or extra-familial. I would also look out for factors identified by the Sexual Offenders Treatment Programme (SOTP) as indicative of high risk, which include a higher level of social inadequacy, a greater lack of empathy for the victims, distorted thinking, a higher level of sexual obsession, and an abnormal emotional congruence.

Given this man's history of repeated sexual offences against children, he clearly has a problem that may or may not be related to a mental illness. One of the possibilities is that his difficulties are secondary to functional disorders such as schizophrenia, schizoaffective disorder, delusional disorder, hypomania and bipolar affective disorder, or due to an organic cerebral disease or a learning difficulty. Substance misuse is another potential contributory factor and an abnormal personality is also a differential diagnosis. It is likely that this man, who is talking to himself in the prison, is currently suffering from a psychotic illness and possibly experiencing auditory hallucinations. My approach would be to review all the available information and liaise with other professionals who have previously been involved in his care, bearing in mind that he might need to transfer to the prison healthcare unit and also to be treated with antipsychotic medication. The next thing would be to decide whether he can be treated continuously in the prison or should be transferred to hospital for further assessment. I would also carry out a detailed risk assessment, which would inform my advice to the court or the prison medical officer who might have to treat him in prison if he ends up with a custodial sentence. I would therefore advise the court on his diagnosis, the anticipated treatment options and the most appropriate psychiatric disposal and treatment setting, if the court deemed fit not to sentence him to prison. The decision on sentencing options is, of course, entirely a matter for the court. I would also advise on the prognosis of the mental disorder and the risk of reoffending in my report.

Since this man might be suffering from a mental disorder of a nature and degree that naturally would warrant treatment in hospital, I would recommend that the court dispose by way of a hospital order, as under Section 37 of the Mental Health Act 1983 in England and Wales. In addition to this I would suggest an order restricting discharge under Section 41 of the same Act in order to protect members of the public. This man might also be transferred from prison to hospital under the appropriate legal framework (Section 47 of the Mental Health Act in England and Wales). In order to advise on the best setting for treatment, I would take into consideration the presence or absence of psychiatric illness such as schizophrenia or affective psychosis, the level of risk this man poses, and in particular the risk of him reoffending. The presence of severe mental illness and/or these risk factors would suggest the need to manage in a secure environment such as a special hospital or a psychiatric medium secure unit with expertise in the treatment of sex offenders. The other option would be to transfer him to a prison with an SOTP, if there were convincing evidence of mental illness or in the event of the court choosing to impose a custodial sentence. The SOTP is also available through the probation service, should the court decide on a non-custodial sentence.

I would suggest a range of biopsychosocial interventions, which would include the use of antipsychotics and antidepressants if indicated. I would arrange for psychometric testing, and a CT scan and EEG to rule out organic cerebral conditions. I would consider penile plethysmography as part of the overall assessment to measure this man's level of sexual arousal when subjected to visual and/or auditory depictions of sexual and violent acts. I would bear in mind the drawback of this investigative technique, which is the criticism it has received regarding the display of pornographic materials to sex offenders. Once settled, he might be able to engage in other psychological treatment programmes, including cognitive behavioural therapy and other approaches to deal with his difficulties. The essential components of CBT include understanding the offending cycle, challenging distorted thinking, understanding the harm done to victims, fantasy and behaviour modification, social skills and anger control, and relapse prevention work. The alternative to this extended programme would be a group of shorter related treatment groups, which would include anger management, stress management, relationship skills and behavioural therapy. The latter would be administered on an individual basis and would include work on sexual fantasies, deviant sexual arousal and impact of offences on victims.

If this man was sentenced to prison, he might be offered similar treatment. The SOTP is based on CBT and consists of four parts: the core programme, the thinking skills programme, the extended programme and the relapse prevention programme. Relapse prevention is aimed at offenders who have already gone through other components of the SOTP. During the programme, offenders are helped to develop strategies for relapse prevention, which they should be able to practise before their release from prison. The other component of care following discharge either from hospital or from prison is psychosocial support. This would focus on ensuring suitable accommodation, social support and a community key worker and/or supervisor who would be able to monitor progress and relapses.

As a last resort, medical treatment using cyproterone acetate would be considered, should this man continue to pose a considerable risk to children. This would, however, only be administered after careful consideration and extensive deliberations with other colleagues and the patient. This treatment would be offered along with the other modalities I have already described.

Note: candidates should avoid being over-inclusive and should tailor the answer to the vignette posed. For example, in this case there is no need to ask for all the information in the bundle of indictment or assess the man's fitness to plead. He has already been convicted and is only awaiting sentencing. Information contained in the bundle of indictment is, however, useful for risk assessment.

ANSWERS TO SUGGESTED PROBES

1. SOTP is a treatment programme introduced in England and Wales in 1992. It is based on CBT. There is an initial assessment which includes psychometric testing, a clinical interview, and in 5 of the 25 prisons where it was introduced, penile plethysmography. The aim of the initial assessments is to:
   - seek the offender's consent for treatment and participation in the programme
   - exclude offenders who are mentally ill, at risk of self-harm, suffering from a severe paranoid personality disorder, low in intelligence (with an IQ of less than 80), or suffering from organic brain damage. These groups are excluded because they are not thought to benefit from such treatment in prison.

   The treatment consists of four parts:
   - the core programme
   - the thinking skills programme
   - the extended programme
   - the relapse prevention programme.

   The core programme consists of a block of 20 sessions, totalling 80 hours, which is essential for all participants. The aim is to increase the offender's sense of responsibility for the offence and decrease denial, to increase the offender's motivation to avoid reoffending, to increase the degree to which the offender has empathy for the victim, and finally, to help the offender develop skills to avoid reoffending.

   The thinking skills programme aims to increase the offenders' ability to see the consequences of their actions and help them consider alternative strategies in the future. The hope is that the skill developed would help the offender to understand, develop and use the strategies of relapse prevention to prevent reoffending in future.

   The extended programme, on the other hand, is a group of shorter related treatment groups, which currently include anger management, stress management, relationship skills and behavioural therapy. The latter is administered on an individual basis and includes work on sexual fantasies, deviant sexual arousal and victimology.

The relapse prevention programme is aimed at offenders who have already gone through other components of the SOTP. During the programme, offenders are helped to develop strategies for relapse prevention, which they should be able to practise before their release from the prison.

SOTP can have several possible unwanted effects. In some offenders, it increases the risk of offending: for example, by 'normalizing' the behaviour if the offender realizes that other group members hold the same views and cognitions as he or she does. The offender may also realize that others have committed much more serious offences, to which his own compare 'favourably or better'. He may think his behaviour will be accepted and not rejected in his pathological peer group.

2. The factors that would increase the risk of recidivism have already been covered in the full answer.

3. The cycle of offending and the components of CBT in the treatment of sexual offending have already been covered in the full answer.

BUZZ WORDS AND USEFUL TERMINOLOGY

Cycle of offending, deviant sexual arousal, victimology, Sex Offenders Treatment Programme (SOTP), risk of reoffending, recidivism, inmate medical record (IMR) and hospital diversion/disposal.

REFERENCES AND SUGGESTED READING

Canter C, Hughes D, Kirby S 1999 Paedophilia: pathology, criminality, or both? The development of a multivariate model of offence behaviour in child sexual abuse. Journal of Forensic Psychiatry 9(3):532–555

Gordon H, Grubin D 2004 Psychiatric aspects of the assessment and treatment of sex offenders. Advances in Psychiatric Treatment 10:73–80

Grubin D 1997 Predictors of risk in serious sex offenders. British Journal of Psychiatry suppl. 32:7–21

Marshall W L, Anderson D, Fernandez Y M 1999 Cognitive Behavioural Treatment of Sexual Offenders. John Wiley, Chichester

Royal College of Psychiatrists 1994 Council Report CR31: the Treatment of Perpetrators of Child Sexual Abuse. Royal College of Psychiatrists, London

You have been asked to see a 43-year-old divorced man for psychiatric assessment. He was recently arrested for pestering his neighbour, who did not acknowledge his 'love letters', but was later released. He has now started following her and keeps trying to take pictures of her. His GP is worried, as he has a history of domestic violence and breaching court orders. The GP has asked you to see the man and advise on his management.

How would you proceed with assessment and management?

SUGGESTED PROBES

1. What is the most likely diagnosis?
2. What are the factors that point to 'stalking' in this case?
3. What are the main risks to the victim and how would you go about assessing them?

PMP PLAN

TASKS TO DO

The following five areas are relevant to this vignette but are not necessarily all-inclusive. The list is also not exhaustive:

a) Recognize this man's behaviour as stalking and set out to look out for evidence and underlying factors.
b) Appreciate the need to conduct a thorough and comprehensive assessment of this man and also seek witness statements (as reported by the victim or others) from the police if necessary.
c) Demonstrate awareness of the need to exclude an underlying psychiatric diagnosis.
d) Demonstrate awareness of risk involved in this case and also the possible impact on the victim.
e) Demonstrate knowledge of the various ways victims might be stalked and the management of such behaviour.

ISSUES

- Recognition that this man might be suffering from a mental disorder

- The psychological distress that his behaviour is causing the neighbour
- The risk of physical harm to the neighbour, given the man's history of domestic violence and his forensic history.

CLARIFY

- Are there risk issues that need immediate attention, such as self-harm or harm to others?
- Is the man due to appear in court following the recent arrest?
- Where is the patient at the present time?
- Is an informant available?
- Is the GP aware of the recent arrest?

SEEK MORE INFORMATION

GP

- How the case came to the GP's attention
- How soon the patient needs to be seen
- What issues the GP wants you to address
- Information on medical and psychiatric history/GP's views based on past experience with the patient.

POLICE

- Details of the arrest and charges, access to the witness statement and previous police involvement with this man.

PROBATION SERVICE

- History of 'breaking court orders' suggesting the man might be known to the probation service.

PSYCHIATRIC/SOCIAL WORK SERVICES

- Details of past psychiatric contact, if known to the local general adult or forensic psychiatric team
- Any social worker involvement. If so, liaison with his social worker for more information on his background, and psychiatric and forensic history.

FAMILY

- Onset of the problem, any link with the recent divorce. How recent was the divorce?

PATIENT

- Full account and background history of the arrest. The letters he wrote and their contents. His feelings about being ignored by his victim. His cognitive and emotional reaction to the situation; what he plans to do about it. Other means used to communicate with the neighbour, i.e. surveillance, loitering and involvement of a third party. Reasons for constantly sending these letters, despite the lack of response to his previous correspondence. Beliefs regarding his victim and whether she is in love or infatuated with him? Encouragement from the victim. Preoccupation with the victim: is it to the exclusion of other interests or producing serious disruption to his life? Depth of his convictions about his victim, suggestion he might have been misinterpreting her actions and words to maintain his beliefs
- Evidence of depression, psychosis, obsessive-compulsive disorder or substance misuse
- History of psychiatric contact and follow-up arrangements. Any evidence of non-compliance with either medication or follow-up plan
- Current family support, bearing in mind his recent divorce
- Past personal or family history of violent behaviour; if present, its exact nature. If history of violence, has he stalked his victims in the past, and were they known to him or total strangers? Has he had a relationship with his current victim in the past?
- Insight into the present problem and motivation to change.

DETAILED RISK ASSESSMENT

- Essential
- Suicidal or homicidal thoughts and sexual fantasies (excluding homicidal thoughts towards the victim's partner and family)
- History of sexual offences
- Patient's views about his ex-wife and whether she is at risk if he bears a grudge and his attention shifts back to her
- Referral for forensic assessment.

Note: the victim may need help but this is not within your remit, as she has not been referred to you. She may need a referral from her GP to the local psychiatric service if there is evidence of psychiatric illness. Otherwise, she could be referred to a victim support officer, or to a police or victim support organization.

DIFFERENTIAL DIAGNOSIS/DIFFICULTIES

- *Functional.* Erotomanic delusion in the context of longstanding mental illness such as paranoid schizophrenia, schizoaffective disorder, delusional disorders (de Clérambault syndrome), bipolar affective disorder, depression with obsessive-compulsive disorder, antisocial personality disorder, adjustment disorder with disturbance of conduct (ICD–10, paragraph F43.24) or disturbance of emotion and conduct (ICD–10, paragraph F43.25)
- *Organic.* Learning disability, brain damage, frontal lobe abnormality.

APPROACH TO TREATMENT

- Carry out a detailed multidisciplinary review of the patient, including a risk assessment.
- Give a detailed report back to the GP, advising on the presence or absence of any psychiatric illness.
- Assess risk issues in relation to the stalking and to the treatability of any mental illness.

WHAT TREATMENT/ADVICE

OFFENDER/PATIENT

- *Medical.* Treat any underlying mental illness with antipsychotics and/or antidepressants or mood stabilizers. Treat drug addiction.
- *Psychological.* Advise cognitive behavioural therapy (CBT) and programmes to manage denial and minimization and to enhance victim empathy.
- *Social.* Support through the criminal justice system, if the case goes to court. Advise a programme to address social and interpersonal skills. Arrange community supervision and referral to the local Multi-Agency Public Protection panel (MAPP) in England and Wales.
- *Legal.* Advise a warning or caution by the police, which has been found to stop stalking in 50% of cases. There may be a need for a court of law to enforce a restraining order. Note that this sometimes makes matters worse, especially in persistent offenders, as it gives them the attention they want.

- More importantly, the victim needs a lot of support and advice: for example, advice on how to protect personal information, and on the protection of relatives and relevant others who may become secondary targets. Arrange referral to a victim support organization, such as the National Anti-stalking and Harassment Campaign and Support Association or the Suzy Lamplugh Trust in the UK.

FULL ANSWER

One of the main issues in this vignette is the possibility that this man might be suffering from a mental illness. The other issues are the psychological distress that his behaviour is causing the neighbour and the risk of physical harm that might follow his behaviour, given the man's history of domestic violence and breach of court orders.

I would clarify whether there are any risk issues that need prompt attention, and if necessary—for example, if this man has made personal threats to harm his neighbour—inform the police. In advising the GP on the management of this man, I would first like to clarify how the case was brought to his/her attention. It might be that this man was arrested or cautioned, or appeared in court following the recent arrest and has been advised to seek medical help. I would also clarify with the GP where the patient is at the moment and whether he is aware of the referral and is willing to see me. I would ask the GP how soon the man should be seen, whether there are any informants available for collaborative information, the details of other professionals involved in the case, and where to contact them for more information.

I would proceed to seek more information about the man and his behaviour, which might legally constitute harassment against a person. I would contact him for his consent to seek information on him from others, but should he not agree to my request, I would still go ahead because of the risk that he poses to his neighbour. I would proceed on a 'need to know' basis to ensure the safety of a member of the public. I would ask for a detailed police record and also talk to his probation officer, if he has one, which is likely given the history of him 'breaching a court order'. I would find out if he has previously been charged under the local harassment legislation (Protection Against Harassment Act 1997 in England and Wales). The information gleaned from the probation officer, GP and local social services department would hopefully shed more light on his background, past psychiatric contacts and forensic history. If he does have a psychiatric history, I would ask the mental health service that managed him to provide information on his diagnosis, current treatment, relapse indicators, risk assessments, the key staff involved in his care and the follow-up arrangements.

The next thing would be to arrange an outpatient appointment for this man or to invite the GP or one of my colleagues to accompany me on a domiciliary visit. If this man should refuse contact, I would consider an assessment under the relevant mental health legislation (assessment order under Section 2 of the Mental Health Act 1983 in England and Wales). When I saw him, I would ask for his account of the alleged behaviour and the circumstances leading to his arrest. I would ask about the letters he has been writing, the content of those letters, his expectations, and how he felt and reacted when his neighbour did not acknowledge his letters. I would ask him to show me a draft, if he has one at home, in order to gain insight into his motives. I would establish why he has kept sending these letters despite being ignored, and what he plans to do about the situation. I would establish whether he has communicated with this lady by any other means, such as by telephone, e-mail or poster, and if he feels she has responded to him in some way or has encouraged him. I would ask him whether he has been loitering in the hope of seeing the neighbour and if he has involved a third party. I would ask him if he thinks his neighbour is in love with him and how he reached that conclusion. I would ascertain whether his beliefs about her are firm, and if there is any suggestion that he has been misinterpreting his neighbour's actions and words to maintain his beliefs. I would exclude the presence of a command auditory hallucination behind his actions. His behaviour might also have an obsessive component, in that the patient might actually see his behaviour as irrational, with attempts to resist stalking the neighbour leading to anxieties, which he eventually has to relieve by following his neighbour repeatedly. I would ask if he finds himself thinking about her most of the time, if these thoughts arouse him sexually, the extent of such arousal and the actions (such as masturbation) that follow. I would find out how far this behaviour has affected his life and what he would eventually do if he later realizes he cannot earn his neighbour's love.

I would then assess his insight into his behaviour, particularly whether he realizes that his actions could cause alarm and distress, provoke anxiety, terrify and intimidate his neighbour, or cause her to fear for her life. I would find out about any past personal or family history of violent behaviour and explore the situation of domestic violence in the past. I would ask about the nature of such violence, which person the violence was directed against, any injury suffered by the victims, and whether he was arrested or charged for these offences. I would find out if alcohol and substance misuse played a significant role in those and the present offences. I would ask if this man found it difficult to let go when previous relationships ended, if he had scores to settle and if he has stalked his ex-partner. If he has a history of previous stalking, I would ask if the victims were known to him or were total strangers. Information from close family members would also be relevant in finding out the exact nature of the problem and helping develop a good understanding of it.

Next, I would assess whether he sees the present situation as a problem and is motivated to change. A detailed risk assessment would also be undertaken, paying particular attention to any suicidal or homicidal thoughts and sexual fantasies. While stalking is the obvious issue in this case, the underlying problem might be a mental illness. The differential diagnoses would include erotomanic delusion in the context of longstanding illness such as paranoid schizophrenia or other schizophrenia-like illnesses (including schizoaffective disorder), moderate to severe depression with obsessive-compulsive symptoms, bipolar affective disorder or a delusional disorder of erotomanic type (de Clérambault syndrome). It is possible that this man is suffering from an adjustment disorder with disturbance of conduct or disorder of emotion and conduct following his marital breakdown. Other differential diagnoses include an antisocial personality disorder or learning disability and I would also consider the possibility of a frontal lobe abnormality from an organic brain damage. I will look for any evidence to suggest the presence of alcohol and substance misuse. I would find out about his current psychosocial situation, including family support, bearing in mind his recent divorce.

In managing this man, I would first like to exclude any underlying mental illnesses in the ways that I have described, and then consider other possible reasons why he might be behaving this way. It is possible that the behaviour is an attempt to take revenge on his neighbour following her rejection or might simply be an attempt to seek intimacy following the breakdown of his marriage.

In determining treatment, I would consider all the information above, the presence of mental illness or an abnormal personality, and the perceived level of risk. I would involve a multidisciplinary team in my approach when reviewing and carrying out a detailed risk assessment for this man. The direction of intervention in this case would depend on whether he has a mental illness or not. If, following a detailed multidisciplinary assessment, he was found not to be suffering from a mental illness of a nature or degree that precluded him from fully understanding his actions, the matter would be for the police to deal with under the relevant harassment laws. In a situation where it was unclear whether he was suffering from a mental illness or not, I would recommend further assessment either as an outpatient or as an inpatient. I would prefer a period of inpatient assessment if there were indications of an underlying mental illness posing significant risk and safety concerns. An admission would provide an opportunity to monitor his mental state and gather as much information as possible on his family and personal background and psychosocial circumstances. We would also have the opportunity to carry out laboratory investigations such as TFTs, a CT scan or MRI, an EEG and further neuropsychological evaluation if the history and preliminary examinations pointed to an underlying organic condition. If there were an underlying mental illness, I would carry out a comprehensive risk assessment focusing on the risks to the patient, his neighbour and others, in particular the neighbour's partner or family.

The treatment that would be offered would depend on the findings of the assessment. Irrespective of the presence or absence of a mental illness, I would educate this man on the implications of his behaviour, which amounts to harassment, and the impact on his neighbour (victim). The aim of clinical management would be to treat any contributory mental disorder, understand what is sustaining the unacceptable behaviour, and confront the patient's self-deception that tends to minimize, justify or deny the behaviour outright. Treatment would also be focused on instilling a sense of empathy and developing appropriate interpersonal and social skills, whilst treating any substance misuse that might be present. I would prescribe for him atypical antipsychotic medication if there were an underlying psychotic illness, and also an antidepressant if necessary. Antimanic drugs and a mood stabilizer might be required if there were an underlying manic or hypomanic condition. I would give consideration to cognitive behavioural therapy aimed at modifying any abnormal beliefs he holds about himself or his victim. In the short term, efforts would be made to optimize his response to both the psychological and the biological treatment. Given the recent separation from his wife, he might also need some counselling and social support.

I would also consider the need to refer this man to the forensic psychiatric services for further advice and an intensive community psychiatric nurse's input, should this be necessary on discharge from the hospital. I would focus long-term management strategies on relapse prevention and regular monitoring for any re-emergence of his stalking behaviour. If he turned out to be suffering from a mental illness of severe and enduring nature, I would recommend that he should be subject to an enhanced care programme approach (in England and Wales) for close supervision. In the event that this behaviour continued despite these interventions, a court injunction might be used by his victim to bring the stalking to an end. It is sometimes useful if the offender is warned or cautioned by police, as stalking has been found to stop in about 50% of cases following this intervention. There might be a need for a court of law to enforce a restraining order but this sometimes makes matters worse, especially in persistent offenders, as it gives them the attention they want.

The victim might also need help, but as she has not been referred to me I would advise that she sees her own GP, who could refer her to the local psychiatric service if there were evidence of psychiatric illness. Treatment for the victim might take the form of education and supportive counselling, cognitive behavioural approaches to allay unreasonable fears and other strategies tailored to the need of the individual. The neighbour might also seek assistance from the Victim Support Scheme and also advice on how to avoid confrontation and how to alert those who are in charge of the stalker's care to any continuing transgressions. She might receive advice on how to protect personal information, relatives and relevant others, as they might become secondary targets. Information could also be given on victim support organizations such as the National Anti-stalking and Harassment Campaign and Support Association and the Suzy Lamplugh Trust in the UK, or CyberAngels and Survivors of Stalking (SOS).

Note: 'stalking' is a colloquial term, and the action is usually interpreted in law as 'harassment against a person'. Neither is a psychiatric diagnosis but both may point to an underlying mental illness.

ANSWERS TO SUGGESTED PROBES

1. The most likely diagnosis is delusional disorder of erotomanic type (erotomanic delusions or de Clérambault syndrome).
2. Diagnostic criteria that point to 'stalking' were laid down by Mullen and Pathé (1994) and require that:
   - The stalker is convinced he/she is in love or infatuated.
   - The victim has done nothing to encourage the stalker.
   - The 'love' preoccupies the stalker to the exclusion of other interests.

- The stalking produces serious disruption to stalkers' lives.
- The stalker is convinced that his/her feelings are genuine.
- The words and actions of the victim are reinterpreted to maintain the stalker's beliefs.
- The stalker repeatedly attempts to follow and approach the victim, creating distress or at least embarrassment.

3. The main risks to the victim are:
   - physical harm: homicide can be a serious consequence.
   - psychological distress: mainly anxiety symptoms, which occur in up to 83% of victims, and post-traumatic stress disorder, experienced by up to 37% of victims.

Stalking could also have other distressing impacts on the victims and their families, including the need for the victim to modify his or her life in terms of work, commuting, relationships, leisure, social life and home security.

The various typologies of stalkers, as described by Mullen et al (2001), are:

- *Rejected stalker*. The relationship went wrong. The stalker therefore either wants revenge or reconciliation.
- *Stalker seeking intimacy*. The stalker desires a relationship, usually with someone who has engaged his/her attention. There is then a delusional interpretation that the person is in love with them.
- *The incompetent stalker*. The stalker lacks the ability to conduct a courtship due to problems such as social or learning difficulties. They make inept approaches and communications.
- *The resentful stalker*. The stalker stalks to frighten the victims. This may be due to a desire for retribution on the part of the individual, or of a group that the victim represents. Usually, satisfaction is gained from the distress caused to the victim. The stalker feels justified in the cause.
- *The predatory stalker*. The stalker stalks as a prelude to a sex attack.
- *The false victim stalker*. The stalker pretends to be stalked.

BUZZ WORDS AND USEFUL TERMINOLOGY

Stalking, relapse indicators, risk assessment, erotomania, erotomanic delusions, de Clérambault syndrome, protection from harassment.

REFERENCES AND SUGGESTED READING

Mullen P E, Pathé M 1994 Stalking and the pathology of love. Australian and New Zealand Journal of Psychiatry 28:469–477

Mullen P, Pathé M 1994 The pathological extension of love. British Journal of Psychiatry 165:614–623

Mullen P, Pathé M, Purcell R 2000 Stalkers and Their Victims. Cambridge University Press, Cambridge

Mullen P E, Pathé M, Purcell R 2001 The management of stalkers. Advances in Psychiatric Treatment 7:335–342

Pathé M, Mullen P E 1997 The impact of stalkers on their victims. British Journal of Psychiatry 170:12–17

Pathé M, Mullen P E, Purcell R 2001 Management of victims of stalking. Advances in Psychiatric Treatment 7:399–406

9

Mental impairments

A 33-year-old man with an IQ of 61 has been brought to your clinic by his mother after a referral by his GP. He has been cautioned by the police for exposing himself in public. He believes young schoolgirls find him attractive and he wanted to show them how 'sexy' he is.

How would go about assessing him and what diagnoses would you consider?

SUGGESTED PROBES

1. What information would you require to complete your assessment?
2. Are there clinical features that would increase your concern about his level of risk?
3. What is the likelihood that this man will reoffend?

PMP PLAN

TASKS TO DO

The following five areas are relevant to this vignette but are not necessarily all-inclusive. The list is also not exhaustive:

a) Assess the implications of this man presenting for the first time and the association of learning disabilities with sexual offending.
b) Discuss the need to obtain information from medical and legal sources.
c) Include functional conditions not related to learning disabilities in your differential diagnosis: for example, frontal lobe abnormalities, hypomania, psychosis, depression and substance misuse.

d) Discuss the man's risk of reoffending and the factors that would increase that risk.

e) Include medical, psychological, social and day-care options in your management plan.

ISSUES

- Underlying factors for this man's unacceptable behaviour
- The risk he poses to others, particularly young girls
- Management of exposure in public to forestall reoffending or more serious crime
- Possibility of a dual diagnosis.

CLARIFY

- Is the man presenting at this age for the first time and the implications of this?
- Is it a one-off incident or repeated behaviour?

SEEK MORE INFORMATION

POLICE

- Exact details of the incident. Is he is a repeat offender?

GP

- Relevant medical and psychiatric history, any history of mental disorder
- Any referrals to local services.

PARENT

- Mother's opinion of her son's behaviour
- Collaboration on history, help received in the past
- Any previous history of aggression.

PATIENT

- Full history, including forensic history, mental state, neuropsychological testing (excluding IQ) prior to completing whole assessment
- Any particular girl at imminent risk?
- Any behaviour towards boys
- Benefit derived from behaviour, erection, masturbation
- Life stressors, presence of anxiety and depression.

DIFFERENTIAL DIAGNOSIS/DIFFICULTIES

- *Functional.* Conditions not related to learning disabilities, e.g. delusional disorder, paranoid schizophrenia, hypomania, schizoaffective disorder, other schizophreniform psychosis, depression, substance misuse, exhibitionism
- *Organic.* Learning disabilities, frontal lobe abnormalities, chronic organic brain damage.

APPROACH TO TREATMENT

- Investigate further (include relevant routine laboratory tests) and assess using clinical rating scales Psychiatric Assessment Schedule for Adults with Developmental Disability (PAS-ADD) (Moss et al, 1993).
- Carry out a risk assessment: the association of indecent exposure with other more serious sexual offending, and the risk of future offending.
- Consider the setting for treatment.

WHAT TREATMENT/ADVICE

MEDICAL

- Use mood stabilizers to reduce impulsivity.
- Use antipsychotics to treat psychotic illness
- Prescribe an antidepressant.
- Prescribe hormonal treatment to reduce arousal, sexual fantasies and desires: progestins, anti-androgens medroxyprogesterone, cyproterone acetate and a long-acting analogue of gonadotrophin-releasing hormone, e.g. triptorelin.
- Give psychological treatment for impulse control, sexual counselling, cognitive behavioural therapy and group psychotherapy.

SOCIAL

- Arrange training of social skills and daytime activities.

FULL ANSWER

In dealing with this case, I would like to address several issues. First, I would want to find out the factors underlying this man's unacceptable behaviour, which would inform my treatment strategy. Second, I would carry out a comprehensive risk assessment to determine the risk he poses to others. Third, I would determine how to deal with his exposure in public to forestall reoffending or a more serious crime. I would have it at the back of my mind that this man has a form of learning disability with an IQ of 61. However, his learning difficulties may not be the only problem. This man may actually have a dual diagnosis.

I would clarify whether this is a one-off incident or whether this man has a history of this difficult behaviour. I would be concerned if this is the first time that he is presenting this way. Given that he believes that young girls find him attractive, I would think that this behaviour might be longstanding and would therefore explore further. I would ask the police officers who cautioned him for any information they have about this man. I would clarify whether the behaviour is directed at any particular set of schoolgirls and whether the girls have done anything to 'invite' this behaviour from a man with learning difficulties. I would find out if school officials are aware of the situation and whether any of the girls has come to any harm. I would also clarify whether this behaviour has taken place with boys at all.

To enable me to arrive at a diagnosis, I would seek more information from his GP, his mother and other person(s) who could give me useful details. I would find out if there is any history of brain injury or learning difficulties, and whether he suffers from epilepsy. I would also ask if the GP has referred this man to any secondary or tertiary services for assessment, support and/or treatment. I would find out from his mother whether this behaviour has been an issue in the past and whether it took place in their neighbourhood. I would find out if the mother thinks this unacceptable behaviour is escalating. It would also be useful to ask if her son frequently behaves in an impulsive manner. I would take a full psychiatric history from the patient and conduct a mental state examination. In the history, I would be particularly interested in how he formed the belief that young schoolgirls find him attractive, what use he makes of this belief, and whether he actually thinks these young girls are making suggestions to him or inviting him.

I would enquire about the circumstances in which these inappropriate behaviours occur, the triggers, and the benefits he derives from exposing himself in this way. I would ask him whether he has an erection when he is exposing himself and whether this behaviour is associated with masturbation. I would find out if he thought he should have sex with any of the girls, with or without their consent. I would ask him whether he thinks they want to have sex with him and, if so, why he believes that. I would explore further to see how fixed he is in this belief, with the hope of being able to do some cognitive work to deal with his difficulties. I would find out from him whether he knows the legal implications of his actions. I would also enquire whether he is in a relationship now or has had one in the recent past. If there has been a relationship, I would enquire about its quality. I would ask him sensitively how he has let out his sexual feelings in the past and how he does so at the current time. I would ask him whether he masturbates regularly. I would examine whether there are any underlying life stressors or life event that may be predisposing him to behave this way.

In addressing this man's difficulties, I would consider what might be wrong with him and why he is behaving in this way, considering that he may have a dual diagnosis. In the differential diagnosis I would consider the possibility that he is suffering from a psychotic illness such as paranoid schizophrenia, delusional disorder, schizoaffective disorder or depression, hypomania and substance misuse disorder, including alcoholism. I would also consider the possibility of him having an organic brain syndrome, such as frontal lobe abnormalities and epilepsy, in addition to his learning difficulties. The diagnosis of a paraphilia, such as exhibitionism, would also be considered, but I am aware that he probably was not exposing himself to a 'complete stranger'. In order to confirm the diagnosis, it would be useful to carry out further neuropsychological assessment and to ascertain his IQ. At a later appointment and in conjunction with our clinical psychologist I would use validated instruments such as the PAS-ADD (used in patients with learning difficulties) to assess psychiatry morbidity in this man. It might be necessary to investigate further to rule out intracranial pathology using a CT scan or MRI. I would also carry out a detailed risk assessment.

My treatment would depend on the findings of my assessment, of the risk assessment in particular. I would determine whether this man could be managed as an outpatient, provided that the behaviour began recently and is of mild to moderate severity, and there is no immediate risk to schoolchildren. I would consider referring him to a specialist unit to deal with the illness, particularly if the behaviour has been long-term and carries a high risk of causing physical and emotional harm to the girls he has been exposing himself to. As far as possible, treatment would be carried out by the multidisciplinary team and I would consider what biological, psychological and social methods to employ in helping him.

As far as medical treatment was concerned, I would use an optimal dose of an atypical antipsychotic if the main problem were one of the psychotic illnesses I have listed. Given his learning difficulties and the need to be careful with the use of psychotropics, I will use as low dose of medication as possible and I would monitor closely for side-effects and follow him up in the clinic. If this man had abnormal sexual (arousal) behaviour or exhibitionism, I would treat with one of the mood stabilizers such as carbamazepine or sodium valproate to reduce impulsive behaviour. This might also be useful in patients with a frontal disinhibition syndrome. I would also explore the use of one of the antidepressant selective serotonin re-uptake inhibitors (SSRIs, e.g. fluoxetine), as these have been found useful in the treatment of some paraphilia. If these measures were not successful, I would consider hormonal treatment to reduce arousal, sexual fantasies and desires in this man. I would use progestins, anti-androgens such as medroxyprogesterone, cyproterone acetate and a long-acting analogue of gonadotrophin-releasing hormone (GnRH), such as triptorelin, to achieve a reduced sexual arousal level. Cyproterone might be preferable as it has specific anti-androgenic action and fewer adverse effects. I would explain the purpose of this treatment option carefully to the patient.

I would give these treatments along with psychological measures, which would include sexual counselling and cognitive behavioural therapy. I would consider using psychotherapy, mainly in groups, to focus on the issues of denial, minimization and responsibility for the offence, harm done to the victim, behaviour consistent with offending and victim awareness. Cognitive behavioural therapeutic approaches using techniques such as covert sensitization, imaginal desensitization, thought-stopping and aversive conditioning have also been found to be useful. In the long term, I would facilitate social and daytime activities for this man to reduce boredom and the tendency to wander around and offend. Where possible, some of the group psychological treatment could be facilitated at a day hospital.

ANSWERS TO SUGGESTED PROBES

1. The information required to complete the assessment is covered in the full answer.
2. The clinical features that would increase my concern about the level of risk are:
   - presence of a schizophrenia-like illness in addition to the learning disability
   - beliefs about girls that are psychotically driven
   - presence of command hallucinations
   - poor impulse and urge control
   - high level of sexual arousal

- past history of violent acts and current propensity to violence
- poor compliance with treatment and management plans.

3. What is the likelihood that this man would reoffend? The rate of reoffending in sex offenders with learning disability is generally quoted as low for serious sex offences and moderate to high for minor offences. Exhibitionists are thought to be at higher risk for recidivism. As well as static factors, more dynamic factors such as treatment (plus compliance with and monitoring of), substance misuse, recent life events and environment need to be considered. An actuarial predictive approach in conjunction with empirically guided clinical assessment is probably best for predicting recidivism in sex offenders.

BUZZ WORDS AND USEFUL TERMINOLOGY

Neuropsychological testing, dual diagnosis, covert sensitization, aversive conditioning.

REFERENCES AND SUGGESTED READING

Klimecki M, Jenkinson J, Wilson L 1994 A study of recidivism among offenders with an intellectual disability. Australia and New Zealand Journal of Developmental Disabilities 19:209–219

Lindsay W R, Smith A H W 1998 Responses to treatment for sex offenders with intellectual disability: a comparison of men with 1- and 2-year probation sentences. Journal of Intellectual Disability Research 42(5):346–353

Moss S C, Patel P, Prosser H et al 1993 Psychiatric morbidity in older people with moderate and severe learning disability (mental retardation). Part 1: Development and reliability of the patient interview (the PAS-ADD). British Journal of Psychiatry 163:471–480

Rosler A, Witztum E 1998 Treatment of men with paraphilia with a long-acting analogue of gonadotropin-releasing hormone. New England Journal of Medicine 338(7):416–422

9.2   MAN WITH DOWN'S SYNDROME

A 52-year-old man with trisomy 21 (Down's syndrome) was admitted following increasing periods of agitation and isolation, after his live-in carer moved on to another town. His mother, who used to care for him, died about a year previously. Staff have noticed that he has become more withdrawn, engages in fewer activities, falls more frequently, and has reduced concentration and poor memory. They are concerned he may be developing Alzheimer's disease.

With the information available to you, how would you go about ascertaining and managing what is wrong with this man?

SUGGESTED PROBES

1. What factors could be contributing to this presentation?
2. What are the differential diagnoses and what further investigations would you do to rule in or rule out Alzheimer's disease?
3. After extensive investigation you decide that he requires an antidepressant and other psychotropics. What pharmacological issues would you consider?

PMP PLAN

TASKS TO DO

The following five areas are relevant to this vignette but are not necessarily all-inclusive. The list is also not exhaustive:

a) Point out that physical symptoms/factors common in Down's syndrome can contribute to the presentation and make it look like dementia.
b) Show an understanding of the neuropathological link/similarities between Down's syndrome and Alzheimer's disease.
c) Demonstrate knowledge of the differential diagnoses and other reasons for the loss of daily living skills in people with Down's syndrome.
d) Demonstrate knowledge of the relevant tests to diagnose dementia and emphasize the need to rule out treatable dementias.
e) Manage in line with the outcome of assessments and consideration of medical, psychological, social and environmental approaches to management.

ISSUES

- Determining whether this presentation is due to Alzheimer's disease and or a physical complication of the Down's syndrome
- Determining the contribution that this man's losses have made to his illness and overall functioning in order to inform treatment strategies
- Getting a clear picture of the temporal event as far as possible.

CLARIFY

- What is the temporal sequence of the symptoms?
- What medication is this man currently on, and have there been any changes recently (e.g. increasing sedation and benzodiazepine use)?
- Are there sensory defects, including hearing loss and cataracts?

SEEK MORE INFORMATION

STAFF

- Symptoms, the patient's response to his losses and bereavement, and the nature of his depressive symptoms.

PATIENT

- Further history, mental state examination
- Physical examination for physical abnormalities, mobility difficulties, infection and cardiac abnormalities that may be incapacitating the patient, and for the exclusion of sensory deficits.

INVESTIGATIONS

- Neuropsychological assessment and laboratory investigations.

DIFFERENTIAL DIAGNOSIS/DIFFICULTIES

- *Organic.* Early-onset dementia of Alzheimer's type, pseudodementia, dementing illness (not of Alzheimer's type; Lewy body dementia), hypothyroidism, reversible dementia

due to B$_{12}$ or folate deficiency, visual impairment, sedation, change in medication
- *Functional.* Bereavement reaction, depression, adjustment disorder secondary to physical symptoms, anxiety disorder, psychotic illness.

APPROACH TO TREATMENT

- Consider medical and psychosocial approaches.
- Treat physical abnormalities and give nutritional support.
- Provide support for identified carers.

WHAT TREATMENT/ADVICE

MEDICAL

- Treat reversible causes, ameliorate irreversible conditions, and treat physical illnesses and disabilities.
- Give antidepressant treatment for depressive disorders and anxiety.
- Consider anticholinesterase treatment for Alzheimer's disease and other dementias. (This should be done in collaboration with specialists.) Treatment should be stopped if benefit is not sustained.

PSYCHOLOGICAL

- Arrange bereavement counselling and counselling for coping with losses.

SOCIAL

- Consider environmental factors, aids, rails and lifts.

FULL ANSWER

This vignette certainly contains many factors that may confound the picture in this man, who may also have difficulties in expressing himself. The main issues that I would like to address are to determine the causation of illness and whether this presentation is due to Alzheimer's disease or the physical complications of Down's syndrome. I would also attempt to assess the contribution of losses and life events to this patient's illness and overall functioning. I would also attempt to form as clear a picture as possible of the temporal sequence of events to enable me to formulate a good treatment strategy.

I would clarify whether his symptoms of agitation, confusion and memory difficulties predate the loss of his mother and carer, or whether the symptoms were worsened or triggered by these life events. I would also clarify whether this man is on any medication, such as sedatives, which may affect the way the man is presently, and whether any change has been made recently. I would also clarify if there is any sensory deficit such as hearing loss or poor sight that may predispose to his present condition. I would determine whether it was necessary to transfer this man to hospital for further assessment and management, or whether this could be carried out at home.

I would arrange to see the patient, take a full psychiatric history, and do a mental state examination in order to seek more information. I would also consider the physical conditions that are relevant to this case. In my history I would be particularly concerned about his experience of bereavement, and what the loss of his mother and his carer meant to him in terms of his functioning and coping. I would look for loss of interest, lack of energy, evidence and biological signs of depression (diurnal variation in mood, weight loss, poor sleep, early morning wakening, loss of appetite), hopelessness and suicidal thoughts, plans and/or intent. In my mental state assessment I would look for evidence of confusion and self-neglect, and carry out a cognitive function assessment (including a Mini Mental State Examination). I would also examine for symptoms that might suggest a dementing illness. I would check for evidence of infection, including that of urinary tract or chest or septicaemia, which might cause a confusional state. The history of inactivity and falls might also be due to a mobility problem caused by osteoarthritis or a cardiac condition, both of which are common in patients with Down's syndrome. I would make sure I look out for sensory deficits, including poor sight due to cataracts, as this is also frequently found in Down's syndrome and may have been contributing to the frequent falls.

I would carry out further assessments and a dementia screen, which would include a full neuropsychological evaluation, blood tests to rule out anaemia, kidney dysfunction, liver abnormalities, hypothyroidism, diabetes mellitus, hypercholesterolaemia, vitamin B_{12} and folate deficiencies, and neuroradiology investigations (MRI or CT scan). In order to reach a baseline objective assessment, I would use the Dementia Scale for Mentally Retarded Persons (DMR) to measure the level of cognitive deficit and possibility of dementia in this man.

In my differential diagnosis, I would consider bereavement and reaction to the losses of his mother and his live-in carer to be very important. I would consider other possible diagnoses, such as depression, pseudodementia due to moderately severe depression, and early-onset dementia of Alzheimer's type. I would also consider other dementias not of Alzheimer's type, particularly reversible ones such as may be caused by hypothyroidism. It might be that this man has an adjustment disorder secondary to multiple physical problems, or he could quite possibly be suffering pain from osteoarthritis, which is common in people with Down's syndrome. It is also possible that increased falls and fewer activities may be due to increased sedation.

In my approach to treatment, I would consider medical and psychosocial approaches, nutrition rehabilitation, and support for identified carers. Treatment would depend largely on what was found during the assessment, and I would pay particular attention to treating reversible causes and ameliorating reversible conditions. As this man might be suffering from a physical disorder that is causing him pain, I would assess this and give appropriate treatment. Since bereavement and losses might be contributing to this presentation, I would offer bereavement counselling using methods that are suitable in a person with learning difficulties. As regards depressive disorder and anxieties, I would employ psychosocial interventions as much as possible, including activity scheduling to improve the mood disorder. I would use antidepressants, if necessary, the choice of which would be informed by the need to avoid side-effects that might worsen the patient's condition. I would also use the optimal dose of medication and avoid higher doses that might cause unnecessary side-effects.

As Alzheimer's disease and other dementias are also possibilities, treatment would be in line with that given to any patient with dementia, albeit with some modifications tailored to the needs of this individual. As there is some possible efficacy in the treatment of symptoms of mild to moderate Alzheimer's disease in people with Down's syndrome (Prasher, Huxley, Haque 2002), I would consider the use of anticholinesterase, particularly donepezil hydrochloride, in this gentleman. I would treat and improve any physical illness that might be contributing to his difficulties, such as hypothyroidism, hypovitaminosis, hearing and visual disabilities, mobility problems and pains from skeletal abnormalities. I would also employ means such as rails and lifts to deal with environmental factors that might be contributing to falls and injuries, and would deal with any other hazards.

ANSWERS TO SUGGESTED PROBES

1. The factors contributing to this presentation have been discussed in the full answer.

2. Differential diagnosis and further investigations have been covered in the full answer.
3. The pharmacological issues of concern are as follows:
   - the need to use smaller doses of medication compared to what is practised in the normal population
   - the risk of precipitating seizures with the use of antidepressants, particularly the tricyclic antidepressants
   - the effect of psychotropic medications on any cardiac abnormalities that may be present
   - the possible prominence of anticholinergic side-effects of some psychotropics in Down's syndrome
   - the possible worsening of mobility problems due to the use of atypical antipsychotics to reduce extrapyramidal side-effects
   - the possible precipitation of disinhibition and worsening of confusion due to the use of benzodiazepines prescribed to reduce agitation.

BUZZ WORDS AND USEFUL TERMINOLOGY

Dementia screen, reversible dementias.

REFERENCES AND SUGGESTED READING

Prasher V P, Huxley A, Haque M S 2002 A 24-week, double-blind, placebo-controlled trial of donepezil in patients with Down's syndrome and Alzheimer's disease. Pilot study

Reiss S, Amman M G 1998 Psychotropic Medication and Developmental Disabilities: the International Consensus. OSU Nisonger Center, Columbus, Ohio

10

Liaison and adult psychiatry

You have received a referral from a local GP, requesting a psychiatric assessment on a 41-year-old hospital porter, who has given up work to look after his 6-year-old daughter. His wife left him about 14 months ago after several family disputes. He has presented to his local accident and emergency department five times during this period, seeking treatment for unexplained bruises on his daughter's body. During the course of two admissions staff have ruled out a haematological or other organic condition and nurses now think he may be causing the child's symptoms himself.

What are your differentials and how would you go about assessing and managing this man? What other advice would you give?

SUGGESTED PROBES

1. Are there risk factors that would make the diagnosis of physical abuse more likely?
2. What personality traits would make the diagnosis of Munchausen's syndrome by proxy more likely?
3. Who else would you involve in the assessment?

PMP PLAN

TASKS TO DO

The following five areas are relevant to this vignette but are not necessarily all-inclusive. The list is also not exhaustive:

a) Demonstrate the ability to assess risk issues in the man and child.
b) Explore and assess in a multidisciplinary way. Demonstrate knowledge of the nature of the injuries in physical abuse of a child.

c) Discuss and back up your differential diagnosis, including that of Munchausen's syndrome by proxy.
d) Appreciate the need to protect the child, including the involvement of child and family services and the local child protection committee.
e) Draw up a management plan for the patient and give support. Arrange management and supervision of the child, particularly if the father retains custody.

ISSUES

- Causes of this child's symptoms and her father's frequent presentation to hospital
- Risk this man poses to his daughter and strategies to reduce it, if the man is found to be the cause of symptoms
- Establishing the underlying cause of this man's distress to minimize risk to himself, the child and others.

CLARIFY

- What is the child's situation and how safe is she? What are the child protection issues and procedures?
- Is there any legal or factual information?
- Would this man abscond with his child?

SEEK MORE INFORMATION

GP

- Past medical and psychiatric history.

PAEDIATRICIAN

- Investigations and features suggestive of child abuse.

CHILD SOCIAL WORKER

- Detailed assessment of the social situation
- Child protection conference.

ESTRANGED WIFE

(The patient's consent is required.)

- Any other children involved
- Any history of mental illness and domestic violence.

PATIENT

- History, mental state examination, appraisal of psychosocial situation and family support
- History of alcohol and illicit drug use
- Reasons for stopping work
- Examination of the child.

PREVIOUS EMPLOYER

(The patient's consent is required.)

- Problems at work, sickness record.

DIFFERENTIAL DIAGNOSIS/DIFFICULTIES

- *Functional.* Depressive disorder, Munchausen's syndrome by proxy, alcohol abuse and substance misuse disorder, psychotic illness such as a delusional disorder, a schizophreniform psychosis
- *Organic.* Organic brain disorder, including epilepsy.

APPROACH TO TREATMENT

- Be sensitive in your approach.
- Carry out a multidisciplinary assessment and seek the advice of the local child protection liaison personnel or committee.
- Present a planned, objective and coordinated response from all the professionals involved.
- Consider the interests and safety of the child to be paramount.

WHAT TREATMENT/ADVICE

MEDICAL

- Prescribe an antidepressant if necessary.
- Give treatment for addiction.

PSYCHOLOGICAL

- Address issues of loss (marital relationship, job, social role and finances) and the need to regain lost ground.
- Use a psychodynamic, insight-orientated approach, in combination with behavioural techniques.

SOCIAL

- Involve child and family services, consider removal of the child and the use of a child protection order; consider her placement on the 'At Risk' register, in the UK. (This is a list of names of children in the area who are considered to be at considerable risk of harm—physical, emotional, sexual or through neglect. The aim of the register is to ensure that children do not suffer further harm and that all the agencies working for the child do so in a coordinated way. The Child Protection Register is kept at the social services department, with a copy at police headquarters. Only authorized people within the health, police, education and social services can obtain information from the register. A check is made to ensure enquiries are genuine before any information is given out. The information kept on the register includes basic factual details about families—names, ages and addresses; date and reason for registration; names and telephone numbers of other people working with families (e.g. health visitor, schoolteacher, doctor); the decision and recommendations made at the child protection conference; date of the next meeting.)
- Arrange practical help to lessen the burden of childcare, along with parental education and help for the father to go back to work.

FULL ANSWER

While it is possible that this girl might have an as yet undiagnosed condition, I would consider child abuse and non-accidental injury caused by the father, given the extensive investigations that have been carried out and his psychosocial situation. He has recently separated from his wife and is now caring for his 6-year-old daughter alone. The main issues that I would like to address are ascertaining the causes of the child's symptoms and the man's frequent presentation to hospital, determining the risk that the father poses to his daughter, and also addressing the underlying cause of his distress in order to reduce the risk he poses to the child, himself and to others.

I would clarify the child's exact situation at the time of referral and find out whether the appropriate social services (child and family) have been informed and have instituted a child protection procedure. I would also clarify whether there are any legal proceedings involved, and whether there has been a trial of fact concerning the cause of the child's symptoms. I would suggest an emergency protection order if I considered the child to be at immediate risk of harm. The safety of the child would be paramount, and it would also be important to establish causative factors and a diagnosis in this man, who might be deliberately feigning illness in his child.

For the sake of clarity, I would first deal with the man who has actually been referred to me, and then, after liaison with other parties, make the necessary suggestions for the management of the child. I would seek more information about the father and about the situation as a whole to enable me to arrive at a safe diagnosis. I would ask his GP for his past medical and psychiatric history, looking for any evidence of past hospitalizations, extensive investigative procedures and surgery. It would also be important to examine for evidence of brain damage and learning disabilities. I would ask whether the GP suspected the patient had a factitious disorder or illness at any time in the past, or whether there was anything to suggest a history of anxiety, depression or psychotic illness. I would ask the team's social worker to conduct an assessment and to find out who else is involved in the child's care, whether other children are being cared for by this man, and whether there have been concerns about them too. I would attempt, with this man's consent, to obtain a corroborative account of what has been happening from other family members or neighbours. His estranged wife would also be in a good position to give information about the access she and others have to the child or children, and any concerns she might have. I would seek the opinion of the paediatrician involved on the evidence for a non-accidental injury, and to find out whether clinical or laboratory findings (including radiological) have revealed any evidence of burns, bites, fractured ribs and/or sexual abuse. It would be important to know if the child's symptoms are limited to one system and if the clinical description of child's illness is consistent with the clinical and laboratory findings. I would make sure conditions such as a vascular, collagen and/or other haematological disorder have been ruled out. I would find out whether the onset of the illness and its progress (or lack of it) have been clearly witnessed by others. If there were conclusive evidence of child abuse, I would ask whether there is a child protection procedure or measure in place. I would enquire about the child protection team's findings and the degree of cooperation the team has received from the father.

When I saw the gentleman, I would quickly clarify whether he knows who referred him and the purpose of the referral. I would be mindful of the sensitivity of the case, involving a man confronted directly or indirectly with the possibility that he is abusing his own child. I would ask him whether he has been assessed by any other official, including staff from the local child and family services department. In his history, I would be particularly interested in past and present psychiatric or emotional problems, particularly fallout from his wife's departure and the divorce proceedings. I would ask questions about the quality of the marital relations between the estranged couple, and whether there is any history of emotional, physical or sexual abuse and domestic violence. I would ask how he has adjusted to this new situation and find out about the level of support he has been receiving from others as regards childcare. I would ask him if he uses alcohol and illicit substances to help him cope with childcare and other difficulties. I would ask him why he has decided to keep the child rather than provide support for her to live with her mother. I would ask him the main reason why he resigned from his work. It would be useful to obtain his sickness record from his employers, but I would seek his permission before doing so. I would ask about his financial situation, including debts, and whether he has been under any pressure to return to work. I would examine for anything that might motivate this man to adopt a sick role and also whether there are possible external incentives and secondary gains for him if his daughter presents in hospital as sick on several occasions. These might include the return of his estranged wife's affection or financial incentives for childcare.

If there were a clinical suggestion of deliberate child abuse in this case, I would find out from the social worker whether the family is known to services and whether any issues of domestic violence have been reported. I would ask whether any child in the family has been subject to a child protection order or placed on the 'At Risk' register with the services, recently or at any time in the past. In order to arrive at a safe working diagnosis, I would consider Munchausen's syndrome by proxy as a differential diagnosis, particularly if the bruising started soon after his wife's departure. This would be most likely, considering the possibly intentional production of physical symptoms to feign illness in this child, risk factors for motivation to assume the sick role, and the likelihood of external incentives such as economic gain from unemployment and childcare support benefits. I would also consider the diagnosis of an adjustment disorder, depressive disorder, substance misuse disorder, psychotic illness or a schizopreniform psychosis in this man.

My approach to treatment would be to be extremely sensitive, involving other members of the multidisciplinary team and working in conjunction with child protection workers. I would advise a planned, objective and coordinated response to this man from the different professionals who would be involved. I would carry out a full risk assessment and advise the child protection team and the GP accordingly.

The treatment options would depend largely on whether there was clear evidence of abuse or whether abuse could be ruled out beyond reasonable doubt. If a diagnosis of Munchausen's syndrome by proxy were made, treatment would consist mainly of preventing the continued abuse of the child, advice on the care of the affected child and the treatment of the father. As far as the child is concerned, I would advise child and family services to remove her from the family, at least temporarily, while her father is undergoing treatment. To minimize disruption to the child's life, she should be placed with an appropriate family member. I would call a meeting where this man could be confronted, directly but in a non-threatening manner, in the hope that he would admit his involvement in the child's presentation. It might also be necessary to inform the police, but this would be done by the child protection committee in accordance with local protocols. I would be mindful that this man might become more depressed and even acutely suicidal after such a confrontation. As there might be moderate to severe problems of adjustment, depression, substance misuse disorder and borderline personality difficulties in this man, I would recommend further intensive outpatient or inpatient evaluation. I would suggest psychodynamic, insight-orientated approaches, in combination with behavioural techniques to deal with psychopathology related to issues of loss and sick role. I would also consider specific treatment for other differential diagnoses mentioned above. I would only give an antidepressant if necessary.

I would also advise social support for this man, if returning his daughter to him were an option. I would suggest that the services facilitate practical help to lessen the burden of childcare. If he remained the main carer, I would advise access to parental education to help him with the various issues involved in bringing up a child on his own. The child would also need closer monitoring and a child protection order might be necessary. I would also consider advising the placement of this child on the 'At Risk' register kept by the social services department in the UK. If it were possible to give assistance concerning childcare, efforts would be made to assist this man to go back to work.

ANSWERS TO SUGGESTED PROBES

1. The risk factors that would make the diagnosis of physical abuse more likely are:

- lack of social support
- use of alcohol and illicit substances
- social isolation
- presence of mental illness in the child's carer
- history of domestic violence
- presence of a learning disability in the child
- feelings of insecurity and low self-esteem in the child's carer
- attention-seeking behaviour in the carer.

2. Borderline and antisocial personality traits would make the diagnosis of Munchausen's syndrome by proxy more likely.
3. I would involve the following people in the assessment:
   - other family members, including the estranged wife
   - professional colleagues (physicians and paediatricians), team psychologist, social workers
   - previous employers (consent of the patient would be required)
   - police and other law enforcement agents, if necessary.

BUZZ WORDS AND USEFUL TERMINOLOGY

Child protection measures/procedures/team, the sick role, external gain or incentives, factitious disorder, child protection order, emergency protection order, 'At Risk' register, trial of fact concerning causation, full risk assessment.

REFERENCES AND SUGGESTED READING

HMSO 1991 Introduction to the Children Act 1989. HMSO, London

McClure R J, Davis P M, Meadow S R et al 1996 Epidemiology of Munchausen syndrome by proxy, non-accidental poisoning, and non-accidental suffocation. Archives of Disease in Childhood 75(1):57–61

Meadow R 1982 Munchausen's syndrome by proxy. Archives of Disease in Childhood 57:92–98

Morley C J 1995 Practical concerns about the diagnosis of Munchausen's syndrome by proxy. Archives of Disease in Childhood 72:528–530

Pasqualone G A, Fitzgerald S M 1999 Munchausen by proxy: the forensic challenge of recognition, diagnosis and reporting. Critical Care Nursing Quarterly 22(1):52–64

Rosenberg D A 1987 Web of deceit: a literature review of Munchausen's syndrome by proxy. Child Abuse and Neglect 2: 547–563

10.2 49-YEAR-OLD MAN, WHOSE PARTNER DIED OF HIV, WHO IS MOODY, IRRITABLE AND LOSING WEIGHT

You have been asked to see a 49-year-old married man with two grown-up children, who has recently become moody and increasingly irritable and is losing weight. He discloses to you that for 3 years he was having an extramarital affair with another man, who died of pneumonia and AIDS 6 months ago. His GP is almost sure that the patient has contracted HIV infection. The man is ambivalent about having an HIV test and is very worried he has contracted the disease, fearing that this will destroy his family.

How would you manage the situation and his symptoms?

SUGGESTED PROBES

1. What procedures would you follow if you had to do an HIV test?
2. The HIV test comes back positive but the patient insists you do not tell anybody. What would you do?
3. What symptoms and signs would suggest deterioration in this man's mental health if he tested positive for HIV?

PMP PLAN

TASKS TO DO

The following five areas are relevant to this vignette but are not necessarily all-inclusive. The list is also not exhaustive:

a) Comment on the sensitivity of the case at hand, confidentiality, the need to protect others and reasons for breach of confidentiality if necessary.
b) Demonstrate awareness of the implications of HIV testing and the local procedure for carrying out such a test.
c) Show an understanding of the psychiatric presentations of persons with HIV infection, the differential diagnoses, and the emotional issues involving disclosure to their family and significant others.
d) Take a multimodal treatment approach for psychiatric disorders. Discuss the need to work with other professionals, e.g. infectious disease specialists, HIV/AIDS mental health nurse or practitioners, physicians, social workers and counsellors. Demonstrate an understanding of the pharmacological issues involved in the use of antidepressants and other psychotropics.

e) Advise social support, practical problem-solving and support networks for the patient and the family.

ISSUES

- Determining whether the cause of the weight loss and the depressive symptoms in this man is HIV infection and AIDS
- Importance of HIV screening
- Confidentiality and the need to protect others from harm
- Management of physical and psychological symptoms, and disclosure to the family and significant others if HIV infection and AIDS are confirmed.

CLARIFY

- Was HIV confirmed in the deceased partner?
- Does the patient have suicidal thoughts, plans or intent?

SEEK MORE INFORMATION

GP

- Patient's presentation and the results of investigations carried out to date.

PATIENT

- Continuity of heterosexual relationship with his wife or other women while in the homosexual relationship
- Symptoms of unexplained illness in the wife or any other member of the family
- Onset of psychiatric symptoms, physical symptoms such as headache, dizziness and tiredness, thoughts about the future and of dying or taking his own life, thoughts of harm towards his family
- Look for other neuropsychiatric complications such as anxiety, mania, memory loss and obsessional features.

DIFFERENTIAL DIAGNOSIS/DIFFICULTIES

- *Functional.* Adjustment depressive reaction, acute depressive episode, recurrent depressive disorder
- *Organic.* Organic affective disorder.

APPROACH TO TREATMENT

- Be very sensitive and ensure confidentiality.
- Seek advice from colleagues, seniors and other experts such as hospital legal advisers.
- Carry out appropriate investigations, ascertain the diagnosis and draw up a risk assessment. (Candidates should be aware that procedures and rules governing consent to and testing for HIV/AIDS differ from one jurisdiction to another.)
- Involve a multidisciplinary team and consider a biopsychosocial approach.

WHAT TREATMENT/ADVICE

MEDICAL

- Give treatment for psychiatric illness; use an antidepressant for major depressive illness.
- Treat medical illness using retroviral therapy.
- The genitourinary clinic may carry out contact tracing and treatment.

PSYCHOLOGICAL

- Give support on emotional issues and for disclosure to others, family support and therapy, cognitive behavioural therapy (CBT) for emotional and psychiatric problems, practical problem-solving, liaison with other professionals.

SOCIAL (INCLUDING MARITAL)

- Arrange social help, socialization, and support and interest groups.

SEXUAL HEALTH COUNSELLING

ALTERNATIVE PRACTICES

- Suggest relaxation techniques and massage.

FULL ANSWER

I think this must be a difficult situation for this man to be in. The main issues I would address in this case are determining whether the weight loss and depressive symptoms in the patient are due to HIV infection or AIDS, and also explaining the importance for this gentleman to undergo HIV screening if we are to proceed to address his difficulties and concerns in a meaningful way. There is also the issue of weighing the duty to maintain confidentiality against the need to protect members of his family and others from harm. I would also address the management of his physical and psychological symptoms, and the disclosure of his problems to his family and significant others if HIV infection or AIDS were confirmed.

I would clarify whether the patient was aware of any specific laboratory diagnosis of HIV infection in his deceased partner. I would ask how much he has told his GP and what information he has obtained. I would inform him that I would need to ask other people's advice on his medical illness and test results if I strongly suspected he had HIV and AIDS, and would emphasize the difficulties that would arise were I not able to seek information from people such as his GP. In view of the nature of the possible diagnosis, I would also emphasize that, where I thought he might pose a continuous risk to his wife or others, I would have a public duty to notify the appropriate authorities. I would reassure him that if I had to do this, I would be sensitive and disclose only relevant issues.

Once he understood and agreed to the issues of consent, confidentiality and disclosure, I would proceed to seek more information by taking a detailed history, carrying out a mental state examination and reviewing the relevant physical factors. In the history, I would be particularly interested in the onset of his psychiatric symptoms. I would look for evidence of depression in the past few months and ask him when he started feeling depressed. In addition to the low mood, tiredness and loss of interest, I would enquire about biological symptoms such as early morning wakening, diurnal variation in mood, poor sleep, poor appetite and loss of libido. As many biological symptoms of depression may be present in medical illnesses, I would specifically enquire about associated symptoms such as wishes and thoughts about the future, thoughts of dying or taking his own life, thoughts of harm towards his family (including ideas, plans and intent to end his life or that of others), excessive guilt feelings and hopelessness. I would check for the presence of physical symptoms such as headache, dizziness, tiredness, blurring of vision, nystagmus and ataxia. I would look out for other psychiatric complications of HIV infection, such as anxiety, mania, memory loss and obsessions. I would ask if he had ever involved himself in other high-risk situations, such as intravenous drug use and the sharing of needles.

I would ask him how much his wife and children know about his illness and clarify whether he continued his sexual relationship with wife or other women while involved in the homosexual relationship. I would find out if there are any unexplained symptoms/illness in his wife or any other member of the family. If there are symptoms similar to his own in his family or other acquaintances, then he has probably contracted HIV infection through his homosexual activities. As he would be a high risk for HIV and AIDS, I would encourage him to undergo HIV testing to enable us to confirm the most likely diagnosis.

He would receive pre-test counselling, and if the test was positive, further counselling, which I will describe later. I would consider admission to hospital for a full assessment and medical work-up. As far as possible, I would confirm the diagnosis of HIV infection and carry out other relevant laboratory tests such as an FBC and differentials, blood film studies, U and Es, LFTs, RFTs, ESR, antibody studies, hepatitis B screening, chest X-ray, CT scan and/or MRI. I would also involve a multidisciplinary team, making appropriate referrals to a haematologist and physicians.

In my differential diagnosis I would consider an adjustment depressive reaction, acute depressive episode, recurrent depressive disorder, organic affective disorder and combined anxiety and depressive disorder. In order to have an objective base line of his depressive symptoms, I would rate his mood using a validated instrument such as Beck's Depression Inventory (BDI), Hamilton Rating Scale for Depression (HAMD) or preferably a Hospital Anxiety and Depression Scale (HADS), which does not include somatic items.

In dealing with and approaching the treatment to be given to this man, I would be extremely cautious and sensitive about the confidentiality issues involved. In line with this approach, I would seek advice from colleagues, seniors and other experts and would discuss this with the patient beforehand. I would consider a biopsychosocial approach in my management and treatment plans. I would carry out a risk assessment and consider factors such as family history of suicidal behaviour, childhood trauma, severe depression and previous attempts to commit suicide that would make him a high suicide risk. If I thought he was at high risk of self-harm or suicide, I would admit him to hospital for further assessment and treatment.

The treatment and other care that would be offered would include psychological support and treatment, family support therapy, an antidepressant and psychological treatment such as cognitive behavioural therapy for depression, practical problem-solving, and if necessary, family therapy. A very important part of the medical management would be antiretroviral therapy, which would be closely supervised by the medical team. I would also treat any medical illness arising de novo or as a complication of the HIV infection. I would monitor for side-effects of the medication, particularly side-effects from antiretroviral drugs, which may predispose to confusional states or drug-induced psychosis. Antidepressants would be prescribed only if he had a major depressive disorder. The genitourinary department treating this man might also carry out the necessary contact tracing and treat any other person who had been in sexual contact with him.

Psychological treatment would form a large component of treatment and would include counselling and support from staff for this man who has to face the possibility of pain, debilitation, stigmatization, discrimination, restrictions to lifestyle and disruption in relationships with friends and family. Through careful appraisal, he would also be given support to help him disclose his situation to his wife and significant others. While he would have a choice as to when to disclose and who to disclose to, I would advise that disclosure should be timely and judicious for the sake of harm minimization and risk reduction. There might be a need for continuous family support and therapy, given the various outcomes of such a disclosure. CBT would also be advised to deal with emotional consequences such as anxiety, anger, guilt and obsessions. The aim of CBT would be to increase the patient's level of activity, monitor and reduce automatic negative depressive thoughts, reattribute the control of the illness from the virus to the patient, prevent or reduce preoccupation with the illness, and encourage a positive adjustment to the diagnosis. Through patient problem analysis, I would help him to solve practical problems by encouraging him to reintroduce a planned approach to doing things.

I would assist in liaising with other professionals to ensure that the necessary social support services can be accessed. I would provide sexual health and marital counselling as part of his overall treatment. This would be useful to address the issues of safer sex, reducing the risk of infecting others, adjustment to sexual behaviour, relationship with partner or partners, and sexual rejection. I would stress that this man should desist from any casual or unprotected sex with others. I would make him realize that behaviour that deliberately exposes others to preventable harm may in fact be a criminal offence.

ANSWERS TO SUGGESTED PROBES

1. If I had to do an HIV test, I would:
   - explain the reason why it is useful to carry out the test

- explain what the test involves and its meaning
- advise a visit to the genitourinary department, if the patient requests further information
- arrange for pre-test counselling
- obtain informed consent from the patient.

2. If the HIV test came back positive but the patient insisted I do not tell anybody, my actions would depend on the risk that I think he poses to others, and in particular to his wife. If he had disclosed that he was continuing to have sexual intercourse with his wife and/or others, he would pose a risk of transmitting a potentially fatal illness. I would take the following measures:

- I would advise he discloses the problem to his wife in a very supportive environment.
- If he refused, I would seek further advice from the hospital legal department, my medical defence or protection union or society, and in England and Wales, the hospital Caldicott Guardian. I would inform him of my duty to protect other individuals from harm.
- I would inform him that I would breach confidentiality if he refused to act to protect others from harm.
- I would act to prevent harm to others (including his wife) by breaching his confidentiality and disclosing information.

3. The following symptoms and signs would suggest deterioration in this man's mental health if he tested positive for HIV:

- *Affective.* Increasing depression, emergence of euphoria and manic symptoms, suicidal thoughts, plans, intent and actions
- *Cognitive.* Confusion and disorientation, reduced attention span and poor concentration, memory loss, loss of abstract thinking, AIDS dementia complex
- *Personality.* Disinhibition and aggressive behaviour.

BUZZ WORDS AND USEFUL TERMINOLOGY

Harm and risk minimization or reduction, antiretroviral therapy, confidentiality, duty of care, Caldicott Guardian.

REFERENCES AND SUGGESTED READING

Ankrah E M 1994 The impact of HIV/AIDS on the family and other significant relationships. In: Bor R, Elford J (eds) The Family and HIV. Cassell, London

Catalan J 1999 Mental Health and HIV infection: Psychological and Psychiatric Aspects (Social Aspects of AIDS Series). Taylor & Francis, London

Hays R B, McKusick L, Pollack L et al 1994 Disclosing HIV seropositivity to significant others. In: Bor R, Elford J (eds) The Family and HIV. Cassell, London

Maj M, Bartoli L 1999 Treatment of depression in patients with human immunodeficiency virus infection. Current Opinion in Psychiatry 12(1):93–97

Roy A 2003 Characteristics of HIV patients who attempt suicide. Acta Psychiatrica Scandinavica 107(1):41–44

Zisook S, Peterkin J, Coggin K J et al 1998 Treatment of major depression in HIV seropositive men. Journal of Clinical Psychiatry 59:217–224

A 24-year-old man with paranoid schizophrenia has continued to be psychotic and unwell despite trials of several different medications. He has now been diagnosed with testicular cancer, for which he adamantly refuses any intervention. Staff thinks he lacks capacity and something needs to be done urgently.

What assessment(s) would you make and what advice would you give?

SUGGESTED PROBES

1. What factors would affect your decision to act?
2. How would you assess his capacity to make a decision?
3. Are you aware of any literature or case laws that would back up your actions?

PMP PLAN

TASKS TO DO

The following five areas are relevant to this vignette but are not necessarily all-inclusive. The list is also not exhaustive:

a) Examine the patient's decision to refuse surgery. Ensure it is not part of a psychotic illness or delusional belief system.
b) Discuss treatment with atypical antipsychotics, including clozapine in the first instance, treat mental illness and then re-seek consent for surgical treatment.
c) Demonstrate the limitations of mental health laws in dealing with physical conditions.
d) Show an understanding of the assessment of mental capacity, common law, duty of care, risk assessment and the right of patients to refuse treatment.
e) Consider the need for widespread consultations with relevant others, e.g. GP, carers/family, surgeons and legal experts/court before any intervention.

ISSUES

- Ascertaining if this man's mental illness is clouding his judgment and his capacity to make decisions
- Examining whether he has the capacity to make decisions or not, and what to do if he does have capacity
- Advice to surgeons if he continues to lack capacity.

CLARIFY

- What is his current medical condition and how urgent is the need to carry out the procedure?
- Is there a risk of fatal complications if action is not taken soon?

SEEK MORE INFORMATION

SURGEONS

- Clarification of the diagnosis, nature of the testicular cancer, potential risk and need for urgency, alternative treatments and success rates
- Any attempt to obtain consent by staff of an appropriate level of skill and seniority?
- Prognosis if the patient refuses treatment.

MENTAL HEALTH TEAM

- Record of past treatment
- Current treatment and compliance. Is this patient treatment-resistant?

PATIENT

- Understanding of his mental illness and physical disorder
- Beliefs about testicular cancer and the proposed treatment
- Capacity to make decisions. Consider using the MacArthur principle: does the patient understand the diagnosis of testicular cancer and the treatment proposed? Does he believe the information given is true and relevant to him? Is he able to retain and recall the information given to him? Can he weigh up the information to arrive at a decision about his own health?

SIGNIFICANT OTHERS/FAMILY

- Awareness of illness and presentation
- Corroboration of relevant information.

DIFFERENTIAL DIAGNOSIS/DIFFICULTIES

Not relevant to this vignette.

APPROACH TO TREATMENT

- Ensure adequate explanation.
- Consult widely with relevant others, e.g. GP, carers/family, surgeons, legal experts/court before any intervention.
- Re-seek consent after ensuring adequate treatment.
- If surgery is a life-saving measure, act in the best interests of the patient.

WHAT TREATMENT/ADVICE

- Attempt to treat the schizophrenia more effectively, if you have time.
- Assess the patient's mental capacity to make decisions about own care, if he has capacity and still refuses treatment, or if he lacks capacity and still refuses treatment.

FULL ANSWER

I would first of all ascertain if this man's mental illness is clouding his judgment and his capacity to make decisions about treatment for a potentially fatal condition. The other issue is to examine whether he has the capacity to make decisions or not, and what to do if he does have capacity but still refuses treatment. I would also consider what advice to give to the surgeons if he continued to lack capacity to make decisions about the proposed treatment.

I would clarify this man's medical condition at the time of referral, the need for urgency and whether the surgical treatment being proposed is a life-saving procedure. I would make the referrer understand that it will not be easy to give advice on treating this man, who has a severe and enduring mental illness and is refusing treatment, and that I would need to carry out a detailed assessment and consult with others. Unless the surgery was an urgent life-saving measure, I would advise that the surgeon withholds treatment while I assess the patient. I would quickly arrange to see him to carry out further assessments, but before this, I would seek details of the diagnosis of his current physical problem and also of his treatment for schizophrenia.

I would seek more information on the testicular cancer from the surgeons and find out if the diagnosis is purely clinical or whether there has been histological confirmation. If there has been a firm diagnosis, I would ask how they obtained consent for the testicular biopsy. It might be that the patient's mental state made him more amenable, and at that time he had the capacity to consent to an invasive investigation. I would find out whether this is a low-grade tumour or not, and how much time the surgeons think they have to carry out the procedure to save his life. I would find out about the proposed treatments for testicular cancer and whether the patient has been given alternative treatment, if that is possible. I would also find out if there has been a full explanation of the need for anaesthesia, what would happen during surgery, possible complications, his probable post-operative condition, analgesia and the implications for future fertility.

I would find out from the mental health team responsible for the patient's care about his past treatment and his compliance on different antipsychotics, including atypical ones. I would also ask about his presentation when he is going through an acute-on-chronic psychotic episode. I would find out about the medication and other treatments he has been using, and also whether clozapine or zotepine has been used or discussed with him. I would review his notes to familiarize myself with his treatment to date, and to check whether he has been prescribed adequate doses of medication, whether he has been complying and if there is a possibility that he has been abusing illicit drugs. I would arrange to see him, take a brief and focused history and carry out a mental state examination. In my assessment, I would be interested in his psychotic symptoms, particularly delusions about his body and what a testicular cancer means to him, delusions about the surgeons treating him, grandiose ideas and delusions about his virility, the treatment proposed and perceived conspiracy or persecution by others. I would find out why he has refused the proposed surgery and assess whether he has unresolved concerns about the diagnosis of testicular cancer and the need for treatment, or fear of surgery, anaesthesia, perioperative and post-operative pain, death, and future complications including infertility. I would find out whether he has a relationship at this time and whether he plans to have children in the future.

I would proceed to assess his capacity to make the decision to refuse surgery and examine whether he understands the implications of having testicular cancer, the nature and details of the proposed surgery, the benefit of the proposed treatment in regard to the cancer and his future health and fertility, and the consequences of not having definitive treatment. I would check to see whether he understands the concerns of the surgeons about the urgency of the situation and that alternative treatments have been explained. I would ask him clearly what his wishes are and establish whether he understands the implications of the decision he is making. I would check whether he is able to remember and retain the information given to him about his illness and the proposed treatment, and whether he believes the explanations offered to him. I would also assess if he has the ability to use the information he has been given, and to weigh it up in order to arrive at a decision. I would ask him whether he involved other people (particularly his partner, parent(s) and/or next of kin) in the attempt to make up his mind about what he wants to do, and if these others supported his decision or were against it. This man either lacks capacity to make a decision to refuse surgery or he has that capacity, but there is a third and more difficult scenario: if he meets only some of the criteria for capacity to make a decision, then it becomes difficult to come to a definite conclusion.

Given the diagnosis of a treatment-resistant schizophrenia, I would think that the reason for his refusal of treatment might be due to his delusions about physical abnormality including the treatment proposed, his lack of insight, a genuine fear of surgery and an unwillingness to have the procedure anyway.

In my approach to treatment, I would bear in mind that there are two main issues: a mental illness and a potentially life-threatening physical illness. Since his belief in and opinion of his physical illness might be coloured by his mental illness, I would focus on treating or improving that, if there were time. I would suggest we use clozapine in this case, since it has been found to give significant improvement of symptoms in 60–70% of patients with treatment-resistant schizophrenia. I would expect his symptoms to improve and that he would be able to make a more rational decision about his own treatment and health. I would expect him to get better after treatment with further antipsychotics, psychosocial interventions and other psychological treatments, and thus be able to make the right decision. It would be necessary to reassess his capacity in that respect. If he still refused treatment and had capacity, it would be unlawful to force physical treatment on him just because he is detained under mental health laws. Of course, if urgent intervention were necessary and he did lack capacity, the surgeons would have a duty of care to act in his best interests to save his life.

A more difficult situation would arise if the patient still did not improve despite treatment with clozapine or another potent antipsychotic, or a combination with a drug such as with amisulpiride. I would consult further with the patient, his family and next of kin (or partner), and the surgeons, and seek the advice of other senior medical colleagues, the medical protection society and the legal department of the hospital. If he lacked capacity and continued to refuse treatment, however, we would have a duty of care to offer him definitive surgery and the surgeons would be well advised to go ahead. In the meantime we would continue to engage him and treat his psychosis. The aim would be to act in the best interests of the patient and it might be necessary to go court to obtain permission from a judge. If the patient continued to lack capacity and needed a life-saving procedure for a potentially fatal condition, it would be appropriate to allow the surgeons to go ahead with treatment. The court would be likely to give direction in this regard and to give legal backing for whatever procedure was in question.

If the patient were found to have the capacity to make decisions yet still refused surgery, it would be wrong to override his wishes just because he is mentally ill. That principle would continue to apply, even in a situation where the medical condition was life-threatening. As difficult as it might be, there would be nothing the surgeons could do. Neither would the court have the power to overrule the man's wishes. In a situation like this, we would have to be clear that continued refusal to accept the recommended treatment might lead to death or to irreversible damage to organs or systems. This would be documented properly in the patient's notes.

ANSWERS TO SUGGESTED PROBES

1. The following factors would affect my decision to act:
   - the best interests of the patient
   - the need to save a life (to carry out a life-saving procedure)
   - complete lack of insight
   - lack of capacity to make decisions.
2. In order to assess the patient's capacity to make decisions, I would ascertain whether he:
   - understands the information given to him, what staff think is right or wrong, the reason for surgery, the benefits, and the possible outcomes if he refuses treatment
   - is able to retain the information given to him
   - is able to recall or remember the information given to him about his medical illness, the need for treatment, the nature and details of the surgical procedure, and the implications of agreeing to or refusing treatment
   - believes that the information given to him is true and relevant to him
   - is able to weigh the information in the balance, as part of the decision-making process.
3. The following pieces of literature and case laws would back up my actions:
   i) Thorpe J in Re C (Adult Refusal of Medical Treatment) [1994] 1 All E R 819

The case of C at Broadmoor Hospital readily comes to mind. C, a patient with paranoid schizophrenia, sought court recognition of his capacity to refuse amputation of a gangrenous foot, which was said to be life-threatening. Although C's general capacity had been impaired by schizophrenia, the court held that C understood and retained the information given to him, believed it and had arrived at a clear choice.

It may sound difficult, but if a patient has capacity, he or she is entitled to refuse treatment and the doctor is bound to respect this. A declaration that it is lawful for the doctor to abide by the patient's refusal is unnecessary (Re J T (Adult Refusal Of Medical Treatment) [1998] 1 F L R 48, Wall J).

ii) St George's Healthcare NHS Trust v S [1998] 3 All E R 673 at 702–704 (Guidelines) Joined cases: R. v Collins ex. p S (no. 2 [1999] Fam. 26)

This is the case of a woman who sued St George's Healthcare NHS Trust after a caesarean section was performed against her wishes. The finding of the Court of Appeal was that an unborn child is not a 'person' in need of protection. The court ruled that a person detained under the Act cannot be forced into medical procedures unconnected with her mental condition unless she is deprived of her capacity to decide for herself.

Richard Jones (2001) suggests that the appeal court's finding could be challenged on the grounds that failure to protect the unborn child constitutes a violation of the child's right to life under Article 2 of the Convention on Human Rights Act 1998.

BUZZ WORDS AND USEFUL TERMINOLOGY

Informed consent, mental capacity, duty of care, common law.

REFERENCES AND SUGGESTED READING

Bellhouse J, Holland A, Clare I, Gunn M 2001 Decision-making capacity in adults: its assessment in clinical practice. Advances in Psychiatric Treatment 7:294–301
British Medical Association and Law Society 1995 Assessment of Mental Capacity: Guidance for Doctors and Lawyers. BMA, London
Jones R 2001 Mental Health Act Manual, 7th edn. Sweet & Maxwell, London
Re C (Adult Refusal of Medical Treatment) [1994] 1 All E R 819

10.4 28-YEAR-OLD MAN WITH UNEXPLAINED ABDOMINAL PAIN

A 28-year-old man, who has been investigated many times by his GP, has presented himself to the local accident and emergency department eight times in the last 3 months. He is feeling desperate and asking for help for his chronic abdominal pain. The doctors have found no organic pathology and want your opinion on the possibility of a psychiatric disorder.

Discuss the differential diagnoses and further management.

SUGGESTED PROBES

1. You suspect very strongly that this man has an underlying psychopathology. What evidence in his premorbid adjustment supports this assertion?
2. You are concerned that the treatment you are offering is not going according to plan. What factors would you look for?
3. What is the basis for cognitive behavioural therapy for chronic pain?

PMP PLAN

TASKS TO DO

The following five areas are relevant to this vignette but are not necessarily all-inclusive. The list is also not exhaustive:

a) Appreciate the need to seek relevant information from the GP and from others who may have treated this patient in the past. Mention the need to engage this patient.
b) Discuss the relevant differential diagnoses in this case, including the remote possibility of an as yet undiagnosed physical ailment.
c) Emphasize exploration of the psychosocial dynamics that may underlie the way the patient feels, rather than undergoing further futile searches for a physical cause.
d) Discuss the setting, situation and conditions conducive to successful treatment.
e) Discuss the relevant psychological and behavioural treatment approaches and the role of antidepressants, the pain clinic, CBT and other forms of treatment.

ISSUES

- Ascertaining that the chronic abdominal pain is definitely not due to an organic problem
- Consideration of the fact that it may be an expression of internal distress or a functional illness
- Establishing whether there is an underlying abnormal personality or illness behaviour
- Ensuring that the treatment offered does not perpetuate the disorder.

CLARIFY

- What is it that the patient is desperate about?
- Are there depressive symptoms, and/or suicidal thoughts and behaviour?

SEEK MORE INFORMATION

GP

- Previous diagnosis, investigations, treatment and interventions, current medication.

PATIENT

- Further history, including the chronology and onset of pain, mental state assessment and review of relevant physical findings, reinforcements by family and frequent medical attention, extent of disabilities
- Any legal proceedings related to the illness.

FURTHER INVESTIGATION

- Assessment of the extent of emotional overlay using the MADISON Scale for Markers of Considerable Emotional Overlay. See Table 10.1 for the acronym's significance/ description.

DIFFERENTIAL DIAGNOSIS/DIFFICULTIES

- *Functional.* Psychogenic pain disorder, depressive disorder, hypochondriasis, somatoform pain disorder, somatization disorder, delusional disorder, substance misuse disorder (particularly opiate/narcotic addiction), factitious disorder, malingering, abnormal personality
- *Organic.* Possibility of an as yet undiagnosed organic problem.

Table 10.1 MADISON Scale for Markers of Considerable Emotional Overlay

M = Multiplicity: Pain is either in more than one place or of more than one variety; when treated, may recur elsewhere

A = Authenticity: More interested in clinician's acceptance of pain as genuine than in a cure.

D = Denial: Especially exaggerated marital or family harmony; when admitting depression or anxiety, no impact on pain is admitted.

I = Interpersonal relationship: Although the connection to the presence of any particular person's company as worsening the pain may be denied, observation of the patient's nonverbal and interactive behaviour indicates otherwise.

S = Singularity: When the pain is described as unlike that of anyone else, ever.

O = "Only you": When the patient immediately idealizes the physician as saviour, despite numerous failures by other competent experts.

N = Nothing helps, or no change: When there is no relief whatsoever from any type of intervention, although all are tried (including narcotics) and there is no hour-to-hour or day-to-day fluctuation under a variety of circumstances.

Adapted from Hackett TP, Cassem NH: Massachusetts General Handbook of General Hospital Psychiatry. Mosby, St. Louis, 1978.

APPROACH TO TREATMENT

- Take a non-judgmental approach and try to understand the situation from the patient's point of view.
- Engage the patient to avoid 'doctor shopping'.
- Disapprove of further futile laboratory investigations.
- Make your treatment multidisciplinary and multidimensional.
- Consider the appropriate setting, situation and timing for treatment.

WHAT TREATMENT/ADVICE

MEDICAL

Give antidepressant treatment for depression (consider a sedative antidepressant for insomnia). Treat opiate and benzodiazepine addictions.

PSYCHOLOGICAL

- Arrange CBT for chronic pain and access to the pain clinic.

SOCIAL

- Arrange daytime activities.

OTHER

- Propose physiotherapy, supervised exercise and transcutaneous electrical nerve stimulation (TENS).

Note: candidates should be aware of the task required by the examiner. You are asked in this vignette to give the differential diagnoses first.

FULL ANSWER

The difficulty here is that of a man who has been frequenting his local accident and emergency department and whose GP has not found an organic problem despite extensive investigations. As part of the differential diagnosis I would consider psychogenic pain disorder, a depressive disorder, hypochondriasis, somatization disorder and delusional disorder. I would also consider the possibility of a substance misuse disorder (particularly opiate or narcotic addiction), for which the patient is seeking opiate analgesics and/or hypnotics. A factitious disorder, malingering and an abnormal personality are other differential diagnoses to be considered. These would be important if there were anything to suggest that this man might be deriving a secondary gain from the attention he receives for his pain. Finally, an unlikely possibility is that he has an as yet undiagnosed medical condition despite the 'extensive' medical investigations.

The first issue I would like to address is ensuring that this man's chronic abdominal pain is definitely not due to an organic problem. The other points to consider are that his pain might be an expression of internal distress or a functional illness such as depression, and there might also be an underlying abnormal personality or illness behaviour. One other important issue is to ensure that whatever treatment is offered to this man does not perpetuate the disorder.

When I saw the patient, I would clarify what exactly is making him desperate. I would examine for the presence of depressive symptoms, biological signs of depression, and suicidal thoughts and behaviour. Once I was sure that he was not in any immediate danger of harming himself or others (whom he may consider to be not helping), I would proceed to assess him as soon as possible.

While making preparations to assess him, I would seek more information from his GP on the previous diagnosis, investigations, treatment and interventions. I would take a further history from the patient on the chronology and onset of pain, and personal past psychiatric histories, carry out a mental state assessment and also review the relevant physical findings. Concerning the pain, I would ascertain as far as possible whether it was the cause of a coexisting psychiatric disorder or the result of another psychiatric syndrome. I would examine whether the pain distribution and quality conformed to known anatomical and physiological patterns. I would also find out whether the quality and location of the pain vary from time to time, particularly with any life events. I would ask whether he thinks the pain is due to a particular condition or disease, despite the condition not being diagnosed. I would also find out whether the onset was related to an injury at work or elsewhere. If there were a preceding injury, I would find out if this man has sought or is seeking compensation for his injury.

I would assess his mood for depression, evidence of anxiety mixed with depression, and insomnia, for which the patient might be seeking or using excessive amount of narcotics, sedative hypnotic agents and/or alcohol. I would also check whether there is an associated loss of appetite, energy and interests. As already stated, I would ask about biological symptoms of severe depression and thoughts, ideas, plans and/or intent to self-harm or harm others. I would examine the basis for his complaints to see whether there is a delusional quality or there are any other abnormal beliefs. I would assess the extent of the disability that the pain has caused, in particular with relation to work and employment opportunities, leisure, social interactions and family life. I would ask questions about any breakdown in family dynamics and the role played by reinforcements on the part of the family and by frequent medical attention. I would examine for any evidence suggesting that the patient might be deriving secondary gains that might reinforce his presentation. These would include monetary gains, opportunities for seeking human relationships and exemption from societal and/or civil roles, manipulation and control of others, particularly family members, and the prospect of compensation for an injury or payment of pension and retirement benefits. Where possible, I would ask our psychologist to assess the extent of emotional overlay concerning his symptoms using the MADISON Scale for Markers of Considerable Emotional Overlay. Although not rigorously validated the scale (as in Table 10.1 on page 338) can prove very useful.

In my approach to treatment, I would not underestimate the experience of this patient, who has been suffering from 'chronic pain'. I would ensure that I engaged him and let him know that I understand the way he is feeling and will try to relieve his symptoms as far as possible. Irrespective of what I consider to be the differential diagnoses, I would suggest that there might be other psychological and psychosocial factors contributing to his symptoms, since investigations, tests and interventions have not revealed any pathology. I would suggest that these factors be explored to end this cycle of 'doctor shopping'. I would clearly disapprove of further extensive investigations and referrals to specialists or subspecialists. I would therefore suggest that we concentrate on the issues in his life that might be making the experience of pain more difficult to bear or the psychosocial factors perpetuating his illness.

Concerning the treatment to be offered, I would consider biological, psychological and psychosocial issues in this case and treat accordingly in a multidisciplinary and multidimensional way. Most of the treatment would be given in an outpatient setting, with the patient being seen on a regular basis, usually by the same person or persons, if that were possible. I would suggest that we continue treatment for as long as there is an improvement. If there were pending litigation issues to be resolved, I would plan the interventions for after the outcomes of the court proceedings. I would suggest that as part of the medical management of his condition, we should try using antidepressants, some of which have been found useful in patients with chronic pain linked to depression. If opiates have been used in the management of this man's chronic pain, he might have already developed an addiction to them, and to any benzodiazepines that have been given for insomnia associated with pain. I would seek to discontinue the drugs very gradually. I would consider the use of tricyclic antidepressants (TCAs), which have been found useful in patients with pain disorders, even in the absence of a frank depressive disorder. I would also consider other antidepressants such as the selective serotonin re-uptake inhibitors (SSRIs), or other sedative antidepressants such as trazodone or venlafaxine to help him to sleep better. This would also help to reduce dependence on hypnotics used for insomnia.

The other treatment options are psychological and take the form of counselling, cognitive behavioural therapy and supportive psychotherapy. Group therapy appears to yield better outcomes than individual therapy. In planning psychological treatment, I would lay down guidelines for continuing and discontinuing treatment. If there were no improvement after 6 months, I would seek to terminate the treatment. The other approaches would be forms of social treatment to engage this gentleman in useful and safe activities, possibly at a day centre or hospital. He might also benefit from other treatments such as physiotherapy and safe, graded, supervised exercises. I hope that, with this combination of multidisciplinary strategies, he would get better and be less dependent on medications that are potentially addictive. I would think, with these measures, he would be better able to tolerate his symptoms.

The other major part of management of this case would consist of advice to his GP. I suggest that the GP see him regularly rather than giving symptom-prompted appointments. He or she should not carry out further investigations unless needed after a new and major development. Similarly, unnecessary specialist consultations should be avoided, as they would only serve to perpetuate the problems. The GP should also maintain the stance of believing the patient's symptoms are 'real and not in the patient's head'. During consultations enquiries should also be broadened out into psychosocial areas to encourage improved functional outcome.

Note: the vignette starts by asking the candidate to give the differential diagnoses. This should always be kept in mind.

ANSWERS TO SUGGESTED PROBES

1. Evidence to support the assertion that this man has an underlying psychopathology would include:
   - alcohol and/or drug abuse
   - sexual difficulties
   - multiple relationships and marriages
   - poor employment history.
2. If I were concerned that treatment was not going according to plan, I would look for:
   - evidence of 'doctor shopping'
   - sourcing and use of drugs or medications not agreed in the treatment plan
   - increasing use of drugs and alcohol
   - an overwhelming psychosocial situation
   - ongoing litigation that had to do with the abdominal pain
   - presence of a depressive disorder.
3. The basis for using CBT for chronic pain is as follows:
   - Individuals with similar physical pathologies experience pain differently.
   - Individuals experiencing pain have negative assumptions and beliefs.
   - Negative assumptions, such as catastrophizing (expecting or worrying about major negative consequences from a situation, even one of minor importance), affect cognition of pain.
   - Events relating to pain are interpreted through this 'perpetual negative' lens.
   - Individual pain-related cognitions and coping responses affect adaptation to pain.
   - This interpretation affects the way individuals respond to pain and the environment (see Fig. 10.1).

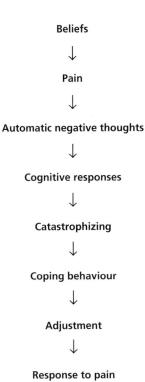

Beliefs

↓

Pain

↓

Automatic negative thoughts

↓

Cognitive responses

↓

Catastrophizing

↓

Coping behaviour

↓

Adjustment

↓

Response to pain

Fig. 10.1 How individuals respond to pain and the environment.

- The aim of CBT is to challenge dysfunctional assumptions and beliefs, attempt a cognitive restructuring and to modify maladaptive behaviour in response to pain.

BUZZ WORDS AND USEFUL TERMINOLOGY

'Doctor shopping', sick role, secondary gain, dysfunctional assumptions, automatic negative thoughts, negative reinforcement.

REFERENCES AND SUGGESTED READING

Guggenheim F G 1999 Somatoform disorder. In: Sadock B J, Sadock V A (eds) Kaplan & Sadock's Comprehensive Textbook of Psychiatry, vol. 2, 7th edn. Lippincott, Williams and Wilkins, Philadelphia, pp 1504–1532

Jenkins P L G 1991 Psychogenic abdominal pain. General Hospital Psychiatry 13:27

Turner J A, Jensen M P, Romano J M 2000 Do beliefs, coping, and catastrophising independently predict functioning in patients with chronic pain? Pain 85:115–125

10.5 24-YEAR-OLD MAN WHO HAS A TONIC-CLONIC SEIZURE DURING A PSYCHIATRIC ADMISSION

A 24-year-old unemployed male has been admitted to your ward for depression. Four days into his admission, he has a tonic-clonic seizure. He is due in court in 2 weeks for possession and supply of amphetamines. There are suggestions within the team that he is 'putting it on' to avoid the criminal justice system.

What are your differential diagnoses and how will you manage this situation?

SUGGESTED PROBES

1. What are the differential diagnoses?
2. What other information would you need to arrive at a safe diagnosis?
3. How would you manage the situation?

PMP PLAN

TASKS TO DO

The following five areas are relevant to this vignette but are not necessarily all-inclusive. The list is also not exhaustive:

a) Discuss the relevance of clinical examination and laboratory investigations in distinguishing between epileptic and non-epileptic pseudoseizures.
b) Describe clearly the organic and non-organic aetiological factors, particularly dissociative convulsions.
c) Show awareness of the risk of brain injury and brain abscess secondary to a thromboembolic phenomenon following drug injections.
d) Demonstrate an understanding of the use of psychotropics in a patient with seizure disorder, and the use of anticonvulsants in patients with mental disorders.
e) Address the issue of support for the patient, the different opinions within the team and avoidance of 'splitting'.

ISSUES

• Determining whether this man is suffering from an epileptic seizure disorder or a non-epileptic seizure, otherwise called 'pseudoseizure' or dissociative convulsions.

CLARIFY

- Is there any immediate risk or life-threatening situation?
- Is the seizure under control?
- Have staff ensured the removal of any potential source of injury to prevent further harm?

SEEK MORE INFORMATION

WARD STAFF

- Witnesses to any of the seizures
- Timing, duration and characteristics of the seizures. Associated features such as foaming at the mouth, incontinence, degree of loss of consciousness. Patient's control over the seizures. Does the patient remember the event, or did he try to stop himself falling?
- Reason that some staff think he is faking.

MEDICAL NOTES

- Review of illicit drug intake, medication history
- Detoxification from substances.

GP

- Past medical history, history of febrile convulsions, head injury and seizure disorders, including treatment
- Anticonvulsant therapy.

PATIENT

- Full history, review of medical history (previous head injury and/or epilepsy), compliance with antiepileptic medication, if prescribed
- Drug and alcohol history, benzodiazepine or barbiturate abuse
- Mental and physical state examination. Septic injection sites or cellulite. Focal neurological deficits. Patient's recall.

INVESTIGATIONS

- Routine bloods: prolactin levels, FBC, U and Es, LFTs, RFTs, urine drug screen (for benzodiazepines and barbiturates), CT scan, MRI, EEG, telemetry and ECG.

DIFFERENTIAL DIAGNOSIS/DIFFICULTIES

- *Organic.* Organic epileptic seizure (?drug-induced, infection), organic non-epileptic seizure, organic seizures secondary to thromboembolic phenomena, brain abscess, substance misuse/withdrawal state from drugs (particularly benzodiazepines and barbiturates) and alcohol, medication-induced
- *Functional.* Dissociative convulsions, non-epileptic seizures (pseudoseizures), acute depressive episode/recurrent depressive disorder with hysterical conversion, factitious disorder, malingering, personality disorder.

WHAT TREATMENT/ADVICE

See Table 10.2.

FULL ANSWER

In dealing with this man, I would like to consider broadly organic and non-organic causes. I am aware there has been a suggestion

Table 10.2 Management plan for patients with seizure

	Biological/ medical	Psychological	Social
Immediate	Terminate seizures using benzodiazepines Oxygen	Nurse in calm, quiet environment	Support for carer
Short-term	Treat any organic cause Treat withdrawal reactions Medical referral	Detailed psychological evaluation	Support in attending court case
Long-term	Antidepressant, anticonvulsant	Psychological treatment for addiction	Assistance with further education and training, vocational activities or gainful employment

within the team that the gentleman might be faking his symptoms. The main issue for me would be to determine whether he actually suffered a true seizure or had a 'pseudoseizure' or 'non-epileptic fit', but I would go ahead and carry out an objective assessment to rule out any treatable conditions.

Concerning the differential diagnoses, I would consider organic and non-organic causes for this problem, bearing in mind that the presentation might be due to both. For the organic causes, I would consider epileptic and non-epileptic seizures, organic seizures secondary to a thromboembolic phenomenon, brain abscess, and substance misuse or withdrawal state from drugs and substances, particularly benzodiazepines, barbiturates and alcohol. The fit might also be medication-induced, possibly caused by antidepressants. I would consider functional causes such as dissociative convulsions (or non-organic pseudoseizures), hysterical conversion, malingering and also factitious disorder.

In addressing this case, I would first clarify what medical condition the patient was in at the time of referral, and ask whether appropriate help had been summoned. My immediate priority would be to terminate the seizure using intravenous benzodiazepines or rectal administration of diazepam, if necessary. I would also advise staff to nurse the patient in a safe position while I quickly made my way to the ward. On getting there, I would deal with anything that could pose a further risk or cause a life-threatening situation. I would remove the patient from potential sources of injury in order to prevent further harm. I would advise staff to check his oxygen saturation pressure (SPO_2) in order to rule out hypoxia.

In order to arrive at a safe diagnosis, I would want to seek further information from the GP, review the medical notes and speak to staff and the patient himself. I would ask the GP for any previous history or treatment suggestive of an epileptic disorder or brain injury, including brain damage due to alcohol or drug use. I would enquire whether he has been prescribed any anticonvulsants or benzodiazepines by the practice. I would ask ward staff whether the seizures were witnessed by anyone and about their timing, duration, characteristics and nature. I would ask about associated features such as foaming at the mouth, incontinence, degree of loss of consciousness and whether the patient appeared to have control over the seizure. I would find out if the patient remembers events surrounding the seizure, if he tried to stop himself falling, and why some staff think he is faking.

I would see the patient to take a further relevant history, and carry out mental state examination, physical assessment and further investigations. I would be particularly interested in the evolution of his depression and its relationship to his alcohol and/or drug use. I would take a detailed alcohol and drug history (amphetamines, benzodiazepines and barbiturates), particularly exploring dependence on these substances. I would ask about any previous consequences of his drug use and any previous complications such as seizures and blackouts. In the meantime, I would suspend the antidepressant, which itself might have lowered the seizure threshold in a person who is predisposed to the development of fits. In my mental state assessment I would explore the patient's depression and would later explore with our unit psychologist the meaning of these experiences for this man. I would explore his anxieties and worries about the impending court case and check whether the fit was a plot by him to evade a court appearance. In order to assist with my assessment I would examine his mood using a Beck's Depression Inventory (BDI) and also assess him on a Malingering Scale. I would check carefully whether he had obsessive symptoms and was in a post-ictal confusional or psychotic state.

I would examine this gentleman for signs of head injury, localized and focal neurological lesions, withdrawal state or intoxication, foaming at the mouth and/or injury to any of the oral structures, track marks of intravenous drug use and evidence of localized and/or systemic infections. I would arrange for him to have his serum prolactin levels measured within 20 minutes of any seizure and review his investigations. In addition to these, I would ensure that baseline blood investigations were normal (FBC, U and Es and ECG). I would ask staff to keep a chart to monitor the pattern and frequency of fits and would refer the patient for an urgent EEG. This would be to check whether he has a positive EEG suggestive of epilepsy, a diffuse or global cerebral abnormality or localized intracranial pathology. It might be necessary to carry out a CT scan, an MRI, sleep EEG or telemetry to make sure we do not miss an organic disorder. I would also liaise with the local neurology registrar or consultant to assess and give a specialist opinion on the management of this man.

In my approach to treatment, I would endeavour to establish whether this man has true seizures or not, bearing in mind that this might prove difficult. The three main things that I would focus on in planning treatment would be centred around treatment for the seizure disorder, depending on whether these are epileptic seizures, seizures due to another organic psychopathology or dissociative convulsions; the cause and treatment of his depression; and last but not the least, his problematic illicit drug use for which he is being brought to court. The strongest possibility is that a predisposing seizure disorder state, pre-existing epilepsy or an organic condition is the aetiological factor for the seizures. Once I was clear in my mind, I would deal with the issue of addiction, if the patient agreed. Then we would be able to assess the depression better. If the man were depressed, I would treat him with an antidepressant. If he had an epileptic seizure or an organic condition, I would treat accordingly.

I would call a team meeting to iron out differences in opinion and review the findings of the investigations and assessments. We would then agree on a care plan based on these findings and on the patient's needs, in order to minimize division within the team. Concerning treatment, the immediate management would be to ensure that the seizure was terminated using one of the benzodiazepines. I would also advise oxygen by face mask while awaiting further medical help to treat any organic causes and withdrawal reactions, and the making of the appropriate medical referral. In the short term I would advise that he is nursed in a calm and quiet environment. I would investigate any organic illness and treat it accordingly, and also give antidepressants and anticonvulsants as necessary. I would prescribe only antidepressants with low pro-convulsive effects, such as citalopram, trazodone or nefazodone. (Nefazodone carries the risk of hepatotoxicity and is no longer available on the UK market.) Other modalities for treating depression in this man include cognitive behavioural therapy. A detailed psychological evaluation would be carried out in order to pinpoint the main cause of this man's problems. If this man had a factitious disorder, then specialized CBT would be advised. There is some preliminary evidence that CBT may be effective in dissociative convulsions.

In the long term, I would advise that this man be given treatment for his addiction and assistance with the criminal justice system, such as support in attending the court case. As he is unemployed, longer-term measures would include assistance with further education and training, vocational activities (including a day centre) and even gainful employment at the appropriate time.

ANSWERS TO SUGGESTED PROBES

The answers to the suggested probes have been given in the full answer. It is advised that candidates answer questions relevant to the specific scenario rather than being over-inclusive.

While it is advised that candidates stick to a structure that they find convenient and useful, they should note that, in this particular vignette, the examiner has asked for the differential diagnoses first. The answer should therefore begin with the differential diagnosis.

BUZZ WORDS AND USEFUL TERMINOLOGY

Telemetry, post-ictal confusion, pro-convulsive effect.

REFERENCES AND SUGGESTED READING

Iriarte J, Parra J, Urrstarazu E et al 2003 Controversies in the diagnosis and management of psychogenic pseudoseizures. Epilepsy and Behaviour 4:354–359

Lesser R P 1996 Psychogenic seizures. Neurology 46(6):1499–1507

Prueter C, Schultz-Venrath U, Rimpau W 2002 Dissociative and associated psychopathological symptoms in patients with epilepsy, pseudoseizures, and both seizure forms. Epilepsia 43(2):188–192

10.6 27-YEAR-OLD MOTHER OF THREE REFUSING LIVER TRANSPLANTATION

The medical team has referred to you a 27-year-old divorced mother of three young children, who has refused to have a liver transplant. She recently took an overdose of 100 tablets of paracetamol with the intention of killing herself.

How would you go about assessment and what advice would you give to the medical team?

SUGGESTED PROBES

1. You conclude that this patient now lacks capacity but discover that she gave an advance directive before she became unwell that 'under no circumstances should she be given an organ transplant'. What would be your advice?
2. What strategies would you use to improve this patient's capacity if you conclude that she lacks it?
3. You decide to admit this woman to a psychiatric ward under mental health legislation. Is there any need to assess her capacity at this stage? If not, when would it be necessary?

PMP PLAN

TASKS TO DO

The following five areas are relevant to this vignette but are not necessarily all-inclusive. The list is also not exhaustive:

a) Try to clarify why a psychiatric opinion is being sought and correct any misconception at an early stage.
b) Establish the possible reasons why the patient does not want to have treatment. For example, patient may be poorly informed, or have an inability to make decisions because of anxiety or an underlying mental disorder affecting her capacity.
c) Demonstrate awareness that, in an emergency, common law can be used to treat this patient.
d) Attempt to explore the reasons why the patient declined medical intervention.
e) Be conversant with assessment of the patient's capacity.

ISSUES

- Establishing whether this lady has the capacity to decline treatment or not
- Establishing whether she is currently suffering from a mental illness that may affect her capacity to make decisions about her treatment.

CLARIFY

- Does the medical team think the patient is suffering from a mental illness and/or lacks capacity?
- Is the patient conscious enough to be interviewed?
- Is there any relevant psychiatric history and is this related to her current decision to refuse treatment?

SEEK MORE INFORMATION

REFERRER

- Seriousness of the patient's condition at present, without medical intervention; how long is she expected to survive without treatment?
- Nature of the operation, in terms of procedures and prognosis
- Whether the patient's decision is related to any underlying depressive or psychotic illness.

PATIENT

- Circumstances surrounding the overdose in terms of planning, seriousness and attempts to conceal the act
- Evidence of an underlying mental illness, such as psychosis or depression
- Any particular reason why she is refusing treatment: feelings of hopelessness about getting better, reaction to a social stressor, given that she is divorced and having to cope with three children on her own, or, in the case of psychosis, delusions or hallucinations that are behind her decision
- Detailed assessment of her capacity: i.e. awareness of the relevant facts about the operation, understanding of the nature and purpose of the intervention, risks and benefits of the intervention, risks of not carrying out the intervention, ability to retain and recall the information given, belief that the information given is true and relevant to her, ability to weigh the information in the balance as part of the process of arriving at a decision.

DIFFERENTIAL DIAGNOSIS/DIFFICULTIES

- *Functional.* Decision related to feelings of hopelessness in the context of depression, psychotic illness with command hallucination telling her not to accept treatment, no underlying mental illness
- *Organic.* Acute confusional state, information too complex to understand or process, language barrier, hearing difficulty.

APPROACH TO TREATMENT

- Arrange to assess this patient at the earliest opportunity, preferably in the presence of the treating physician or surgeon.
- Explore and consider the various issues in the presentation, including reasons for refusing treatment.
- Make a decision on whether she has capacity or not.
- Whatever the outcome of the capacity assessment and should time permit, consider seeking advice from the trust or hospital's solicitor or medical indemnity body.

WHAT TREATMENT/ADVICE

IF SHE LACKS CAPACITY AND REFUSES TREATMENT

- If time permits, try to improve her capacity, depending on what the problem is: for example, improving language or communication difficulties, or presenting the information in a simpler way.
- If there is an underlying psychiatric illness, treat with appropriate psychotropic medication in the hope that, if her condition improves, she would agree to the medical intervention.
- Treat any acute confusional state.
- If she continues to lack capacity, advise the physicians to offer the necessary treatment to save her life. Bear in mind that the decision to treat is that of the treating doctor and that the doctor should take the decision in the best interests of the patient, i.e. under common law.

IF CAPACITY IS PRESENT AND SHE REFUSES TREATMENT

- Advise the referring team to provide written information on treatment in the hope that she will reconsider her stance.
- Continue to see her and give her the opportunity to ask questions rather than getting angry with her for refusing treatment.

- Offer her the best available treatment in keeping with her wishes.
- Abide by her wish to refuse treatment.

FULL ANSWER

The history raises several issues. First is whether this lady, who is refusing liver transplantation following a massive overdose, has the capacity to decline treatment or not. Second is the issue of whether she is currently suffering from a mental illness that might affect her capacity to make decisions about her treatment.

To begin with, I would like to clarify with the referring team whether they think the patient is suffering from a mental illness or lacks capacity, and how they came to their conclusion. I would ask if they knew of any relevant psychiatric history and if they thought this is related to her current decision to refuse treatment. I would try to correct at an early stage any misconception they might have about the use of mental health laws (Mental Health Act 1983 in England and Wales) to enforce medical treatment, which in this case happens to be a liver transplant. I would also clarify with the referrer whether the patient is sufficiently conscious and medically fit to be interviewed.

I would then proceed to seek more information from the referrer and the patient. I would ask about the seriousness of her condition and how long she is expected to survive without treatment. I would use the opportunity to familiarize myself with the nature of the operation, in terms of procedures and prognosis, prior to assessing the patient's ability to use such information to arrive at a decision and communicate her choice. I would arrange to see her on the ward, preferably with the operating surgeon, as he or she would be best informed about the nature of the treatment proposed and the risks and benefits of receiving or refusing treatment. When I saw this woman, I would make sure that she was not confused and was able to engage in the interview and make informed decisions. I would ask about the circumstances of the overdose in terms of planning, seriousness and attempts to conceal her actions. I would assess the seriousness of the suicide attempt and find out how she eventually got to hospital. I would ask her why she is refusing treatment and if she feels hopeless about getting better. I would ask if she finds it difficult to cope with three children on her own and if she has considered what would happen to them if she dies. I would find out if there are other psychosocial stressors, which is likely, given that she is recently divorced and may be in financial difficulties or engaged in child custody proceedings. As the care and safety of these three children might be at risk, I would ask whether staff have made the necessary referral to the local social services department for foster placement, if there are no close family members to look after the children.

I would look for evidence of any underlying mental illness such as adjustment disorder, depression or psychosis, and whether any of the differential diagnoses are contributing to her feelings of hopelessness. I would check for any associated delusional or hallucinatory experiences that might be interfering with her capacity to make decisions. I would be particularly concerned about any delusional interpretation of her illness and intended treatment. I would ask about command hallucinations prompting her to refuse treatment. In assessing her capacity to make decisions, I would like to know if she understands the relevant facts given to her, the nature of her illness, the purpose of the proposed treatment, the risks and benefits of the intervention, and whether she understands the risk of not having a liver transplant. I would assess whether she is able to retain and recall the information given to her, and if she believes that the information is true and relevant to her situation. I would also assess whether she is able to weigh all the information in the balance as part of the process of arriving at a decision. Whilst not directly relevant to the assessment of her capacity, I would bear in mind that the presence of a mental illness could affect this woman's decision-making capacity. I would therefore give consideration as to whether she is suffering from a mental illness such as depression or psychosis, or perhaps whether she has no mental illness at all. I would assess whether her decision to refuse treatment is related to the complexity of the information she has been given or to the presence of language or communication difficulties, or if she has made this decision with full capacity.

In advising on the above issues, my approach would be first to review all the available information, to consult with relatives and other professionals, and then decide whether or not this woman has the capacity to make a decision on the proposed treatment. Given the complexity of the situation, I would advise the treating clinician or surgeon to contact his or her hospital or trust legal department or even the medical defence union for advice and guidance. In addition to the above, due to the contentious nature of issues relating to capacity and thus the propensity for such cases to be subjected to a high degree of medical and legal scrutiny, I would ensure that any records on this patient were clear, precise and legible. Also, the final decision and opinion and the rationale behind them would be clearly documented in accordance with all the formalities of correct note-making.

I would ensure that the diagnosis of any mental disorder was stated clearly, or the fact that there is none and what steps have been taken to exclude it. In a situation where this patient lacked capacity, I would document clearly whether treatment of her mental disability might restore her capacity to make the decision and how long this might be expected to take. All these factors would influence the decision as to whether she should be treated under common law, should she lack capacity at that particular point.

It would be much easier if a decision could be made as to whether this woman has capacity or not, but in reality things might not be so clear-cut. If her capacity remained in doubt and she continued to refuse treatment, I would advise the medical team to consult her relatives to ask if they know of her wishes before she became ill. If time permitted, I would suggest that the medical team attempt to improve the patient's capacity by attending to any language or communication problems, presenting information in a simpler form and, if there was no contraindication, treating an acute confusional state or any underlying mental illness. If there were a desperate need to act to keep this patient alive, she would have to be treated under common law in her best interests, but the least invasive procedure should be considered when such a decision is taken. Obviously, if she lacked capacity to make decisions about her own treatment, that treatment would have to be given under common law against her wishes. In this case I would advise the team to go ahead with the necessary treatment to save her life.

A more difficult situation would be if she had capacity but was refusing treatment. If she clearly understood, retained, believed and was able to weigh the relevant information, I would assume she had capacity, no matter how irrational I might think her decision. If this were the situation, I would advise the medical team to document clearly the various consultations that have been made and how they arrived at the decision. I would also advise them to provide written information on the proposed treatment, in the hope that she would reconsider her stance. The medical team should also continue to see her and give her the opportunity to ask questions, rather than getting angry about her decision not to comply with their treatment advice. They would have to offer her the best available treatment in keeping with her wishes, even if this might mean abiding by her refusal of treatment in the face of death.

ANSWERS TO SUGGESTED PROBES

1. If the patient had made an advance directive prior to becoming mentally unwell, I would unfortunately have to respect that, but I would seek the opinion of senior colleagues and my medical defence union.
2. Strategies to improve this patient's capacity are covered in the full answer.
3. Admission under a section of the Mental Health Act—for example, Section 3—does not require capacity assessment as the decision only takes into account the combined criteria of presence of a mental disorder (status), the initial severity of the disorder, and the perceived outcome without intervention (risk). However, if treatment of the mental disorder were to go beyond 3 months under Section 3 of the Mental Health Act, this would require either the patient's consent or the opinion of a second doctor appointed by the Mental Health Act Commission.

BUZZ WORDS AND USEFUL TERMINOLOGY

Capacity assessment, common law.

REFERENCES AND SUGGESTED READING

Bellhouse J, Holland A, Clare I, Gunn M 2001 Decision-making capacity in adults: its assessment in clinical practice. Advances in Psychiatric Treatment 7:294–301

British Medical Association and Law Society 1995 Assessment of Mental Capacity: Guidance for Doctors and Lawyers. BMA, London

Jones R 2001 Mental Health Act Manual, 7th edn. Sweet & Maxwell, London

Re C (Adult Refusal of Medical Treatment) [1994] 1 All E R 819

10.7 51-YEAR-OLD MAN WITH ERECTILE DYSFUNCTION

A GP has referred to you a 51-year-old man who has been having erectile problems. He wants a prescription for sildenafil (Viagra), an anti-impotence drug, but the GP thinks there are underlying psychological problems.

How would you go about assessing and managing this patient?

SUGGESTED PROBES

1. What are the possible psychological factors that could contribute to erectile problems in this patient?
2. If this man's impotence began following a radical prostatectomy, would he still benefit from sildenafil? Please explain the reason for your answer.
3. What do you know about Masters and Johnson's technique, or sensate focus therapy?

PMP PLAN

TASKS TO DO

The following five areas are relevant to this vignette but are not necessarily all-inclusive. The list is also not exhaustive:

a) Be sensitive and empathic in your approach.
b) Assess systematically, focusing on possible underlying organic and functional factors.
c) Consider the various diagnostic possibilities and differentiate between total and partial impotence and erectile difficulties.
d) Demonstrate awareness of the need to explore the consequences of the man's erectile difficulties.
e) Demonstrate a good knowledge of the various treatment approaches and the rationale behind them.

ISSUES

- Effectively ruling out organic causes of erectile dysfunction in this man
- Identifying the main psychological factors underlying the erectile dysfunction
- Treatment strategies to alleviate the erectile problems.

CLARIFY

- Why is the patient being referred now?

- Is the problem actually erectile dysfunction?
- What is the nature of the problem: erectile or ejaculatory, primary or secondary?
- Was onset sudden or gradual?
- How soon does the GP want the patient to be seen?
- Are there any immediate risk or safety concerns?

SEEK MORE INFORMATION

GP

- Patient's medical and surgical history, with particular attention to neurological disease such as multiple sclerosis, spinal injury; endocrine disorders such as hypothyroidism and diabetes; vascular diseases; traumatic injury to the perineum; use of drugs like beta-blockers that might interfere with endocrine or neurovascular function.

PATIENT

- Full history, including the nature, onset and course of erectile dysfunction. Criteria for male erectile disorder under paragraph F52.2 of ICD–10 (failure of genital response) or male erectile disorder under paragraph 302.72 of the DSM–IV
- His rating of erection quality on a scale of 0 to 10 (with 10 being the best-quality erection) under a variety of circumstances: for example, upon awakening, with fantasy, masturbation, foreplay, intercourse with different partners
- Unusual and/or disturbing life circumstances coincident with the development of the erectile problem
- Other parameters of sexual life, including sexual drive, frequency of lovemaking, orgasmic difficulties and sexual satisfaction
- Performance anxiety and its magnitude
- Detailed sexual development and experience, including attitude to puberty, onset of sexual interest, previous sexual experience and problems, masturbation, traumatic experiences (e.g. sexual abuse)
- Gender orientation and gender identity problems, as conflicts in this area may produce erectile dysfunction
- Details of relationship with partner, including its development, previous sexual adjustments, general relationship, children and contraception, infidelity, commitment to relationship, feelings and attraction towards partner
- Quality of couple's non-sexual relationship

- Family background and early childhood, including relationships with parents, parental relationship and family attitude towards sex
- Presence of organic factors, psychological factors or both in the development and maintenance of this man's problem
- Social aspects of this man's life, including finance- and work-related difficulties
- Detailed mental state examination.

INVESTIGATIONS

- Bloods for glucose, creatinine, lipids, thyroid hormones, testosterone, sex hormone-binding globulin, luteinizing hormone, prolactin
- Possible referral to specialist sexual disorder clinic, where further investigations such as the nocturnal penile tumescence test and/or Doppler colour imaging would be considered (the latter providing detailed information about penile haemodynamics to help distinguish arterial insufficiency from veno-occlusive dysfunction).

PHYSICAL EXAMINATION

- Body fat distribution, facial and pubic hair (gives an estimate of adequacy of androgen)
- Neurological examination with evaluation of the S2–S4 dermatomes by testing perineal sensation, anal sphincter tone and the bulbocavernosus reflex
- Vascular examination with checks on blood pressure, cardiac status and lower extremity pulses
- Evidence of Peyronie's plaque and examination of the testes to confirm their size, location and consistency.

PARTNER

Seek the patient's permission to see his partner.

- Her/his view of and sympathy for the problem
- The couple's expectations about and motivation for seeking further investigations and treatment.

DIFFERENTIAL DIAGNOSIS/DIFFICULTIES

- *Psychological.* Anxiety, depression, alcohol and drug problems. Psychogenic cause if onset is sudden, if the problem occurs only in specific situations and the patient has normal nocturnal and early morning erections. Social problems, marital/relationship difficulties and financial worries

- *Organic*. Endocrine: diabetes, hypogonadism, hyperprolactinaemia secondary to hypothalamic or pituitary disease and possibly alcohol (alcohol can induce liver disease, which in turn can cause secondary hyperoestrogenization)
- *Pharmacological*. Antihypertensives such as beta-blockers and psychotropics such as antipsychotics and antidepressants
- *Neurological*. Peripheral or autonomic neuropathy in diabetes or chronic alcohol abuse and dependence, radical pelvic surgery causing autonomic neurological disruption, spinal cord lesion as in transection of the cord or multiple sclerosis
- *Vascular*. Arterial disease interfering with blood supply to the pelvic organs, incompetent venous valves
- *Local*. Peyronie's disease (progressive fibrosis in tunica albuginea and sometimes also cavernosa, resulting in curvature of the penis on erection), congenital deformities like hypospadias/epispadias, absence of suspensory ligaments, priapism (rare but may result in impotence if not treated within 24 hours).

APPROACH TO TREATMENT

- See Table 10.2.

WHAT TREATMENT/ADVICE

FIRST-LINE TREATMENT

- *Psychological*. Counselling: give practical advice on sexual techniques and ways of reducing performance anxiety. The latter involves teaching on a range of sexual activities that do not require an erection of sufficient rigidity for penetration. This requires the close cooperation of the sexual partner. Consider cognitive behavioural therapy, couple therapy and sensate focus therapy.
- *Pharmacological*. Prescribe psychotropics: antidepressants/anxiolytics for mood and affective disorders. Choose one with less effect on erectile function. Trazodone has been used in the treatment of erectile problems in some patients but priapism occurs in about 0.01% of patients. Discuss the relative sexual side-effects of different psychotropics (see Maudsley Guidelines). Use oral erectogenic agents like apomorphine sublingual and

Table 10.2 Approach to treatment in patients with erectile problems

	Biological	Psychosocial
Immediate	Establish diagnosis Psychoeducation Exclude physical causes Blood investigations: glucose, LFTs, RFTs and endocrine test	Explore psychosocial maintaining factors such as anxiety, depression, drug and alcohol problems, marital, financial and work-related difficulties
Short-term	Modify risk factors Withdraw offending drugs Treat any underlying anxiety, depression, drug and alcohol problem or diabetes mellitus Smoking cessation and cholesterol-lowering tablets Refer to specialist sexual disorder clinic	Address psychosocial issues Consider psychological interventions such as CBT for anxiety or depression Family therapy, if appropriate Consider referral to drug user and alcohol liaison team Psychosocial counselling with the overall aim of decreasing performance anxiety
Long-term	Optimization of short-term treatment plan and relapse prevention	

sildenafil. Explain the indications, contraindications and side-effects of sildenafil, which is a phosphodiesterase inhibitor.
- *Physical/mechanical.* Propose vacuum constriction devices.

SECOND-LINE TREATMENT

- *Physical.* Advise self-injection transurethral therapy with prostaglandin E_1. Alternatives include phentolamine and papaverine hydrochloride, but bear in mind that both are yet to be approved by the Food and Drug Administration Agency.

THIRD-LINE TREATMENT

- Consider implantation of a penile prosthesis.

Note: depending on the way the question is framed, you may have to suggest what other specialists would do when treating impotence and what role there is for the psychiatrist.

FULL ANSWER

The history of erectile dysfunction in this middle-aged gentleman suggests a difficulty that is giving him serious concern. The main issues that I would be concerned with are the need effectively to rule out an organic cause for this man's erectile dysfunction and also to identify the possible psychological factors that may be underlying the erectile difficulties. I will also discuss the treatment strategies for alleviating the erectile problems.

I would clarify from the GP the reason for referral at this particular point and the main reason he or she thinks there are underlying psychological problems. I would find out if it was the couple, the patient or his partner who first had this idea. I would clarify whether the consultation was prompted by their desire to have children or whether there are any difficulties in their relationship. I would also clarify the onset (sudden or gradual) and nature of the problem (erectile or ejaculatory, primary or secondary impotence). I would ask the GP how soon the patient should be seen and whether there are any immediate risk or safety concerns.

I would then proceed to seek more information from the GP regarding this man's medical and surgical history, paying particular attention to any history of neurological disease such as multiple sclerosis and spinal injury, or any history of endocrine disorders such as hypothyroidism and diabetes. I would also ask about the presence of vascular diseases such as arterial sclerosis, traumatic injury to the perineum, and use of drugs such as beta-blockers that might interfere with the neurovascular mechanisms underlying erection. Following this, I would arrange to see the man in the outpatient clinic at the earliest opportunity. While I would encourage him to bring his partner to the clinic, I would ideally see them individually at first and then jointly later. I would take a full history of the nature, onset and course of the erectile dysfunction. An attempt would be made to rate the quality of his erection on a scale of 0–10 (with 10 being the best-quality erection) under a variety of circumstances such as upon awakening, with fantasy, masturbation, foreplay and sexual intercourse. I would also assess his functioning with different people, if he has sexual liaison with anyone else apart from his partner. I would enquire about unusual and/or disturbing life events that might be coincident with the development of his difficulty.

In addition, I would look into the other parameters of his sexual life, including his sexual drive, frequency of lovemaking, orgasmic difficulties and sexual satisfaction. I would estimate the magnitude of any performance anxiety, if present. My assessment would also include a detailed exploration of sexual development and experience, including attitude to puberty, onset of sexual interest, previous sexual experience and problems, masturbation and traumatic experiences such as childhood sexual abuse. I would ask him about his sexual orientation, if he is bisexual or has problems with his gender identity, as conflict in the latter might predispose to erectile dysfunction. I would find out more about his relationship with his partner, paying attention to its development, previous sexual adjustment, general and non-sexual relationship, his feelings and attraction towards his partner and his commitment to their relationship, and also ask if there is any infidelity. In trying to explore further the aetiology of this man's problem, I would also ask about his family background and early childhood, including his relationship with his own parents, parental relationships and his family's attitude towards sex. I would explore the social aspects of this man's life, including financial or work-related difficulties, and the presence of any organic and/or psychological factors in the development and maintenance of his problem. I would talk to his partner, with his permission, to seek relevant collaborative information, assess her level of sympathy towards his problem, assess what problems she is having herself and also to gain an idea of their expectations of and motivation to seek further investigations, treatment and help.

I would conduct a detailed mental state examination to look for evidence of psychological problems such as anxiety, depression, or drug- and alcohol-related problems. I would examine for guilt feelings and performance anxiety, which might make it difficult for him to achieve an adequate erection for successful intercourse. Physical examination would focus on examining his body fat distribution, and facial and pubic hair, which might give an estimate of the adequacy of his androgen level. My initial assessment would also include blood testing for glucose levels, creatinine, lipids, thyroid hormones, testosterone, sex hormone-binding globulin, luteinizing hormone and prolactin levels. Checks on his blood pressure, cardiac status and lower extremity pulses might help to reveal a vascular problem, which could be the underlying disorder. If I suspected a neurological condition, I would suggest a referral to an appropriate clinic which could carry out specialist neurological examination, including evaluation of the S2–S4 dermatomes (by testing perineal sensation), and assessment of anal sphincter tone and the bulbocavernosus reflex. There might also be a need to examine for evidence for Peyronie's plaque, and to check the testes in order to confirm their size, location and consistency. If indicated, I would consider making a referral to a specialist sexual disorder clinic, where further investigations such as the nocturnal penile tumescence test and colour Doppler imaging could be arranged. The latter could provide detailed information about penile haemodynamics and help distinguish between arterial insufficiency and veno-occlusive dysfunction. If an organic cause could be effectively ruled out by these specialist clinics, it would make it easier for us to focus on eliciting the possible underlying causes.

My thoughts on the possible causes of this man's erectile dysfunction include psychological problems such as anxiety, depression, and alcohol or drug misuse. There is also the possibility of serious psychosocial problems such as marital, intrafamilial and financial difficulties. As part of the differential diagnosis I would also consider organic disorders: for example, problems induced by the use of certain medications such as antihypertensives (betablockers), antipsychotics and antidepressants, neuroendocrine problems, neurological conditions affecting the nerve supply to the cavernosus muscles, vascular disease such as arterial sclerosis, incompetent venous valve and local penile diseases.

My approach to treatment in this situation would be to establish a diagnosis of erectile dysfunction, provide psychoeducation for the couple, ensure that physical problems have been excluded by arranging appropriate investigations, and also explore psychosocial maintaining factors that need to be addressed in order to help this gentleman. I would consider immediate, short-term and long-term management, bearing in mind biological and psychosocial issues.

The immediate plan would be to attend to any treatable conditions and this might involve modifying several risk factors by withdrawing any offending medication, treating underlying psychological problems, and achieving good control of physical problems such as diabetes mellitus, hyperlipidaemia (including hypercholesterolaemia) and vascular diseases. If the latter two were problems, in order to improve outcome I would advise smoking cessation and the use of cholesterol lowering medication. I would do this in collaboration with the GP and any specialists that might be involved. As part of the psychoeducation, I would ensure that this couple was well informed about the various therapeutic approaches and the preferred order of treatment. I would refer the patient to the local community drug and alcohol team, as appropriate. Since this man has actually asked to be prescribed sildenafil, I would explore with the urologist whether his condition would be helped by anti-impotence medication. I would look at the indications for sildenafil, its contraindications and the side-effects. Second-line treatment options include self-injected transurethral therapy with prostaglandin E_1. The alternatives to prostaglandin E_1 include phentolamine and papaverine hydrochloride, but unfortunately these are yet to be approved by organizations such as the American Food and Drugs Administration Agency. However, some unlicensed drugs may be used on a 'named-person' basis. Other first-line interventions include the use of psychotropic drugs and vacuum constriction devices. The last option would be the implantation of penile processes and I would not be in a position to offer advice, as this is completely outside my area of specialization. I would therefore refer to a specialist urological clinic.

If the situation persisted, and particularly if I had excluded organic causes, I would consider treating the underlying psychological problem using a combination of psychotropic medication and psychological interventions. A psychological cause of this man's problem is more likely if the onset of erectile dysfunction was sudden or situation-specific and if he continues to have nocturnal and early morning erections. My approach would be to offer, as first-line treatment, psychological measures such as counselling, cognitive behavioural therapy, couple therapy and sensate focus therapy. Sensate focus therapy is a behavioural psychotherapy that involves the couple in graded assignments, which may be modified according to the particular problem. It is used extensively in the treatment of both men and women with sexual disorders. It entails a combination of specified homework tasks together with the setting of specific limits to the extent of sexual contact allowed. It should ideally proceed in stages from non-genital to genital contact, whilst the couple derives some pleasure from the experience. In the long term, the aim would be to optimize the immediate short-term treatment goals and prevent relapse.

1. The psychological factors that might contribute to sexual dysfunction in this man are shown in Box 10.1.

2. Probably not. This type of impotence is related to the failure of nitric oxide release in patients that have undergone radical prostatectomy with inevitable loss or damage to the cremasteric nerve endings that release nitric oxide upon sexual stimulation. As with other oral erectogenic agents, nitric oxide is essential to achieve the erectogenic effect of sildenafil (Viagra). Sildenafil is an orally active inhibitor of phosphodiesterase type 5. It promotes erection by inhibiting the degradation of cyclic guanosine monophosphate (GMP). An increased level of cyclic GMP promotes and amplifies the relaxation of cavernosal smooth muscle that occurs after sexual arousal, thereby facilitating the erectile response.

3. Sensate focus therapy is a behavioural psychotherapy that involves the couple in graded assignments, which may be modified according to the particular problem. It is used

---

Box 10.1 Psychological factors that can contribute to sexual dysfunction

Predisposing factors
Restrictive upbringing (inhibited/distorted parental attitudes to sex)
Disturbed family relationships (poor parental relationship, lack of affection)
Traumatic early sexual experiences (child sexual abuse, incest and poor sex education)

Precipitating factors
Discord in general relationships
Childbirth
Infidelity on the part of either partner
Sexual dysfunction in partner
Anxiety and depression
Traumatic sexual experience
Ageing
Psychological reaction to physical illness/organic factor
Random failure

Perpetuating factors
Performance anxiety
Fear of failure
Partner's demand
Poor communication (especially about each partner's anxieties and sexual needs)
Loss of attraction
Discord in general relationship
Fear of emotional intimacy
Depression and anxiety

extensively in the treatment of both men and women with sexual disorders. It entails a combination of specified homework tasks, together with the setting of specific limits to the extent of sexual contact allowed. It should ideally proceed in stages from non-genital to genital contact, whilst the couple derives some pleasure from the experience:

- *Stage 1*. Touching the partner without genital contact for the subject's own pleasure.
- *Stage 2*. Touching the partner without genital contact for the subject and the partner's pleasure.
- *Stage 3*. Touching the partner with genital contact, but intercourse is prohibited.
- *Stage 4*. Simultaneous touching of the partner and being touched by the partner with genital contact, but intercourse is prohibited.
- *Stage 5*. When both are ready, the female invites the male to put his penis into her vagina. If the female is on top this heightens female control and allows the male to relax. No thrusting. Initial containment is brief, the period of containment lengthening with each session.
- *Stage 6*. Vaginal containment with movement. Different positions are encouraged. This does not inevitably lead to climax. The couple practise stopping before climax. Provided physical contact is pleasurable, orgasm is not necessary.

BUZZ WORDS AND USEFUL TERMINOLOGY

Nature of impotence (primary or secondary, ejaculatory or erectile), sexual history, organic and psychological causes, sensate focus therapy, erectogenic oral medications.

REFERENCES AND SUGGESTED READING

Eardley I, Morgan R, Dinsmore W et al 2001 Efficacy and safety of sildenafil citrate in the treatment of men with mild to moderate erectile dysfunction. British Journal of Psychiatry 178:325–330

Kirby R S 1994 Impotence: diagnosis and management of male erectile dysfunction. British Medical Journal 308:957–961

Nehra A, Steer W D, Althof S E et al 2003 Third international conference on the management of erectile dysfunction: linking pathophysiology and therapeutic response. Journal of Urology 170(2, part 2 of 2):S3–S5

Puri B K, Hall A D 1998 Erectile dysfunction. In: Revision Notes in Psychiatry. Arnold, London, pp 318–321

11

Neurology in relation to psychiatry

A GP has asked you to see a 33-year-old accountant for further advice and management. He has had epileptic fits and also has been making more mistakes at work, 3 months after he slipped and banged his head on a pavement during a night out with his colleagues. At the time of his injury, he was seen at the local hospital, where a deep 5 cm scalp laceration was sutured. He was prescribed analgesics and sent home after 2 days.

How would you go about assessment and management?

SUGGESTED PROBES

1. What parameters would you use to assess the severity of the head injury that this man suffered?
2. What factors would you take into consideration in prescribing psychotropics for him?
3. The MRI shows orbitofrontal lesions. What features would you look for on clinical examination to suggest a frontal lobe abnormality?

PMP PLAN

TASKS TO DO

The following five areas are relevant to this vignette but are not necessarily all-inclusive. The list is also not exhaustive:

a) Demonstrate the ability to take a relevant history in a patient with a closed-head injury to ascertain severity.
b) Elicit relevant neuropsychiatric symptoms that may suggest the most likely diagnosis and other possible differential diagnoses.

c) Show awareness of the clinical, neuropsychological and neuroradiological assessment of patients with closed-head injury.
d) Manage the physical, cognitive and emotional sequelae of head injury in this man.
e) Discuss management options with a view to rehabilitating him and enabling him to return to work.

ISSUES

- Determination of the nature of the epileptic fits and their relationship to the patient's head injury
- Nature of any neurological and cognitive deficits
- Need for treatment and rehabilitation with a view to returning the man to work.

CLARIFY

- Is this man really having epileptic fits?
- Are the fits under control or has the patient had recent fits that might interfere with assessment?

SEEK MORE INFORMATION

GP

- Past medical history: premorbid history of fits or epilepsy, use of anticonvulsants, previous history of epilepsy, syncope, cardiac arrhythmia or diabetes mellitus, which may predispose to hypoglycaemia leading to a fall.

ACCIDENT AND EMERGENCY NOTES

- Glasgow Coma Scale on entry to accident and emergency, associated confusion on presentation
- Diagnosis of head injury, any relationship to alcohol
- Result of CT scan or MRI.

EMPLOYERS

Seek the cooperation and consent of the patient.

- Nature and severity of the fits suffered at work
- Nature of the mistakes, degree of slowness or clumsiness
- Colleagues' views of any personality changes.

PATIENT

- Any loss of consciousness at the time of injury
- How many fits since the injury
- Length of the period of post-traumatic amnesia (PTA)
- Headache, mood change and forgetfulness
- Affective symptoms, such as depression, dysphoria, anxiety and mania
- Cognitive deficit, including memory difficulties, clumsiness, and dysexecutive syndrome with problems in organizing, planning, scheduling, prioritizing and monitoring cognitive activities
- Memory impairment, confabulation and communication difficulties
- Self-depreciation or guilt, apprehension, emotional lability
- Symptoms suggestive of post-traumatic stress disorder (PTSD) and post-concussional state
- Psychotic symptoms, including delusion of misidentification
- Behavioural abnormality and personality changes, sexual disinhibition, apathy and impairment of motivation and ambition
- Psychosocial stressors, including financial difficulties and family stress.

INVESTIGATIONS

- MRI
- EEG.

DIFFERENTIAL DIAGNOSIS/DIFFICULTIES

- *Organic.* Cerebral contusion, post-concussion syndrome, post-traumatic epileptic phenomenon, comorbid depression and anxiety, organic mood disorder
- *Functional.* PTSD, depression and anxiety disorder.

APPROACH TO TREATMENT

- Advise on sick leave.
- Carry out minimal investigation, and then only if absolutely necessary.
- Arrange an occupational therapy assessment.
- Refer to a specialist brain injury unit or department, if available.
- Assess risk of self-harm or suicide.

WHAT TREATMENT/ADVICE

Treatment would depend on the outcome of assessment and investigations.

MEDICAL

- Treat any organic condition.
- Treat depression with an antidepressant.
- Consider carbamazepine for aggression and impulsivity.
- Treat epilepsy with carbamazepine or another anticonvulsant.
- Treat psychosis with low-dose antipsychotics. Consider atypical antipsychotic medication to reduce the risk of extrapyramidal side-effects, but remember that some atypical medication may reduce the seizure threshold.
- Give a prophylactic anticonvulsant only if necessary.

OCCUPATIONAL

- Arrange a back to work scheme (graded exposure) and graded physiotherapy.

PSYCHOLOGICAL

- Give supportive psychotherapy, and cognitive behavioural therapy (CBT) for post-concussional syndrome.

SOCIAL

- Ensure a supportive social network for the family, and prevent social isolation.

FAMILY

- Give support to the family.

FULL ANSWER

This 33-year-old accountant appears to have developed some neuropsychiatric complications and cognitive deficits following his injury. The main issues that I would like to address are ascertaining the nature of the injury that this man suffered, the associated neurological deficit and the degree of cognitive deficit, with a view to suggesting appropriate management. I would also discuss his rehabilitation and return to work once he had improved.

First of all, I would want to assess whether this man's epilepsy is under control and I would also find out if he has had a fit recently that might interfere with my assessment. I would clarify whether he has a premorbid history of fit or epilepsy, and if so, what relationship this has with the current presentation. I would also clarify whether this man has any major neurological deficit following the injury or any other medical condition such as headache that needs treatment. If this gentleman were medically fit for assessment, I would arrange an appointment for him to be reviewed in the outpatient clinic at the earliest opportunity.

I would seek more information and talk to the patient's GP, review the accident and emergency department notes, talk to his employers with his permission, and assess the patient himself. I would focus on the history, mental state examination, cognitive assessment, physical examination and assessment of psychosocial factors that might be perpetuating his illness. I would ask the GP about the patient's relevant medical history, such as a history of epilepsy disorder, severe liver disease and other conditions that might predispose to unconsciousness or falls. I would ask for the history of any cardiac condition and of diabetes mellitus. I would reassure myself that this man does not have a skull fracture that has gone undetected. I would review the medical and nursing entry notes in the records, looking at the severity of injury as assessed by the Glasgow Coma Scale. I would ask about his diagnosis and ascertain whether staff think there is a relationship to alcohol or not. I would find out why he was kept in hospital for 2 days, to ascertain whether this related to the severity of his injury or to the instability of his physical status. I would review the result of the CT scan and MRI, and of the EEG if one was carried out. I would seek permission from the patient to speak with his employer about the nature of the mistakes he has been making at work, when the mistakes were first noticed, the nature of any fit witnessed at work and if there is any problem of strange behaviour or personality changes.

I would arrange to see this patient in the outpatient clinic or, if necessary, at home, either alone or with a colleague such as our clinical psychologist or occupational therapist. I would find out if he had a history of alcohol misuse or dependence prior to this time, if he had been drinking on the day of the accident, how much he had been drinking before the fall, the actual event and the circumstances surrounding it on the day of his injury, and whether he lost consciousness following the fall. I would ask about the presence of headache, dizziness and pain at the time of the accident, and whether these have improved or worsened since the injury. I would ask if the headache or dizziness has persisted and if he has mood changes and forgetfulness, which might suggest a post-concussional syndrome. I would look specifically for affective, cognitive and psychotic symptoms, and evidence of changes to his personality. I would find out if this patient feels perplexed or low in his mood, and would look for evidence of dysphoria, anxiety, apathetic state, anhedonia and loss of self-esteem. I would also look for emotional lability, apprehension and intrusive thoughts about the event, and also rule out phobic avoidance, hyper-arousal state avoidance and other symptoms that might suggest a post-traumatic stress syndrome. I would find out if he is depressed or whether he has had thoughts of harming himself or any other person. I would ask whether he blamed anybody on the day of the incident for his falling and banging his head on the pavement. I would ask specifically if there are any ongoing legal proceedings or compensation issues in the aftermath of the above injury.

With regard to cognitive deficit, I would seek more information about the duration of post-traumatic amnesia (PTA) in this man, as this could give an indication of the severity of the injury. Amnesia of less than 1 week's duration is less severe than that of more than 1 week's duration. Amnesia of greater than 1 month would suggest a very severe injury. I would find out from the patient or from others when he started noticing memory difficulties and when he found out that he was becoming clumsy in his job. I would ask about the mistakes he has been making at work and would look specifically for symptoms such as poor organizing, planning, scheduling, prioritizing and monitoring of cognitive activities, all of which are suggestive of a dysexecutive syndrome. I would particularly look for specific memory impairment and confabulation and assess for abnormality of communication, visuospatial impairment and language difficulties. I would also look for symptoms suggestive of perplexity, derealization and depersonalization, and of paranoia, persecutory ideas and delusion of misidentification. I would specifically enquire about symptoms of impulsivity, sexual disinhibition, apathy, impairment of motivation and control, and aggression, all of which might suggest a frontal lobe abnormality leading to personality changes. I would ask specifically about symptoms suggestive of misuse of or dependence on alcohol or any other drug since his head injury. I would find out about any physical impairment, disability or handicap that this man suffers from as a result of the injury, and how he has been coping since it occurred.

In order to explore further what might be wrong with this man, I would suggest that our clinical psychologist carried out further neuropsychological assessment, including a test of IQ and the

Behavioural Assessment for Dysexecutive Syndrome (BADS), particularly if I suspected that he might have suffered a moderate to severe closed-head injury. I would refer him to a specialist brain injury unit for assessment, if there were one locally. Concerning his psychosocial situation, I would find out about any financial problems that the patient might have, and family stressors such as relationship problems or difficulties with children. If he has continued to have fits, I would find out their nature and whether they are clonic or tonic-clonic, and their duration and frequency. It would be necessary to carry out a CT scan or an MRI and perform an EEG to further assess him. I would also find whether he has been placed on any medication.

Once I had carried out all these tests and assessments, my thoughts on differential diagnosis would include organic problems like cerebral contusion, post-concussional syndrome, post-traumatic epileptic disorder, organic mood disorder and comorbid functional disorders such as depression, anxiety and PTSD. My approach to treatment would be to carry out minimal investigations, and then only if absolutely necessary and if they are likely to yield a positive or significant negative result that would influence decisions about treatment. I would suggest that the patient take sick leave, to allow adequate recuperation before considering going back to work. I would carry out a comprehensive risk assessment of accidental injury, self-harm or suicide, and harm to others.

I would offer treatment along medical, psychological, social and occupational lines, the details of which would depend on my findings. Treatment would include support for his carer and family. Concerning medical treatment, I would treat any organic or functional condition present, and this might include using low doses of psychotropics to treat agitation, impulsivity and aggression. I would prescribe an anticonvulsant such as carbamazepine for the epilepsy, and this would also have a positive effect on cognition. Although it is no longer thought necessary to give prophylactic anticonvulsants following head injury, I would consider putting this man on a maintenance anti-epileptic drug if his seizures continued at an unacceptable frequency. I would prescribe a low dose of an antipsychotic medication if there were distressing psychotic symptoms, and also a low-dose antidepressant for any depressive disorder. I would choose one of the selective serotonin re-uptake inhibitors (SSRIs) over the traditional tricyclic antidepressants. In prescribing psychotropics, I would be guided by the need to give smaller doses of any medication. I would avoid drugs that tend to reduce seizure thresholds, such as clozapine and chlorpromazine, or drugs with high anticholinergic activity in order to minimize confusion. I would also avoid drugs with a tendency to cause extrapyramidal side-effects such as akathisia, parkinsonism and neuroleptic malignant syndrome, and also drugs that would interact adversely with the other medications prescribed. I would avoid the use of benzodiazepine, which may cause severe withdrawal or a tendency to addiction or unwanted aggressive behaviour.

Psychological treatment in the form of supportive psychotherapy and counselling would be necessary in order to help the patient come to terms with the nature of his injury. This would also go a long way towards helping the family to cope better with their difficulties. Cognitive behavioural therapy would be offered for neurobehavioural problems, PTSD, depression and also personality changes following the head injury. Concerning social support, I would suggest that this man be put on sick leave for at least 6 months, so as to enable him to undergo the necessary assessment and rehabilitation programme. A detailed occupational therapy assessment would reveal the deficit and what needs to be done. I would refer him to an appropriate local day centre to enhance his social network and avoid social isolation. I would enrol him on a back to work scheme in order to accelerate his return to employment and also match him with work that suits his current ability. I would suggest graded physiotherapy to reduce fatiguability, and to increase his energy and ability to cope with stress. I would hope that, with all this treatment from a multidisciplinary team supported by a specialist brain injury unit or advice from them, this man would get better and be able to return to work in a few months' time.

ANSWERS TO SUGGESTED PROBES

1. I would use the following parameters to assess the severity of the head injury:
   - *Glasgow Coma Scale (GCS)*. This may suggest mild, moderate or severe injury. Mild—GCS = 13–15; moderate—GCS 9–12; severe—GCS 3–8.
   - *Duration of post-traumatic amnesia (PTA)*. This is a rough guide and cases may vary depending on individuals and on whether injury is closed or open. PTA < 1 hour—mild; PTA > 20 minutes and < 24 hours—moderate; PTA > 24 hours but < 1 week—moderately severe; PTA > 1 week to 1 month—very severe. It is likely that a patient in the latter category will suffer a global and far-reaching disability.
   - *Period of unconsciousness*.

- *Neurological evidence of cerebral injury.* Abnormality on neuroimaging or EEG.
- *Duration of retrograde amnesia.* The period leading up to the injury, for which the patient has no memory. This is probably the least useful parameter.

2. The factors I would take into consideration in prescribing psychotropics for this man are as follows:
   - Prescribe small doses of medication for him at all times.
   - Give medication only if necessary. The routine prescription of anticonvulsants for prophylaxis against seizures is no longer acceptable.
   - Avoid drugs that reduce seizure thresholds, such as chlorpromazine and clozapine.
   - Avoid drugs with a high level of anticholinergic activity in order to minimize confusion.
   - Avoid drugs with a tendency to cause extrapyramidal side-effects such as akathisia, parkinsonism, neuroleptic malignant syndrome, dystonia and tremor.
   - Avoid drugs with a high tendency towards pharmacological interaction.
   - Avoid drugs with a tendency to cause addiction or severe withdrawal symptoms.
   - Avoid drugs such as benzodiazepines that may predispose to unwanted aggressive behaviour.

3. The following clinical features would suggest a frontal lobe abnormality:
   - impulsivity
   - disinhibition, including sexual disinhibition and reduced social control
   - elevated mood
   - perseveration
   - problems with initiation, switching attention and concentration
   - irritability
   - lack of concern for the needs or feelings of other people
   - symptoms related to poor organizing, planning, scheduling, prioritizing and monitoring cognitive activities
   - emotional lability and aggressive behaviour.

BUZZ WORDS AND USEFUL TERMINOLOGY

Retrograde amnesia, post-traumatic amnesia, concussional syndrome, dysexecutive syndrome, post-traumatic stress disorder, paradoxical confusion, neurocognitive deficit, neurobehavioural syndrome.

REFERENCES AND SUGGESTED READING

Bishara S N, Partridge F M, Godfrey H P et al 1992 Post-traumatic amnesia and Glasgow Coma Scale related to outcome in survivors in a consecutive series of patients with severe closed-head injury. Brain Injury 6:373–380

Lishman W A 1998 Organic Psychiatry: the Psychological Consequences of Cerebral Disorder, 3rd edn. Blackwell Science, Oxford

Master C A, Ruff R M 1990 Effectiveness of behaviour management procedures in the rehabilitation of head-injured patients. In: Wood R L (ed.) Neurobehavioural sequelae of traumatic brain injury. Taylor & Francis, New York, pp 277–302

Ruff R M, Buschbaum M S, Troster A I et al 1989 Computerised tomography, neuropsychology, and positron emission tomography in the evaluation of head injury. Neuropsychiatry, Neuropsychology and Behavioural Neurology 2:103–123

Schierhout G, Roberts I 1998 Prophylactic antiepileptic agents after head injury: a systematic review. Journal of Neurology, Neurosurgery and Psychiatry 64:108–112

Teasdale T W, Engberg A 1997 Duration of cognitive dysfunction after concussion, and cognitive dysfunction as a risk factor: a population study of young men. British Medical Journal 315:569–572

You work as the registrar in a local community mental health team. A GP has referred a 37-year-old woman with multiple sclerosis (MS) to you. She has complained of increasing low mood, forgetfulness and loss of interest in normal activities. She has also been very tearful in the past week. She has difficulties having sex with her partner who looks after her, and she fears that he will leave her.

How would you go about assessment and treatment?

SUGGESTED PROBES

1. What physical symptoms due to her MS would contribute significantly to the development of depression in this lady?
2. Three months into treatment for depression and her MS symptoms, the patient becomes elated and euphoric. What three things may account for this development?
3. What laboratory investigations would support the diagnosis of MS in this lady?

PMP PLAN

TASKS TO DO

The following five areas are relevant to this vignette but are not necessarily all-inclusive. The list is also not exhaustive:

a) Demonstrate an ability to identify clearly the main issues regarding the patient's mental and physical health and the interplay between them.
b) Show awareness of the causation of depression and other affective symptoms in a patient with MS.
c) Appreciate that assessment of patients with MS should include the impact of the disease on their lives in general.
d) Demonstrate knowledge of the pharmacological interventions for physical and psychiatric symptoms in MS.
e) Plan systemic management, including psychological treatment and social support.

ISSUES

- Determining whether this lady's mood disorder is typically endogenous, or related to her MS and disability or factors in her sexual relationship
- Determining to what extent her MS and other issues in her relationship have a bearing on her overall functioning and mental state.

- Is the patient at immediate risk of self-harm or suicide?
- Is there any acute pain or spasticity requiring immediate medical attention?

SEEK MORE INFORMATION

GP

- Medical and psychiatric history: is the MS a recent diagnosis or something the patient has lived with for some time?
- Onset of mood and sexual problems
- Treatment given so far (for mood and physical symptoms)
- Any other symptoms.

PATIENT

- Full history and mental state
- Review of physical and laboratory findings
- If the MS is recently diagnosed, ask about:
  - *Mood*. Onset and duration of the mood disorder. Associated loss of interest in activities, lack of energy. Associated biological symptoms, elevation of mood, other hypomanic symptoms, euphoria, lability of affect, and suicidal thoughts, plans or intent
  - *Fatigue*. Worsening of symptoms of fatigue as the day progresses or with physical exertion and stress. Activities completed in the morning or abandoned altogether because they exacerbate fatigue?
  - *Cognition*. How severe is the cognitive deficit? Look for poor memory for recent events, poor abstracting, poor problem-solving and slow information processing. Assessment on Category Test and Wisconsin Card Sorting Test (CST) to detect impairment in abstraction and problem-solving ability (perseverative responding). Assessment of IQ and further cognitive deficits on neuropsychological testing (Mini Mental State Examination (MMSE) is not usually sensitive). Language problems (rare) and intellectual deterioration. Visual processing task impairment shown on performance test. Confabulation and presence of subcortical dementia
  - *Personality changes*. Evidence of frontal lobe disinhibition (Symptoms and signs suggestive of a frontal lobe abnormality are listed under 'Answers to suggested probes' in PMP vignette 11.1, p. 376)

- *Physical symptoms.* Onset of physical symptoms, any blurred vision, spasticity, pain and paraesthesiae. Ataxia, ocular signs such as retrobulbar neuritis, deterioration in central vision, diplopia, nystagmus. Urinary incontinence and other conditions that impact on the patient's life—employment, mobility, leisure
- *Sexual problems.* Dyspareunia (pain during sex), which may be due to spasms. Partner's coping and sensitivity. Couple's sexual relationship
- *Other.* Hamilton Rating Scale.

DIFFERENTIAL DIAGNOSIS/DIFFICULTIES

- *Organic.* MS, Huntington's disease and other central nervous system disorders that can affect the integrity of the white matter (myelin): traumatic brain injury (especially closed-head injury), vascular disorders such as Binswanger's disease, AIDS, neurotoxins such as alcohol, volatile inhalants, leucodystrophies (rare)
- *Functional.* Acute depressive episode or adjustment disorder (either independently or as a comorbid condition).

APPROACH TO TREATMENT

- Carry out a risk assessment and decide whether to manage this woman as an inpatient or outpatient.
- Involve other colleagues such as a clinical psychologist, liaise with neurologists, sex therapists and neuropsychiatrists.
- Consider the possibility of drug interactions in your treatment plan.

WHAT TREATMENT/ADVICE

MEDICAL

- Prescribe medication to relieve physical symptoms: spasticity—baclofen, clonazepam; pain—opiates; urinary incontinence—oxybutynin and refer to a continence adviser; fatigue—amantadine, pemoline, corticosteroids—to reduce inflammation and shorten the duration of relapses. Caveat: steroids may affect mood and behaviour significantly.
- Give disease-modifying drugs (treatment that affects the course of the disease), i.e. interferon beta-1a and interferon

beta-1b. Interferon can worsen depression and should be used cautiously.

- Give psychotropics for neuropsychiatric symptoms and conditions: depression—tricyclic antidepressants (TCAs), amitriptyline, nortriptyline, desipramine and imipramine (TCAs are good in patients with emotional lability and bladder control difficulties), SSRIs such as fluoxetine and sertraline; bipolar illness—lithium or other mood stabilizers; psychotic episodes—treat with a low-dose antipsychotic (including clozapine).

Note: due to the risk of overdose in a depressed patient who may be suicidal, it is wise to give small amounts of medication at any one time.

PSYCHOLOGICAL

- Arrange cognitive therapy, CBT and group psychotherapy, family therapy to help relatives cope with the unpredictable and variable nature of the disease, and couple therapy.

SEXUAL PROBLEMS

- Liaise with the sex therapy clinic.
- Consider the use of a muscle relaxant and suggest other coital positions.

SOCIAL

- Arrange social support, support groups, carer's assessment and support for the carer.
- Provide information on the disease and on local resources.

FULL ANSWER

In dealing with the assessment and treatment of this 37-year-old lady, I would bear in mind that different factors might be contributing to the overall picture and to the difficulty in deciding whether symptoms such as fatigue are due to physical illness or to depression. The main issues for me in this case would be to confirm the diagnosis of depression, and determine whether the patient's mood disorder is typically endogenous, related to her multiple sclerosis, or a reaction to the presence of a chronic debilitating illness or the adverse physical symptoms and disability that follow. I would also determine the extent of her MS and examine factors in her sexual relationship that might be contributing to her depression and overall functioning and mental state. I would then carry out the necessary investigations and suggest a treatment plan that would involve different professionals.

To begin with, I would like to clarify whether this lady is at immediate risk of self-harm or suicide. I would also find out if there were any acute pain or spasticity that required immediate medical attention.

Before arranging to see this woman and her partner, I would seek more information from her GP concerning her medical and psychiatric history. I would ask whether MS was diagnosed recently or if the patient has been living with the illness for several months or years. I would find out about the onset of her mood and sexual problems. I would ask about the treatment given so far for her depression, MS, mood disorder, sexual difficulties and other symptoms. I would find out if other specialists (neurologists, pain clinic staff, counsellors or psychologists) are involved and if so, the nature of their role in the overall treatment plan. I would make arrangements to see the patient with one of my colleagues at the outpatient department, and if necessary, would carry out a domiciliary visit to see how she was coping in her home environment.

When I saw the patient, I would focus on the pertinent history, assess her mental state and review the relevant physical and laboratory findings. If the MS were newly diagnosed, I would ask the patient about the onset of the depressive and other mood symptoms. I would look for associated loss of interest in activities, lack of energy, anhedonia and other biological symptoms of depression. I would also look for symptoms suggestive of elevation of mood, hypomania, lability of affect and euphoria. I would ask about suicidal thoughts and whether the patient has entertained any ideas or has a specific intent to harm herself or end her life. I would look for symptoms of fatigue and ask if it worsens as the day progresses or with physical exertion and/or stress. I would find out if the patient is able to carry out activities in the morning or abandons them altogether because of tiredness. I would look for signs of cognitive abnormality, such as poor memory for recent events, abstracting, information processing and problem-solving. If the MS was longstanding, I would look out for any signs that might suggest intellectual deterioration, language problems (rare), impaired visual processing task, confabulation and the presence of a subcortical dementia. There might be a need to consider further neuropsychological tests in order to assess the extent and severity of her cognitive deficits. As the Mini Mental State Examination (MMSE) is not very sensitive, I would ask our clinical psychologist to carry out further testing, including IQ measurement, to detect further cognitive deficits. A Category Test and

Wisconsin Card Sorting Test (CST) might detect impairment in abstraction and problem-solving ability, which might be shown by perseverative responses.

I would ask about recent personality changes and symptoms suggestive of frontal lobe abnormalities. I would enquire about the onset of physical symptoms, such as blurred vision and other ocular signs like retrobulbar neuritis, deterioration in central vision, diplopia and nystagmus, as well as spasticity, pain, urinary incontinence, ataxia and paraesthesiae. I would find out about the onset of the sexual problems, particularly dyspareunia. I would sensitively ask how the woman's partner is coping with this and what the couple has done about it. I would ask the patient what impact this condition has had on her life in the areas of employment, mobility and leisure. In order to reach an objective assessment of the level of morbidity, I might consider the use of rating instruments such as the Beck's Depression Inventory or the Hamilton Rating Scale. I would prefer the latter, as the former might inadvertently conclude that some of the symptoms of MS, such as fatigue and memory disturbance, were due to depression.

Although I have been told that this patient is suffering from MS, I would ensure that Huntington's disease and other central nervous system disorders (differential diagnoses) that can affect the integrity of the white matter (myelin) have been excluded. These would include conditions such as traumatic brain injury (especially closed-head injury), vascular disorders such as Binswanger's disease, AIDS, neurotoxins such as alcohol, volatile inhalants and leucodystrophies. In addition to the MS, this lady may also be suffering from an adjustment disorder or depression either independent of the MS or as a comorbid condition.

Having understood the nature and the cause of this woman's difficulties, I would make my approach to her care multidisciplinary, involving colleagues such as our clinical psychologist, neurologists, sex therapists and a neuropsychiatrist. I would carry out a risk assessment, particularly the risk of self harm, to decide whether to manage her as an inpatient or an outpatient. I would carefully consider the possibility of drug interactions in giving pharmacological treatment.

Concerning medical treatment, I would focus on treating the depression and any psychotic episodes. If a bipolar disorder were present, I would prescribe lithium. I would treat psychotic episodes with low-dose antipsychotics, including clozapine. For the depression, I would consider the use of SSRIs such as fluoxetine and sertraline, or tricyclic antidepressants such as amitriptyline, nortriptyline or desipramine. Imipramine would be particularly useful in this patient if difficulty in bladder control were a problem.

I would consider the use of amantadine, pemoline or corticosteroids, which can reduce inflammation and shorten the duration of relapses in the treatment of fatigue, but I would be mindful of the interactions of these drugs with mood and behaviour. It has been suggested that interferon beta-1a and interferon beta-1b can affect the course of MS, but they can also worsen depression and would therefore be used cautiously and only after consultation with professionals experienced in their use. I would liaise with appropriate specialists to treat the physical symptoms of spasticity, fatigue and pain. Baclofen or clonazepam and opiate analgesics would be useful for spasticity and pain respectively. If this woman suffered from urinary incontinence, I would refer her to a continence adviser and, after consulting with other specialists, prescribe oxybutynin to treat her symptoms. Due to risk of suicide and overdosing, I would advise prescription and dispensing of only small amounts of medication at a time.

The use of psychological approaches such as cognitive therapy, CBT and group psychotherapy might help to alleviate the depression, minimize the stress that causes exacerbations, and cope with fluctuations in the illness and the uncertainty that usually surrounds the short-term and long-term courses of MS. I would also advise couple (or family) therapy to help the patient and her partner cope with the unpredictable and variable nature of the disease. I would liaise with a sex therapy clinic, which would be best placed to advise on treatment of the sexual problems, the use of muscle relaxants or emollients, and the adoption of suitable alternative coital positions.

These treatment measures would be coupled with the necessary social support, including referral to local support groups and the provision of information on the disease and on available local resources for treatment and leisure. I would also advise a carer's assessment and continuous support for the partner and other family members.

ANSWERS TO SUGGESTED PROBES

1. The following physical symptoms would contribute to the development of depression:
   - spasticity and pain
   - urinary and sphincter disturbance
   - paraesthesiae
   - visual impairment (diplopia, nystagmus, retrobulbar neuritis)
   - spastic paraparesis
   - impaired mobility due to ataxia, paraesthesiae, loss of joint position sense and intention tremor.

2. Euphoria and elation of mood may be due to the following factors:
    -   The patient's depressed mood may have been over-treated by antidepressants (iatrogenic factor).
    -   Hypomanic symptoms may be due to treatment with corticosteroids.
    -   Euphoria may suggest a later course of the disease or worsening of illness.
    -   Euphoria and elation of mood may be symptoms of MS.
    -   A predominant lesion in the left temporal area is more likely in patients with euphoria and elation of mood.
3. The following laboratory investigations would support the diagnosis of MS:
    -   MRI: 90% of subjects with a clinical diagnosis of MS have discrete white matter abnormalities disseminated in space, and 98% have periventricular lesions.
    -   CSF studies: IgG, oligoclonal bands.
    -   Visual evoked potentials: delayed or absent response to checker aid patterns.

BUZZ WORDS AND USEFUL TERMINOLOGY

Neuropsychological testing, Wisconsin Card Sorting Test (*note: make sure you know what this involves; there is a computer base test available*), frontal lobe disinhibition.

REFERENCES AND SUGGESTED READING

Beatty W W, Paul R H 2000 Neuropsychiatric aspects of multiple sclerosis and other demyelinating disorders. In: Saddock B J, Saddock V A (eds) Kaplan & Saddock's Comprehensive Textbook of Psychiatry, 7th edn. Lippincott Williams & Wilkins, Philadelphia, pp 299–308

Hotopf M H, Pollock S, Lishman W A 1994 An unusual presentation of multiple sclerosis: case report. Psychological Medicine 24:525–528

Ron M A, Logsdail S J 1989 Psychiatry morbidity in multiple sclerosis. A clinical and MRI study. Psychological Medicine 19:887–995

You have been called to the ward to see a 65-year-old woman who is complaining of a severe headache that started about half an hour ago. She is worried that she is going to die, feels dizzy and has numbness of the lips.

What are your differential diagnoses and how would you assess and manage this complaint?

SUGGESTED PROBES

1. If you suspected that this woman might have suffered a cerebrovascular accident, what would be your line of management?
2. What symptoms would suggest raised intracranial pressure?
3. After extensive assessment, you conclude that this woman has a migraine. What treatment would you give?

PMP PLAN

TASKS TO DO

The following five areas are relevant to this vignette but are not necessarily all-inclusive. The list is also not exhaustive:

a) Exclude acute life-threatening events such as intracranial haemorrhage.
b) Show familiarity with the organic and non-organic causes of headache at this age.
c) Demonstrate an understanding of the systematic evaluation of headache, including physical examination.
d) Demonstrate knowledge of the relevant investigations and expected findings in these specific conditions.
e) Do not restrict treatment modalities to medical and surgical intervention.

ISSUES

- Determining the cause of the severe headache and excluding an acute life-threatening condition
- Determining whether anxiety is a direct consequence of the headache or both are caused by a common condition.

CLARIFY

- What is the patient's BP, if there is an acute problem needing immediate hospitalization?
- Is there any history of a fall, focal neurological deficit or weakness of any part of the body?

SEEK MORE INFORMATION

REFERRER

- History of fall, fever or trauma to the head.

MEDICAL NOTES AND GP

- Past medical history, history or presence of coagulation disorders, high blood pressure, renal dysfunction, diabetes mellitus, liver disease and epilepsy
- Psychiatric and emotional history
- Medication.

PATIENT

- Nature of headache, onset, location, character (throbbing or dull), time (night—hypnic headache, intermittent or constant). Family history of migraine. Association: flashes, aura and visual hallucination. Aggravating factors, e.g. noise, tiredness, depression, nausea/vomiting, insomnia, fever. Induration and tenderness of temporal or occipital scalp (temporal arteritis), diplopia, lethargy
- Risk factors for the development of ischaemic heart disease, cerebral stroke, thromboembolism, head trauma, intracranial aneurysm.

INVESTIGATIONS

- Neuroradiology: CT scan, MRI, EEG
- Routine bloods: FBC, white cell count, coagulation studies
- Full neurological examination: focal neurological, visual impairments, pallor of the optic disc, ataxia
- Neurosurgical assessment to rule out intracranial mass lesion, as above.

DIFFERENTIAL DIAGNOSIS/DIFFICULTIES

- *Organic*. Primary headache disorders: migraine, tension type headache, cluster headache, migraine with or without aura (classic and common migraine). Secondary headache disorders: temporal arteritis, giant cell arteritis, hypnic headache, headache of Parkinson's disease, intracranial lesion, trauma, trigeminal neuralgia (brushing the teeth and chewing cause headache), migraine (less likely at age 65), polymyalgia rheumatica (muscle pain, joint stiffness). Mass lesions: subarachnoid haemorrhage, large intracranial aneurysm, meningitis, cerebrovascular stroke, chronic subdural haematoma, pituitary tumour, craniopharyngioma and cerebellopontine angle tumour, brain abscess, encephalitis (causes cerebral swelling), meningioma; look for signs of raised intracranial pressure (ICP), papilloedema, obstructive hydrocephalus, constant headache in the morning. 'Metabolic headache': medication-induced, anaemia, hypoxia, hypercalcaemia, hyponatraemia, chronic renal failure

- *Functional*. Psychogenic headache, generalized anxiety disorder, 'involutional' depression, agitated depression causing tension headache, chronic involutional hypochondriasis, hysterical conversion.

APPROACH TO TREATMENT

- Deal with emergencies first.
- Tailor treatment to the aetiology of the headache.

WHAT TREATMENT/ADVICE

MEDICAL

- Deal with any treatable conditions, infections, coagulation disorders, high blood pressure and metabolic imbalance.
- Give treatment for stroke or imminent stroke. Transfer to the acute assessment or stroke unit for stabilization. Urgent neuroradiological investigation can usually be arranged. Take steps to reduce the blood pressure, ICP and cerebral oedema, and to ensure adequate cerebral perfusion.
- For migraine, consider symptomatic relief: non-steroidal anti-inflammatory drugs (NSAIDs), e.g. aspirin, indometacin and ibuprofen. Consider risk of bleeding, asthma and peptic ulcer disease.
- Give migraine prophylaxis. Consider beta-blockers, e.g. atenolol or propranolol; calcium channel inhibitors, e.g. verapamil; serotonin antagonists, e.g. methysergide and pizotifen; antidepressants, e.g. amitriptyline and phenelzine;

anti-epileptics, e.g. sodium valproate; and NSAIDs, e.g. naproxen and ibuprofen.
- Consider neurosurgery for a massive space-occupying lesion, intracranial aneurysm and chronic subdural haematoma.

PSYCHOLOGICAL

- Arrange cognitive behavioural therapy (CBT) for chronic headache.

FULL ANSWER

The main issue I would address is the cause of severe headache in this lady, making sure that acute life-threatening conditions are ruled out. I would assess whether the reported anxiety is a direct consequence of the headache or whether both are caused by a common condition. I would consider both organic and non-organic causes as part of the differential diagnosis in this 65-year-old lady. I would consider common organic causes such as subarachnoid haemorrhage, temporal arteritis, large intracranial aneurysm, cerebrovascular stroke, headache due to trauma and meningitis. I would also consider other primary headache disorders such as migraine, tension type headache, cluster headache, and migraine with or without aura (classic and common migraine). I would also think about secondary headache disorders, such as giant cell arteritis, hypnic headache, headache of Parkinson's disease, trigeminal neuralgia (in which brushing the teeth and chewing cause headache) and polymyalgia rheumatica (with muscle pain and joint stiffness). Other causes that might be revealed by appropriate investigations include mass lesions such as chronic subdural haematoma, pituitary tumour, meningioma, craniopharyngioma, cerebellopontine angle tumour, brain abscess and encephalitis (which causes cerebral swelling). I would look for signs of raised intracranial pressure, such as papilloedema, obstructive hydrocephalus, and constant headache in the morning if I suspected a mass lesion. I would make sure I excluded 'metabolic headache', which can be induced by medication, anaemia, hypoxia, hypercalcaemia, hyponatraemia or chronic renal failure. There might also be a functional disorder causing psychogenic headache, such as anxiety disorder, 'involutional' depression, agitated depression (causing tension headache), chronic involutional hypochondriasis and hysterical conversion.

The main issue would be to determine the cause of the headache so as to exclude an acute life-threatening condition. The other issue is to determine whether the anxiety is a direct consequence of the headache, or whether the headache is causing the anxiety. I would also consider the possibility that both conditions are related to an undiagnosed hyperthyroidism, phaeochromocytoma or hypertension.

In attending to the management of this woman, I would be very concerned about her safety and would make sure that there was no acute medical problem needing immediate medical attention or hospitalization. While I was making my way to the ward, I would ask staff to assess her level of consciousness and her blood pressure, and also to check for any signs of trauma to the head, focal neurological deficit or weakness of any part of the body. On reaching the ward I would seek more information and find out if there was a history of fall, fever and vomiting that might suggest raised intracranial pressure. This would be important to exclude a cerebrovascular event or stroke. Once I was reassured that there was no emergency, I would check the medical notes for details of the condition she was being treated for and the medication prescribed. In addition, I would ask her GP about her relevant medical history, including migraine, head injury, intracranial aneurysm, coagulation disorder, epilepsy, high blood pressure, diabetes mellitus and renal dysfunction. I would look for risk factors for the development of ischaemic heart disease, thromboembolism and haemorrhagic stroke, and for symptoms of depression, anxiety and somatization disorder. I would enquire about her medication, including drugs prescribed for the headache.

Once I had familiarized myself with the patient's history and current treatment, I would proceed to see her to ask more questions. I would ask about the onset, location, nature and character of the headache, whether it is throbbing or dull and how severe it is. I would ask if it occurs at any particular time, such as during the night (a hypnic headache), or is intermittent or constant. I would explore any family history of migraine and if the headache is associated with or preceded by flashes, or a particular aura or visual hallucination. If I suspected migraine, I would ask whether the headache is accompanied by nausea and vomiting. I would ask what the relieving and aggravating factors are and whether they include noise, tiredness, depression and insomnia. I would try to examine what role anxiety plays in this presentation, and if that is the cause of the dizziness and lip numbness. I would ask if the headache brings on the anxiety, or whether the patient is anxious because she thinks she might have a life-threatening organic condition. I would ask if she has fever and periods when she has felt unwell. I would also look for induration and tenderness of the temporal or occipital scalp (temporal arteritis), blurring of vision, diplopia and lethargy. I would carry out a full neurological examination to check for any focal neurological deficit, visual impairment, pallor of the optic disc, ataxia and confusion. It might be necessary to refer the woman to a neurologist for an expert opinion. I would carry out various investigations, including a CT scan, MRI, EEG, routine bloods, FBC, white cell count and coagulation studies to exclude any slow intracranial leak. If all these did not lead to a definitive diagnosis, I would refer her for neurosurgical assessment to rule out an intracranial mass lesion. The overall aim of a comprehensive assessment would be to narrow down to a specific diagnosis in order to decide treatment. I would bear in mind that the headache might be due to one of the many differential diagnoses I have listed.

My approach to treatment would be to deal with any emergency first, exclude or confirm an organic disorder and treat appropriately. Treatment would depend on the aetiology of headache. If this were related to an organic condition, I would treat as appropriate or refer to relevant specialists for their input. If I suspected an imminent stroke, I would refer the patient immediately, transferring her to the acute assessment or stroke unit where she could be stabilized and urgent neuroradiological investigation could be arranged. Further measures can also be implemented at these units to reduce high blood pressure, raised intracranial pressure and cerebral oedema and to ensure adequate cerebral perfusion. On the other hand, if this lady were found to have a space-occupying lesion, such as a subarachnoid haemorrhage, intracranial haemorrhage, intracranial aneurysm, chronic subdural haematoma or massive tumour, neurosurgery would be the main option and I would therefore refer her for urgent neurosurgical evaluation.

If the headache were found to be due to another organic condition, I would advise symptomatic relief. I would consider the use of non-steroidal anti-inflammatory drugs such as aspirin, indometacin and ibuprofen for migraine, but would take into account the risk of bleeding, asthma and peptic ulcer disease with these medications. I would consider prophylactic treatment for migraine using beta-blockers such as atenolol or propranolol, calcium channel inhibitors such as verapamil, and serotonin antagonists such as methysergide and pizotifen. The use of NSAIDs such as naproxen and ibuprofen and of antidepressants such as amitriptyline and phenelzine has been found useful in migraine prophylaxis, as has the use of anti-epileptics such as sodium valproate.

If the cause of the headache were purely psychogenic, I would focus my treatment strategies on identifying and treating the underlying psychological problems. These might include depression and anxiety, hypochondriasis or a somatization disorder. I would use antidepressants and suggest appropriate psychological treatments, including cognitive behavioural therapy for the headache symptoms.

ANSWERS TO SUGGESTED PROBES

1. If this patient had had a stroke, management would be as follows:
   - Keep her as calm as possible to prevent any agitation that might worsen raised blood pressure, cerebral hypoperfusion, increased oxygen demand and cerebral oedema.
   - Refer her immediately to the physicians or to a local acute assessment or stroke unit.
   - If the onset of stroke were followed by a seizure, attempt to bring the fits under control.
   - Once she was on an acute medical ward, the attending physicians would arrange the necessary investigations.

Note: the management of acute stroke is usually outside the remit of the attending psychiatrist and no time should be lost in contacting the experts.

2. The features that would suggest a raised ICP are:
   - generalized morning headaches
   - nausea and vomiting
   - gait disturbance, confusion, incontinence
   - reduced pulse rate and increased blood pressure
   - papilloedema (little seen, even in massive space-occupying lesions, as with sterile atrophy of brain tissues space is not consumed).

3. Treatment for migraine would include symptomatic and prophylactic treatment:
   - beta-blockers, e.g. atenolol or propranolol
   - calcium channel inhibitors, e.g. verapamil
   - serotonin antagonists, e.g. methysergide and pizotifen
   - antidepressants, e.g. amitriptyline and phenelzine
   - anti-epileptics, e.g. sodium valproate
   - NSAIDs, e.g. naproxen and indometacin.

BUZZ WORDS AND USEFUL TERMINOLOGY

Hypnic headache, psychogenic headache.

REFERENCES AND SUGGESTED READING

Philips C, Hunter M 1982 Headache in a psychiatric population. Journal of Nervous and Mental Disease 170(1):34–40

Toth C 2003 Medications and substances as a cause of headache: a systematic review of literature. Clinical Neuropharmacology 26(3):122–136

Weatherhead A D 1980 Headache associated with psychiatric disorders: classification and aetiology. Psychosomatics 21(10): 832–833, 839–840

A 57-year-old man was prescribed an SSRI antidepressant by his GP after presenting with symptoms of low mood, poor sleep, lack of concentration and weight loss. Two weeks after starting the antidepressant, he started showing severe tremor and complained of slowing down. Despite stopping the antidepressant over 2 months ago, his mood and motor symptoms have persisted; he has become more agitated and emotionally labile. There is a very strong suspicion that he is developing Parkinson's disease.

How would you assess and manage him?

SUGGESTED PROBES

1. Apart from Parkinson's disease, what other conditions would present with the triad of tremor, rigidity and bradykinesia?
2. What pharmacological issues are important in this case?
3. Following treatment with levodopa, the patient develops increasing paranoia, thought abnormality and auditory hallucinations. How would you manage the situation?

PMP PLAN

TASKS TO DO

The following five areas are relevant to this vignette but are not necessarily all-inclusive. The list is also not exhaustive:

a) Demonstrate an understanding of the physical and psychiatric presentation of patients with suspected Parkinson's disease.
b) Show adequate knowledge of the necessary investigations to confirm diagnosis, assist management and monitor disease progression.
c) Recognize the need for multidisciplinary working and liaison with other specialists.
d) Demonstrate an understanding of the pharmacological issues involved in managing affective and psychotic illness in Parkinson's disease.
e) Include psychoeducation, psychological treatment and support for both patient and carer in your treatment plan.

PATIENT MANAGEMENT PROBLEMS IN PSYCHIATRY

ISSUES

- Determining whether the patient has Parkinson's disease or a drug-induced parkinsonism
- Possibility of the depression being an early manifestation of Parkinson's disease
- Treatment of the depression and the parkinsonian symptoms.

CLARIFY

- What is the basis for the GP's suspicion of Parkinson's disease?
- Has the patient sought a neurological opinion of the diagnosis?
- What is his present mental state?
- Is there a risk of self-harm and/or suicide?

SEEK MORE INFORMATION

GP

- History of falls and motor symptoms
- Past medical and psychiatric history.

NEUROLOGIST

- How the diagnosis was reached; the results of the various investigations and assessments done to date.

PATIENT

- Onset of low mood, history of depression: reactive, endogenous or drug-induced
- Affective symptoms: sleep disturbance (insomnia, sleep fragmentation and daytime somnolence), anhedonia, loss of appetite, psychomotor retardation, apathy, agitation, anxiety, guilt feelings, sexual disturbances, anorexia, fatigue, facial masking. Use Beck's Depression Inventory (BDI) to screen and monitor for depression
- Motor symptoms: bradykinesia, tremor, rigidity, postural imbalance, drooling, festinant gait (small shuffling steps, bent posture, decreased arm swing), 'lead pipe' or 'cog wheel' rigidity, dysarthria
- Cognitive symptoms: delirium (fluctuation in symptoms, confusion and deterioration), subcortical dementia characteristic of Parkinson's disease, slow information

processing, memory deficit, difficulty in manipulating acquired knowledge, attentional difficulties, loss of intellectual aspects of language, aphasia, agnosia
- Psychotic symptoms: mild illusions, visual hallucination, vivid dreams, nightmares, paranoid ideation, delusion, paranoia
- Physical symptoms: sex/urinary function, sweating.

INVESTIGATIONS

- Only if necessary: FBC, U and Es, biochemistry (including LFT), thyroid function, folate, vitamin B_{12}, brain CT scan/MRI, lumbar puncture.

DIFFERENTIAL DIAGNOSIS/DIFFICULTIES

Not particularly relevant in this PMP but it is important to be clear about the presence of depressive illness and underlying or superimposing dementia and to rule out other organic causes. The deterioration in quality of life imposed by parkinsonism may be more closely related to psychosocial adjustment than to physical disability.

Drug-induced parkinsonism can be caused by antihypertensives such as alpha-methyldopa and captopril, and by metoclopramide, phenothiazines, fluphenazine, trifluoperazine.

Other conditions that may present with tremor, rigidity and bradykinesia are listed in 'Answers to suggested probes' below.

APPROACH TO TREATMENT

- Work with other specialists such as neurologists, clinical pharmacists, physiotherapists and occupation therapists.
- Establish the diagnosis of Parkinson's disease.

WHAT TREATMENT/ADVICE

Treatment should aim to be protective, symptomatic and restorative.

MEDICAL

- Liaise with neurologists and other specialists in the management of neurological and motor symptoms.
- For tremor, rigidity and other motor symptoms, give dopamine agonists such as bromocriptine, pergolide and cabergoline.

- Ensure that poor mobility is not the cause of incontinence. Exclude multiple system atrophy, if bladder symptoms occur early. Give oxybutynin and tolterodine for moderate detrusor instability or hyper-reflexia.
- Treat constipation with increased fluids, fruit and fibre, then laxatives.
- For symptomatic treatment, use levodopa in slow- or modified-release formulations such as Madopar CR and Sinemet CR. Delay the use of levodopa for as long as possible.
- Give tricyclic antidepressants (TCAs) for depression (some clinicians would give an SSRI). They may increase the risk of extrapyramidal side-effects (EPSE), but data on the use of antidepressants in Parkinson's disease are few and of poor quality. Moclobemide, a monoamine oxidase inhibitor, may also be useful.
- Try propranolol and valproic acid for agitation.
- To control psychotic symptoms, slowly withdraw any anti-parkinsonian medication that may be the precipitant. Give medication only when necessary. Some patients may tolerate mild and occasional illusions and visual hallucination that is not distressing in the early stages. Avoid typical antipsychotic medication. Olanzapine, quetiapine and risperidone are useful. Clozapine (less than 100 mg per day) is useful to avoid EPSE but weekly blood monitoring is necessary.
- Small trials with the anticholinesterases donepezil and rivastigmine have shown promising results in the management of cognitive deficits.

PSYCHOLOGICAL/BEHAVIOURAL

- Arrange supportive psychotherapy and CBT for depression.

SUPPORTIVE

- Propose physiotherapy to maximize activities of daily living and minimize secondary complications with exercises and balance training.
- Add occupational therapy to include support in adjusting daily routine, learning new skills for alternative and adaptive methods of doing things, and provision of advice on specialist equipment and resources.

- Facilitate help from support groups such as the UK Parkinson's Disease Society, care-giver education and information leaflets.
- Arrange visits by a Parkinson's disease specialist nurse in the community.

FULL ANSWER

In addressing the assessment and management of this 57-year-old gentleman, I would first want to clarify the basis for the GP's suspicion of Parkinson's disease and whether a neurological opinion on the diagnosis has been sought. The main issue in this case would be to establish whether the patient's illness is due to a mental disorder or organic condition, or both.

I would clarify the man's present mental state to make sure there was no risk of self-harm and/or suicide, given that he might be very shocked about the diagnosis of an incurable and deteriorating condition. Once he was stable, I would arrange to see him as soon as possible to assess his motor symptoms, establish the impact of the motor abnormalities on his mental state, determine whether a mental illness is present or not, and then suggest appropriate treatment.

Prior to seeing him, I would seek more information from various sources to arrive at a diagnosis and also to formulate my treatment strategies. I would ask his GP about any history of falls, past presentations with motor symptoms, past medical and psychiatric history, and details of the treatment he has received so far. If a neurological opinion had been sought, I would ask how the diagnosis of Parkinson's disease was reached and what attempts were made to exclude other possible organic causes. I would proceed to see the patient to ask for his own account of the onset of low mood and to clarify the chronology of the depressive symptoms. As far as possible I would try to understand whether the depression is endogenous, drug-induced or a reaction to his present condition. I would check for affective symptoms, including sleep disturbance (insomnia, sleep fragmentation and daytime somnolence), anhedonia, loss of appetite, psychomotor retardation, apathy, agitation, anxiety, guilt feelings, sexual disturbances, anorexia, fatigue and apparent anhedonia, which might be portrayed as facial masking due to parkinsonism. It might be useful to use validated instruments such as the Beck's Depression Inventory to screen and monitor depressive symptoms.

I would look for cognitive symptoms such as slow information processing, memory deficit, difficulty in manipulating acquired knowledge, attentional difficulties, loss of intellectual aspects of language, aphasia, agnosia, delirium, dementia, forgetfulness and symptoms suggestive of a subcortical dementia which are characteristic of Parkinson's disease. The patient might also show evidence of psychotic symptoms such as mild illusions, visual hallucinations, vivid dreams, nightmares, paranoid ideations or delusions. The presence of delirium might be heralded by fluctuation in symptoms, confusion and deterioration. In addition to these symptoms, I would enquire about motor difficulties such as bradykinesia, tremor, rigidity, postural imbalance, drooling, 'lead pipe' or 'cog wheel' rigidity, features of dysarthria, and festinant gait (small shuffling steps, bent posture, and decreased arm swing), which may occur as the disease is progressing. Other physical symptoms to explore include incontinence, which might in fact be due to poor mobility, abnormality of sexual and urinary function, and profuse sweating.

In addressing the problem, my approach would be to establish the diagnosis of Parkinson's disease and, as far as possible, exclude the presence of other organic conditions. I would bear in mind that the parkinsonian symptoms might be drug-induced by antihypertensives such as alpha-methyldopa and captopril, or by metoclopramide, phenothiazines, fluphenazine and trifluoperazine, which the patient might be using for other reasons. I would carry out further investigations only if necessary and would consider a routine full blood count (FBC), blood biochemistry, including LFTs, TFTs and U and Es, folate, vitamin B_{12}, lumbar puncture and a brain CT scan or MRI. I would work with other specialists such as neurologists, physiotherapists, occupational therapists and clinical pharmacists in formulating an appropriate treatment plan. I would ensure that this included the necessary support, as the deterioration in quality of life imposed by parkinsonism may be related more closely to psychosocial adjustment than to physical disability.

The aim of treatment in this man would be to address the distressing symptoms, restore lost function, prevent or minimize complications and also to protect the integrity of the central nervous system, if possible. I would consider treatment along biopsychosocial lines and would involve a multidisciplinary team.

Concerning medical treatment, I would liaise with neurologists and other specialists in the management of neurological and motor symptoms. I would consider giving dopamine agonists such as bromocriptine, pergolide or cabergoline to treat tremor, rigidity and bradykinesia. As constipation is a frequent problem with parkinsonism, I would suggest an increase in fluid intake and consumption of fruit and fibre, and then the use of laxatives if these options did not work. I would ensure that poor mobility was not the cause of any incontinence, and also exclude multiple system atrophy, if bladder symptoms occurred very early. I would consider oxybutynin and tolterodine for moderate detrusor instability or hyper-reflexia. I would also consider symptomatic treatment, using levodopa in slow- or modified-release formulations such as Madopar CR and Sinemet CR. The use of levodopa would be delayed as long as possible to avoid short- and long-term complications such as dyskinesia, dystonias and the emergence of psychiatric symptoms like delirium and frank psychosis. The use of levodopa might, however, be necessary if the patient developed significant functional disability.

I would consider the use of low-dose tricyclic antidepressants or a selective serotonin re-uptake inhibitor (SSRI) for the treatment of any depression, although SSRIs may increase the risk of extrapyramidal side-effects (EPSE). The data on the use of antidepressants in Parkinson's disease are few and of poor quality, so choosing one might not be easy. Moclobemide, a monoamine oxidase inhibitor, may also be useful in treating depression in this patient. Agitation in this patient might be treated with propranolol or valproic acid, which have been tried by some doctors. If psychotic symptoms emerged as a result of treatment or deterioration of the disease, I would slowly withdraw any antiparkinsonian medication that might be the precipitant. I would prescribe other medications only if and when necessary, as some patients may tolerate mild and occasional illusions and visual hallucinations that are not distressing in the early stages. I would avoid typical antipsychotic medication but use olanzapine (2.5 mg daily), quetiapine or risperidone, which have been found useful. Clozapine at a dose of or less than 100 mg per day has also been found useful for avoiding EPSE but would require mandatory weekly blood monitoring. For cognitive symptoms, small trials with the anticholinesterases donepezil and rivastigmine have shown promising results.

Other treatment for this man would include psychological modalities such as behavioural and supportive psychotherapy. Cognitive behavioural therapy would also be useful to address the man's depression. Other supportive treatment such as physiotherapy would help maximize activities of daily living and minimize secondary complications with exercises and balance training. Occupational therapy would support the patient in adjusting his daily routine, learning new skills for alternative and adaptive methods of doing things, and for the provision of advice on specialist equipment and resources. This treatment would be complemented by social assistance and help from support groups such as the UK Parkinson's Disease Society, care-giver education and information leaflets. Visits by a Parkinson's disease specialist nurse in the community, provided by some services, have also been found useful. I would hope that once all these options were explored, the patient could be helped to cope with an illness that can progress slowly without the prospect of a cure.

ANSWERS TO SUGGESTED PROBES

1. Other conditions that may present with the triad of tremor, rigidity and bradykinesia are:
   - drug-induced movement disorder
   - dementia pugilistica
   - post-traumatic encephalopathy ('punch-drunk' syndrome)
   - post-encephalitic state
   - progressive multisystem degeneration (Shy–Drager syndrome)
   - progressive supranuclear palsy
   - Hallervorden syndrome (rare)
   - parkinsonian dementia complex of Guam (rare)
   - multiple system atrophy (suspect this if bladder symptoms occur very early).

2. The following pharmacological issues are important in this case:
   - Doses of medication should be kept as low as possible.
   - Benzodiazepines that may cause or worsen delirium should be avoided.
   - Anticholinergic medication may worsen cognitive symptoms or precipitate psychosis.
   - Typical neuroleptics, such as haloperidol, may worsen motor symptoms.
   - Regular blood monitoring is necessary for the use of clozapine.

3. If, following treatment with levodopa, the patient developed increasing paranoia, thought abnormality and auditory hallucinations, I would:
   - Consider slowly withdrawing the levodopa or other minor agents such as the anticholinergics amantadine and selegiline, which may only have small impact on the motor symptoms.
   - Consider pharmacological and non-pharmacological means to treat psychosis. Pharmacological means include the use of atypical medication: quetiapine, olanzapine, risperidone or clozapine.

BUZZ WORDS AND USEFUL TERMINOLOGY

Functional disability, dyskinesia, bradykinesia, detrusor instability.

REFERENCES AND SUGGESTED READING

Bhatia K, Brooks D, Burn D 1998 Guidelines for the management of Parkinson's disease. Hospital Medicine 59:469–480

Brown R G, MacCarthy B 1990 Psychiatric morbidity in patients with Parkinson's disease. Psychological Medicine 20:77–87

Clarke C E 2001 Parkinson's Disease in Practice. Royal Society of Medicine, London

Klassen T, Verhey F R J, Sneijders G H J et al 1995 Treatment of depression in Parkinson's disease: a meta-analysis. Journal of Neuropsychiatry and Clinical Neurosciences 7:281–286

11.5 54-YEAR-OLD SECRETARY PRESENTING WITH LOW MOOD AFTER STROKE

A 54-year-old woman, who used to work as a secretary, was referred to you by her GP. She suffered a cerebrovascular stroke 6 months ago, and has not made the expected recovery. She has minimal use of her right side and occasionally becomes doubly incontinent. Three weeks after discharge from the local stroke unit, she becomes depressed and suicidal. You suggest a transfer to the local psychiatric unit for further assessment and treatment.

Discuss your assessment and management strategies.

SUGGESTED PROBES

1. What adverse psychosocial situation may have contributed to the development of depression in this lady?
2. You have established that she is suffering from a major depressive disorder following the stroke, but she refuses treatment. What specific adverse outcomes would you warn her about?
3. Following persuasion, she reluctantly agrees to a trial of antidepressants. What medication would you give and why?

PMP PLAN

TASKS TO DO

The following five areas are relevant to this vignette but are not necessarily all-inclusive. The list is also not exhaustive:

a) Seek appropriate information on contributory factors to the patient's illness, such as the extent and anatomical location of the lesion, the extent and nature of her disabilities, the prospect of her going back to work, her financial, relationship and psychosocial difficulties, the loss of her role and job, and any previous history of mental illness.
b) Discuss relevant differential diagnoses and the psychological effect of the cerebrovascular stroke on this woman.
c) Discuss the concerns regarding the use of medication, and the choice of antidepressant and other psychotropic medication.
d) Demonstrate an understanding of the use of multidisciplinary resources in the hospital and outpatient settings.

e) Include medical (treatment and/or alleviation of disability and incontinence, antidepressants), psychological and psychosocial treatment (including referral to support groups for patient and carers) in your management plan.

ISSUES

- Determining whether this woman has widespread infarction, which makes the development of depression more likely
- Determining the role that her current disability, psychosocial support or lack of it, life events and other issues contribute to her illness
- Management with a view to minimizing risks and improving her quality of life
- Ensuring an appropriate treatment and rehabilitation package to aid her recovery.

CLARIFY

- Are there are any safety issues?
- Is this patient able to communicate?
- Does she have suicidal thoughts, intent and/or plans?
- How stable is the condition and is the patient fit enough to be on a psychiatric ward?
- Would there be adequate facilities and skilled manpower on an acute psychiatric ward to nurse this lady, given her physical problems?

SEEK MORE INFORMATION

GP

- Past medical history, including risk factors for cerebrovascular stroke (diabetes mellitus, hypertension, hypercholesterolaemia, cardiac disorders/diseases such as atrial fibrillation and endocarditis, morbid obesity)
- Current treatment: any depressogenic drug, e.g. antihypertensives
- Premorbid adjustment and history of mental illness.

NEUROLOGIST/STROKE UNIT

- Nature, location and extent of injury
- Extent of the recovery and residual disabilities

- Follow-up plan and post-discharge support available
- Prognosis and likelihood of recurrence. Possibility of readmitting the patient to hospital.

PATIENT

- Detailed histories, past history of depression, current mental state examination and review of relevant physical factors
- Recent prescription of an antidepressant
- Biological symptoms of depression and hypomanic symptoms
- Baseline objective assessments
- Feelings about disabilities and double incontinence, loss of role and job, prospect of going back to work, financial burden, relationship and psychosexual difficulties
- Living alone or socially isolated
- Suicidal thoughts, their frequency and distress level. Any plan/intent to self-harm or harm others, and if so, how. Access to tablets or other potential poisons.

CARERS/RELATIVES

- Identifying the main carer
- View of the problems and progress
- Loss or discontinuity of support received on the stroke unit
- Availability of home care and what help is provided.

DIFFERENTIAL DIAGNOSIS/DIFFICULTIES

- *Functional.* Moderate to severe depressive episode, recurrent depressive disorder and adjustment depressive disorder
- *Organic.* Organic mood disorder (depression contributed to largely by the extent and anatomical location of brain lesion).

APPROACH TO TREATMENT

- Consider very strongly the physical problems that may be contributing to the disorder and find solutions to them.
- Involve other professionals: neuropsychiatrist, neurologist, physiotherapist, psychologist, occupational therapist, incontinence nurse, home carers and community physical disability team.

MEDICAL

- Prescribe an antidepressant: nortriptyline or citalopram as first-line but trazodone has been found useful.
- Consider the side-effects of medication, particularly of the tricyclic antidepressants.
- Consider ECT as a final option if definite contraindications to medication use or if medications cannot be tolerated.
- Address the treatment of incontinence, pain and discomfort.
- Prevent bed sores/pressure ulcers and contractures following stiffness. Physiotherapy and specialist stroke nurses are very useful.

ENVIRONMENTAL

- Propose home improvements and adaptations, including bath rails and alarms.

PSYCHOLOGICAL

- Arrange cognitive behavioural therapy, family therapy, practical problem-solving therapy and rehabilitation counselling.

SOCIAL

- Give support to carers and family (e.g. transport, home carers and CPNs), provide information leaflets and educational materials, refer to and link up with the local support group or association.

FULL ANSWER

In assessing and managing this lady, I would concentrate on ascertaining the nature of her depression and whether it is organic or functional, and whether she has a widespread lesion that would make the development of depression more likely. The other issues are to determine the nature of the psychosocial factors contributing to her illness, how to minimize the risk of self-harm and suicide, and how to improve her quality of life. All these would aim to ensure that she receives an appropriate treatment and rehabilitation package to aid her recovery.

In the first instance I would like to clarify the current position as regards her safety and the stability of her medical condition. I would ask whether she is currently expressing suicidal thoughts and/or plans or intent to harm herself. I would make sure there are no acute medical concerns and that she is medically fit to be discharged to an acute psychiatric ward. In view of the possibility of this transfer, I would also clarify whether there would be adequate facilities and skilled manpower to nurse this lady.

While making arrangements for transfer to the psychiatric unit, I would seek more information to guide my assessment and management. I would ask the patient's GP about her past medical history, including risk factors for cerebrovascular stroke (diabetes mellitus, hypertension, hypercholesterolaemia, cardiac disorders or diseases such as atrial fibrillation and endocarditis, and morbid obesity). I would also ask if her current treatment includes any potentially depressogenic drugs, such as antihypertensives. I would enquire about premorbid adjustment and previous history of and treatment for mental illness, in particular depression. I would establish with the neurologist the extent and anatomical location of her lesion, as a larger lesion on the left side of the brain, particularly the anterior left hemisphere, is more likely to cause a depressive illness after a cerebral event. I would also want to know about the extent of her disabilities, the treatment that she has received so far and the likelihood of the event recurring. I would also find out what future role or roles the other professionals would be playing once she was on the ward.

Once the patient was transferred, I would see her to take a detailed history, ask about any past history of depression or psychiatric illness, and find out if she is living alone or is socially isolated. I would carry out a mental state examination, review the relevant physical factors and elicit her views on the treatment she has received so far. I would ask if her GP has ever prescribed an antidepressant for her. In the history, I would be particularly concerned with the onset of depressive features, in particular in relation to the cerebrovascular accident. I would examine for loss of interest and lack of energy, bearing in mind that some of the physical factors due to a neurological lesion, such as weakness, might be mistaken for lack of energy. I would examine for biological signs of depression and other features such as anxiety, insomnia, hyper-emotionalism, catastrophic reactions, hopelessness, guilt, feelings of unworthiness and suicidal thoughts, plans and/or intent. I would quickly assess for episodes of confusion and any cognitive impairment, and other features such as forgetfulness, slowing, inattentiveness and motor impairment that might point to a subcortical lesion. I would also check for elation of mood at any time (more likely after a right cerebral lesion) and for psychotic illness (hallucinations, paranoid and persecutory delusions, ideas of reference, misidentification phenomena and personality changes such as excessive irritability, aggression, abnormal eating behaviour and hypersexuality). I would enquire about the type and amount of support she has at home and her living arrangements. I would seek her opinion of her disabilities, look for exaggerated abnormal feelings about her body and ask how she is coping with incontinence. I would find out about other psychosocial stressors such as family tensions, financial difficulties, psychosexual difficulties, and negative feelings about her loss of independence and her role as a mother, wife and secretary.

High on my list of differential diagnoses would be depression to which functional impairment and disabilities due to the stroke have contributed, depressive illness to which the extent and anatomical location of the brain lesion have contributed, and a prolonged adjustment depressive disorder. In order to monitor treatment and progress, I would use validated instruments such as the Hamilton Rating Scale or Hamilton Anxiety and Depression Scale/Montgomery–Asberg Depression Rating Scale (MADRS) to carry out a baseline objective assessment.

In my approach to treatment, I would consider very strongly the physical problems that might be contributing to the disorder, aim to find solutions to them, and involve other professionals such as the neuropsychiatrist, neurologist and/or neuropharmacologist, physiotherapist, incontinence nurse or continence adviser, speech therapist, home carers and the community physical disability team. I would invite these different professionals to the ward to provide treatment and support, based on the needs of the patient. Some of these assessments would be carried out in the patient's home, in a way that avoids duplication and extra stress to the patient and her family.

Treatment would hinge on a multimodal approach and would include medication in the form of antidepressants. In using antidepressants or other psychotropics, I would consider the need to avoid unnecessary side-effects and give the lowest optimal dose possible. I would consider nortriptyline or citalopram as first-line treatment, although trazodone has also been found useful. In order to minimize physical discomfort and side-effects, I would make sure there were no contraindications to tricyclic antidepressants, such as heart block, cardiac arrhythmias, narrow angle glaucoma, sedation or postural hypotension, or to citalopram, such as allergy. If the patient were deteriorating or at risk of self-harm or suicide but there were definite contraindications that would preclude the use of these medications or if the medication were not tolerated, I would consider electroconvulsive therapy as a final option.

Treatment would also include the alleviation of disabilities by physical and other means, treatment of her incontinence and assistance with practical problem-solving. I would also address the treatment of pain and discomfort, and prevent the bed sores or pressure ulcers and contractures that might follow stiffness. I would liaise with a physiotherapist and specialist stroke nurse, and ask them to see the patient whilst she was on the psychiatric unit.

In addition, I would consider psychological treatment, including cognitive behavioural therapy for the patient's depression and disabilities, and support for the family and carers. I would also refer her for rehabilitation and counselling under the appropriate specialists to enhance her ability to maintain a positive sense of direction and purpose in her life, to help her to adapt to change and to improve her long-term psychosocial adaptability. Family therapy might also be useful in addressing many of the concerns and expressed emotions that might have been generated since this woman became ill, and would also help the main carer and the family to cope with her day-to-day care. I would consider referral and link-up with a local support group or association that might be able to provide further social support for carers and family in the form of transport to and from appointments, provision of advice on home carers, and provision of information leaflets and educational materials. I would also explore avenues for increasing the patient's opportunities for social interactions, if possible through a befriending scheme.

ANSWERS TO SUGGESTED PROBES

1. Adverse psychosocial factors that may have contributed to the development of depression in this lady include:
   - past personal history of depression and psychiatric illness
   - moderate to severe functional disability
   - dysphasia
   - living alone and social isolation
   - discontinuation of services following discharge from acute stroke services
   - need to depend on others to do basic tasks, particularly toileting and grooming.
2. If this woman refused treatment for a major depressive disorder, I would warn her about:
   - failure and impairment of cognitive recovery
   - impairment of physical recovery
   - increased risk of death.
3. Regarding antidepressant medication, I would consider the use of citalopram and nortriptyline as first-line treatment. Trazodone has also been found useful.

   If these were not tolerated or helpful, I would consider the use of fluoxetine, although some studies did not find it useful in such cases.

BUZZ WORDS AND USEFUL TERMINOLOGY

Adjustment reactions, activities of daily living (ADL), hyper-emotionalism, post-stroke depression.

REFERENCES AND SUGGESTED READING

Gonzalez-Torrecillas J L, Hildebrand J, Mendlewicz J et al 1995 Effects of early treatment for post-stroke depression on neuropsychological rehabilitation. International Psychogeriatrics 78:547–560

Lincoln N B, Flanagan T, Sutcliffe L et al 1997 Evaluation of cognitive behavioural treatment for depression after stroke: a pilot study. Clinical Rehabilitation 11:114–122

Ouimet M A, Primeau F, Cole M G 2001 Psychosocial factors in poststroke depression: a systematic review. Canadian Journal of Psychiatry 46(9):819–828

Robinson R G 1998 Relationship of depression to lesion location. In: The Clinical Neuropsychiatry of Stroke: Cognitive, Behaviour, and Emotional Disorders following Vascular Brain Injury. Cambridge University Press, Cambridge, pp 94–124

Robinson R G 2000 Poststroke depression: prevalence, diagnosis, treatment, and disease progression. Biological Psychiatry 54(3):376–387

12

Perinatal psychiatry

12.1 37-YEAR-OLD SINGLE MOTHER BEHAVING STRANGELY FOLLOWING CHILDBIRTH

You have received a referral from your hospital maternity unit about a 37-year-old single mother whose first child was delivered by caesarean section 8 days ago. She has had problems sleeping and has been hearing voices telling her to give her baby away. She has started to run around the ward, believing this will save her baby and the world from harm.

Discuss your most likely differential diagnoses. How would you go about assessment and management?

SUGGESTED PROBES

1. What immediate risks would you be concerned about?
2. What prenatal, perinatal and immediate postnatal factors would predispose this woman to the risk of developing postpartum psychosis?
3. You have decided to prescribe an antipsychotic medication. What would you choose if this lady were breastfeeding?

PMP PLAN

TASKS TO DO

The following five areas are relevant to this vignette but are not necessarily all-inclusive. The list is also not exhaustive:

a) Address safety and risk issues regarding the mother, the child and others on the ward.
b) Discuss psychosocial and other risk factors that may predispose to the development of illness.
c) Mention puerperal (or postpartum) psychosis as the most likely diagnosis. Discuss the need to exclude organic conditions that may cause this presentation.

d) Demonstrate knowledge of the pharmacological interventions for postpartum psychosis and the implications of such interventions in a breastfeeding mother.
e) Discuss the multidisciplinary management of postpartum psychosis in different settings.

ISSUES

- Safety and risk issues with regard to the mother (patient), the newborn child and others
- Diagnosis and management of postpartum maternal illness.

CLARIFY

- Is the patient medically fit?
- Is the baby safe with the mother? Is there a need to take the baby away?

SEEK MORE INFORMATION

MIDWIVES AND OBSTETRICIAN

- Description of the pregnancy
- Prenatal, perinatal and immediate postnatal factors; complications and anxieties surrounding pregnancy, labour and delivery; post-operative complications
- Current medication
- Risk to the patient and to the baby
- Patient's suspicion of health professionals and the care they provide for her and the baby. Refusal or misunderstanding of any of the procedures or interventions given.

GP

- Past psychiatric history, e.g. manic depression, schizoaffective psychosis, paranoid schizophrenia or depression
- Any physical illness
- Prescribed medication.

PATIENT

Arrange to see the patient once she has settled down, take a full history, carry out a mental state assessment and review any physical factors that may be contributing to her presentation.

- History of this particular pregnancy
- Any family history of psychiatric illness

- Manic symptoms: elation, pressure of speech, irritability, disorganization, grandiosity and other hypomanic symptoms
- Depressive symptoms: low mood, low energy, anhedonia, irritability, negative emotions, depressive thoughts, thoughts of self-harming, or harming the baby or others
- Schizophreniform symptoms: look out for perplexity, thought disorder, delusional beliefs, passivity phenomenon and presence of auditory hallucinations (command hallucinations to harm the baby), visual hallucinations, derealization and depersonalization. Whose voice(s) is she hearing?
- Insight: does she realize she has a mental illness? What would she do if she found out she was 'not able to protect the baby'? Would she give the baby away and if so, how?
- Social circumstances, partner and family support.

INVESTIGATIONS

- FBC including white cell count and differentials, blood and urine for microscopy, culture and sensitivity tests, U and Es, LFTs, TFTs and a chest X-ray.

DIFFERENTIAL DIAGNOSIS/DIFFICULTIES

- *Functional.* Postpartum psychosis, severe postpartum depression, bipolar disorder, anxiety disorder, previous diagnosis of schizophrenia
- *Organic.* Delirium state, acute confusional disorder possibly due to organic conditions such as infection, complications of drug therapy, thromboembolic phenomenon, eclampsia (some cases do occur after birth), Sheehan syndrome (pituitary infarction following postpartum haemorrhage), chronic subdural haematoma following anaesthesia.

APPROACH TO TREATMENT

- Rule out organic causes before assuming the problem is due to a psychiatric disorder.
- Assess the risk of suicide and infanticide.
- Manage jointly with maternity services, health visitors and CPNs as a multidisciplinary team.
- Arrange supervision by a registered mental health nurse to ensure the safety of the mother, child and others. If the ward is in a multistorey building, nurse the mother with care away from windows.

- Arrange treatment in a mother and baby unit, if one is available locally.
- A period of separation of the mother and baby may be inevitable.

WHAT TREATMENT/ADVICE

MEDICAL

- Give sedation and treatment with antipsychotics.
- Choose antipsychotic medication carefully, if the mother plans to breastfeed. The use of newer atypical antipsychotics during breastfeeding has not been well studied.
- Electroconvulsive therapy is useful in severe conditions.
- Arrange joint mother–baby psychiatric hospitalization. Transfer them both to a mother and baby unit, if available, to maintain mother–child bonding and relationship.

PSYCHOLOGICAL

- Arrange supportive counselling when the patient is settled, along with psychoeducation and relapse prevention work.

SOCIAL

- Arrange supervised care and visits to mother and child, initially by midwives and health visitor or CPN.
- Enrol the mother on outpatient and day programmes.
- Supply health education and information.
- Arrange support for the woman's partner and other family members.
- Provide information on contraception and the planning of subsequent pregnancies.
- Suggest the patient attends a postnatal women's support group.

FULL ANSWER

The woman's presentation would suggest the development of a postpartum psychotic illness. The main points in this case are safety and risk issues with regard to the mother (or patient), the newborn child and others on the ward. I would also focus on the diagnosis and management of what appears to be a postpartum maternal mental illness. My immediate considerations would be to ensure that this patient, her baby and others were safe on the ward. I would advise staff to separate the baby from its mother immediately, if they thought her behaviour would put the baby at risk. While I was making my way to the ward, I would advise staff to arrange for supervision of the mother by a registered mental health nurse in a quiet environment separated from others. I would then address risk and safety issues, establish a diagnosis, formulate a safe treatment plan in an appropriate environment, and aggressively treat this woman before arranging a post-treatment follow-up plan.

I would carry out a detailed assessment and seek more information about this lady from staff, particularly the midwives and the obstetrician. I would ask about the pregnancy and about the prenatal, perinatal and immediate postnatal factors that might be involved in this particular case. I would find out if there were complications such as antepartum haemorrhage, pre-eclampsia or eclampsia during the pregnancy, labour or delivery, or any post-operative complications such as haemorrhage or systemic infection. I would examine the patient's current medications and explore whether any of them could have caused an acute confusional state or a psychotic episode. I would ask staff whether they have reason to believe that the patient is putting herself, the baby or others at risk and whether the baby is safe and properly looked after. I would ask if the mother has become suspicious of the health professionals caring for her and the baby, and if she has misunderstood any of the procedures or interventions that might have been carried out. Before seeing the patient, I would ask her GP or one of my colleagues about her psychiatric history, to see whether it is suggestive of manic depression, schizoaffective psychosis, paranoid schizophrenia or depression. I would also ask about the presence of any medical conditions such as epilepsy and the medication prescribed for them.

I would then proceed to see the woman (once she had settled down), to take a full history, carry out a mental state assessment and review any physical factors that might be contributing to her presentation. I would clarify with her the information given to me about her pregnancy and delivery. I would be particularly interested in how she coped during the pregnancy and the extent of her psychosocial support. I would ask about any family history of psychiatric illness. Concerning her mental state, I would look out specifically for hypomanic symptoms such as elation, pressure of speech, irritability, disorganization and grandiosity. I would also look for depressive symptoms, including depressed mood, agitation, anxiety, or thoughts of harming herself, the baby or others. I would check whether she had psychotic symptoms, which might take the form of perplexity, delusional beliefs, thought disorder, passivity phenomenon, auditory (including command hallucinations) or visual hallucinations, derealization, depersonalization and lack of insight. I would ask whether she realizes that she has a mental illness, and what she would do if the symptoms persisted and she found out she was 'not able to protect the baby'.

As it has been suggested that the insomnia, auditory hallucinations and bizarre behaviour started a few days after delivery, I would consider postpartum or puerperal psychosis as the most likely diagnosis. I would bear in mind the possibility of other functional disorders, such as paranoid schizophrenia or another schizophrenia-like illness, severe postpartum depression, bipolar disorder and generalized anxiety disorders. I would also consider (as part of the differential diagnoses) organic conditions such as acute confusional state due to systemic infection, complications of drug therapy, thromboembolic phenomenon, eclampsia (some cases do occur after birth), Sheehan syndrome (pituitary infarction following postpartum haemorrhage), chronic subdural haematoma following anaesthesia or another obstetric condition.

In order to rule out possible organic causes for this presentation, I would carry out relevant investigations, including an FBC, white cell count and differentials, blood culture for microscopy, culture and sensitivity tests, U and Es, LFTs, TFTs and a chest X-ray. If the diagnosis pointed to a neurological disorder, I would order a CT scan or MRI to exclude any intracranial pathology.

My approach to the treatment of this lady would be first to exclude organic causes before assuming the problem is due to a psychiatric disorder. I would assess what risk of suicide and infanticide she poses. I would manage jointly with maternity services, health visitors and CPNs. I would ask for the patient to be continuously supervised by a registered mental health nurse to ensure her own safety, and that of the child and others. If the maternity ward were in a multistorey building, I would advise that the mother be nursed with care away from windows, through which she might attempt to escape her perceived persecutors. I would consider arranging for her treatment to be carried out in a mother and baby unit, if one were available locally. A period of separation might be inevitable if she had to be admitted to an acute psychiatric bed. I would suggest that staff liaise with the appropriate family members to ensure that the baby was taken care of during this time. An alternative temporary placement with a foster carer might become necessary if the mother were hospitalized.

I would offer treatment along medical, social and psychological lines. In the first instance, I would advise appropriate sedation in the early stages to reduce agitation. I would prescribe low-dose antipsychotic medication to treat the psychotic component of her illness. Joint mother–baby psychiatric hospitalization would be advisable to ensure that the baby remained close to its mother for bonding purposes. This, of course, would be carried out with the highest regard for the safety of the mother and the baby. As far as possible, efforts would be made to maintain mother–child bonding and relationship. I would consider arranging supervised care and visits to the child initially for the mother, and later, as she got better and regained insight, I would allow unsupervised care. As most antipsychotics are expressed in breast milk, my advice would be to avoid breastfeeding at the time of acute treatment. If the mother still decided to breastfeed, the benefits would have to be weighed against the risk of exposure in the infant. Where possible, the lowest optimum dose of medication would be given and I would avoid neuroleptics with a very long half-life. One other practical option would be to time feeds so as to avoid peak drug levels in the milk. I would keep this woman on a low dose of sulpiride, which has a low excretion in breast milk. An alternative would be to prescribe stelazine, which has been used successfully in some units. If this lady did not improve with time as expected, I would consider the use of electroconvulsive therapy, which has been shown to give good results in puerperal psychosis.

Once this lady was more settled, I would consider offering psychological treatment in the form of supportive counselling, psychoeducation about the illness and relapse prevention work. This would be coupled with social assistance, particularly if she lacked support from her partner or immediate family. The patient would also be monitored through outpatient clinics and day programmes. She would also benefit from attending a postnatal women's support group, which could be accessed via a day hospital in the community. As part of the holistic care, I would offer health education, information and support for her partner and other family members. The patient would also be given information and advice on planning subsequent pregnancies in order for her to receive more support from different professionals.

ANSWERS TO SUGGESTED PROBES

1. In the immediate term I would be concerned about:
   - risk of harm to the child and to others on the ward
   - risk of suicide
   - risk of infanticide.

2. The prenatal, perinatal and immediate postnatal factors that would predispose this lady to the risk of developing postpartum psychosis are:
    *   primiparity
    *   previous psychiatric history
    *   presence of stressful life events during pregnancy
    *   antenatal complications, e.g. antepartum haemorrhage, pre-eclampsia
    *   delivery by caesarean section
    *   perinatal death
    *   lack of support from family or partner
    *   female birth (associated with an increased risk of postpartum psychosis by researchers from India and parts of Asia).
3. My choice of antipsychotic medication if the patient were breastfeeding would be sulpiride or stelazine in the lowest optimal dose. Risperidone has also been used.
    Most antipsychotics can be given with caution but there is a paucity of research. Sulpiride has a very low excretion in breast milk, while two case reports in which the infants were exposed to risperidone did not suggest any developmental abnormalities.

BUZZ WORDS AND USEFUL TERMINOLOGY

Perinatal factors/complications.

REFERENCES AND SUGGESTED READING

Brockington I F, Cernik K F, Schofield E M et al 1981 Puerperal psychosis: phenomena and diagnosis. Archives of General Psychiatry 38:829

Klompenhouwer J L, van Hulst A M 1991 Classification of post-partum psychosis: a study of 250 mother-and-baby admissions in the Netherlands. Acta Psychiatrica Scandinavica 84:255

Ratnayake T, Libretto S E 2002 No complication with risperidone treatment before and throughout pregnancy and during the nursing period. Journal of Clinical Psychiatry 63:76–77

Reed P, Sermin N, Appleby L et al 1999 A comparison of clinical response to electroconvulsive therapy in puerperal and non-puerperal psychoses. Journal of Affective Disorders 54:255–260

Terp I M, Engholm G, Møller H et al 1999 A follow-up study of post-partum psychoses: prognosis and risk factors for re-admission. Acta Psychiatrica Scandinavica 100(1):40–46

Terp I M, Mortensen P B 1998 Post-partum psychoses: clinical diagnoses and relative risk of admission after parturition. British Journal of Psychiatry 172(6):521–526

A 25-year-old mother has been referred to you, who suffered febrile episodes as a child. She began to have tonic-clonic seizures 4 months into her second pregnancy and was noticed to be confused on occasion. Her blood pressure is normal and pre-eclampsia has been ruled out. Her obstetrician is certain that she has a seizure disorder and has asked for your expert advice and management.

What advice would you give for management of this woman, both during pregnancy and after she has delivered?

SUGGESTED PROBES

1. What factors may influence seizure activity in this woman?
2. What factors would you take into consideration in establishing her on an effective anti-epileptic drug?
3. At 29 weeks she goes into status epilepticus. What advice would you give on her management?

PMP PLAN

TASKS TO DO

The following five areas are relevant to this vignette but are not necessarily all-inclusive. The list is also not exhaustive:

a) Demonstrate adequate knowledge of the differential diagnoses, including psychogenic causes.
b) Carry out a systematic evaluation and investigation of a pregnant epileptic patient. Mention the need to rule out organic causes.
c) Discuss the need to work with other professionals and specialists.
d) Show a good knowledge of teratogenic issues related to anti-epileptic medication and to the safe management of the patient and the pregnancy.
e) Include psychosocial support in your management options.

ISSUES

- Establishing the cause of seizures and their management in this pregnant woman
- Balancing the need to treat the seizure disorder in pregnancy against the teratogenic risk to the fetus.

- What is the woman's present location?
- What control does she have of her seizures?
- Are there any psychological symptoms?

SEEK MORE INFORMATION

GP

- Past medical and psychiatric history.

OBSTETRICIAN AND MIDWIVES

- History of the current pregnancy and management of complications to date
- History of the previous pregnancy.

NEUROLOGIST

- Knowledge of the patient and opinion on seizures.

PATIENT

- History of seizures before pregnancy
- Onset of the present seizures, before and after pregnancy started
- Presence of aura, frequency, witnesses, aggravating factors
- Factors that might influence seizure activiy, such as non-compliance with anti-epileptic medication (fear of teratogenicity), hyperemesis leading to electrolyte imbalance (particularly hyponatraemia), psychological stress and sleep deprivation
- Association with headaches or vomiting
- Need to rule out psychogenic causes as far as possible
- History of pregnancy: planned or not
- Marital status/partner
- History of mental illness and previous treatments.

INVESTIGATIONS

- EEG, telemetry, abdominal ultrasound, 3-D fetal ultrasonography at 18 weeks to exclude neural tube defects (NTDs), MRI, urinary protein, serum anti-epileptic drug level, alphafetoprotein at 18 weeks.

DIFFERENTIAL DIAGNOSIS/DIFFICULTIES

- *Organic.* Primary generalized or partial epilepsy, idiopathic epilepsy, eclampsia, syncope, hypoxia, hyponatraemia, hypoglycaemia, hypocalcaemia, drug withdrawal, drug-induced seizures, intracranial tumour, e.g. cavernous angioma or other space-occupying lesion
- *Non-organic.* Non-epileptic pseudoseizures, psychogenic epilepsy, conversion disorder.

APPROACH TO TREATMENT

- Focus management on maintaining a seizure-free state.
- Minimize harm to mother and fetus.
- Consider the pregnancy high-risk, and manage jointly with obstetrician and midwives.

WHAT TREATMENT/ADVICE

DURING PREGNANCY

- Prevent hyperemesis.
- Offer psychosocial support and counselling: the importance of medication, the possibility of an increase in seizure frequency during pregnancy, the need for compliance with medication, the risk of congenital malformation due to anti-epileptic medication and the need to monitor the level of drugs. Discuss likely events in late pregnancy, during labour and after the birth. Discuss the need to treat the seizures and to balance this against the risk of teratogenicity.
- Establish the patient on suitable anti-epileptic medication.

DURING LABOUR

- Avoid prolonged labour and maternal exhaustion; avoid pethidine and the infiltration of high doses of local anaesthetics (both potential convulsants).
- Prepare for seizures in labour; exclude eclampsia, ensure early involvement of paediatric, medical and anaesthetic specialists, ensure adequate airway and oxygenation, ensure intravenous access. Be ready.

POSTPARTUM

- Reduce the dose of medication, and monitor levels on day 7, at 4 weeks and monthly for a further 3 months.
- Avoid phenobarbital and diazepam in breastfeeding mothers.

- Give postpartum prophylaxis.
- Consider the safety of the mother and care of the infant during bathing.
- Advise on contraception.

FULL ANSWER

I think the main issue in this case would be to establish the cause of the seizures and how to manage them in this pregnant lady. The other important issue is the need to balance the treatment of a seizure disorder against the teratogenic risks to the fetus that might arise from such treatment. In dealing with the case, I would bear in mind that this woman might have had a history of seizures before the pregnancy, or the seizures might have developed for the first time during this pregnancy. They could also be non-epileptic seizures or dissociative convulsions (otherwise called pseudoseizures), which have developed in response to the pregnancy. I would focus on clarifying and understanding the nature of this woman's epilepsy, excluding any treatable organic causes, and determining whether the seizures are of a psychogenic nature. I would then carry out the appropriate investigations, and advise on or institute an appropriate management plan.

First of all, I would clarify whether the patient is in hospital or at home, whether the seizures are under control, and if any further investigations are planned. I would also clarify whether she is on any medication, and if so, what it is being used for.

Before seeing her, I would seek further information from her GP about her medical and psychiatric history. I would ask when her childhood febrile episodes stopped and whether she has had seizures or episodes of epilepsy recently. If she had had a recent episode, I would ask whether she is on any medication. I would be particularly interested in anticonvulsants and would ask if she stopped her medication because she became pregnant. I would ask the obstetrician and midwives about this pregnancy, the well-being of the fetus and the management of any complications so far. If the patient had seen a neurologist recently, I would ask his or her opinion about the seizures and the likely causes.

I would then proceed to assess this woman. I would ask her about the onset of the seizures and whether it was before or after the pregnancy started, the presence of aura, the nature and the frequency of the seizures, and whether there have been any witnesses. I would enquire about associated features such as foaming at the mouth, incontinence and loss of consciousness. I would ask what she thinks aggravates the seizures, and would also look for factors that might influence seizure activity. These would include non-compliance with anti-epileptic medication due to her fear of teratogenicity, hyperemesis leading to electrolyte imbalance (particularly hyponatraemia), psychological stress and sleep deprivation. While it might be difficult to be sure that this presentation has an emotional cause, I would ask other questions to exclude a psychogenic cause as far as possible. I would assess from the accounts of witnesses whether the patient appears to have control over the seizures and if she remembers events surrounding them. I would also ask if she is able to respond to instructions during the episodes and attempts to stop herself falling. I would find out about her pre-morbid state and whether she thinks being pregnant has made her symptoms worse. I would ask if the pregnancy was planned, and if not, what her reaction was when she found out about it. I would ask about her partner and the kind of support she is receiving at this time from her family.

As part of the assessment process, I would carry out investigations such as an EEG, telemetry, abdominal ultrasound, (including 3-D fetal ultrasonography at 18 weeks to exclude a neural tube defect) ECG, MRI of the brain, urinary protein and serum anti-epileptic drug level, serum alphafetoprotein at 18 weeks and routine blood investigations including LFTs and U and Es. I would suggest a referral to a neurologist to seek expert medical advice on the clinical presentation and comments on the results of the various investigations.

I would consider an organic and non-organic aetiology in the differential diagnosis and this would inform my decisions on treatment. I would consider primary generalized or partial epilepsy, idiopathic epilepsy, eclampsia, syncope, hypoxia, hyponatraemia, hypoglycaemia, hypocalcaemia, drug withdrawal and drug-induced seizures (caused by medication such as antidepressants) as possible differential diagnoses. Other possible organic causes include intracranial tumours such as a cavernous angioma or other space-occupying lesions (associated with headache, vomiting and signs of raised intracranial pressure). I would consider the possibility of non-epileptic seizures, otherwise called pseudoseizures, psychogenic epilepsy or dissociative convulsions.

In my approach to management, my priority would be to maintain a seizure-free state in order to minimize harm to the mother and the fetus. I would consider the pregnancy a high-risk one and would suggest joint management with the obstetrician, midwives and medical specialists, including a neurologist or an epileptologist. Treatment would depend on the causative factors and I would focus on measures for during pregnancy, labour and the postpartum period. These would include medical treatment, psychosocial support and counselling. I would also offer psychoeducation about the likely events and implications of seizures in late pregnancy, during labour and after the birth. I would also counsel on the importance of medication, the possibility of an increase in frequency of seizures during pregnancy, compliance with medication, the risk of congenital malformation due to anti-epileptic medication, and the need to monitor anti-epileptic drug levels. I would initiate folate therapy at a dose of 5 mg per day throughout pregnancy to reduce the risk of neural tube defects (NTDs). I would advise that serum alphafetoprotein be measured at 18 weeks, particularly if the patient were on a high dose of sodium valproate. As far as possible treatment would be given to prevent hyperemesis, electrolyte imbalance and other factors that might affect seizure episodes and frequency.

I would aim to establish this pregnant lady on suitable anti-epileptic medication following advice from a neurologist or an epileptologist. This would help reduce the risk of maternal and fetal complications such as pre-eclampsia, intrauterine growth retardation, antepartum haemorrhage, and an increased rate of instrumental delivery with its attendant consequences. I would discuss how to balance the need to give treatment for the seizures against the risk of teratogenicity, and would make sure the patient and her partner fully understand this so as to give informed consent. I would bear in mind that all common and standard anti-epileptic medications are potentially teratogenic and would plan to treat with only one anticonvulsant. I would give the lowest effective dose and monitor the level of the drug periodically. As anti-epileptic medications induce hepatic enzymes, I would give oral vitamin K supplements to the patient in the last week of pregnancy to prevent haemorrhagic disease of the newborn (HDN). A dose of about 10 mg per day from the 36th week of pregnancy would be recommended.

As labour was drawing near, I would prepare for the eventuality of a seizure during labour and ensure the early involvement of paediatric, medical and anaesthetic specialists. I would advise staff to monitor closely for pre-eclampsia by frequently checking blood pressure and urinary protein. I would ensure adequate airway and oxygenation and check that intravenous access was ready. I would suggest that staff avoid a prolonged labour and maternal exhaustion, and also did not use pethidine or infiltration of high doses of local anaesthetics, which are both potential convulsants.

Following delivery, I would suggest monitoring the postpartum level of anti-epileptic medication as this might have risen to toxic levels. It might be necessary to reduce the dose, and to monitor drug level on day 7, at 4 weeks and then monthly for a further

3 months. If there were a need to stop anti-epileptic medication in the postpartum period, I would consider withdrawing it carefully, especially if this patient suffered from an epileptic syndrome, had a structural brain abnormality or had a history of prolonged seizure or status epilepticus. Too rapid withdrawal of anti-epileptic medication may precipitate seizures in the postnatal period. Careful counselling about the danger of seizures and status epilepticus would also go a long way towards bolstering her compliance with medication. I would avoid phenobarbital and diazepam if the woman decided to breastfeed.

I would ask the obstetrician and midwives to advise on appropriate contraception, bearing in mind that anti-epileptic medication may induce enzymes that can metabolize oestrogen-based oral contraceptives. Despite all these measures, it is possible that this lady might still suffer from largely uncontrolled epilepsy and this might raise the issue of the safety of the mother and the care of the infant during bathing, changing of nappies and feeding. If this were the case, I would suggest that further support and assistance were provided by the midwives and the health visitor. As there might be a psychogenic component to the illness, I would advise support for the new mother from a community mental health worker, preferably a community nurse or a social worker. I would also refer her for psychological assessment and treatment, if necessary. Finally, if she desired to have more children in the future, I would advise pre-pregnancy counselling and adequate monitoring of symptoms and drug levels. Pre-pregnancy planning would also afford the opportunity for her to commence low-dose folate in order to reduce the risk of a neural tube defect significantly.

Note: if a very knowledgeable maverick examiner 'corners' you, be aware that phenobarbital seems to have the slightest adverse effect on fetal development, but unfortunately is probably the least effective medication for most women.

ANSWERS TO SUGGESTED PROBES

1. The following factors might influence seizure activity in this woman:
   - non-compliance with anti-epileptic medication (fear of teratogenicity)
   - decreased absorption of anti-epileptic drugs in the gut
   - changes in the pharmacokinetics of anti-epileptic medication
   - increased blood volume in pregnancy, which reduces the effective serum concentration of anti-epileptic drugs

- metabolic changes in pregnancy
- hyperemesis leading to electrolyte imbalance (particularly hyponatraemia)
- psychological stress
- sleep deprivation during pregnancy.

2. I would take the following factors into consideration in establishing this patient on an effective anti-epileptic:
   - There is a need to control epilepsy, as it may predispose to maternal complications such as pre-eclampsia, intrauterine growth retardation, antepartum haemorrhage, and an increased rate of instrumental delivery with its attendant consequences.
   - All common and standard anti-epileptic medications are potentially teratogenic.
   - Polytherapy increases the risk of teratogenesis and the practice is best avoided.
   - Monotherapy should be the goal of treatment.
   - The lowest effective dose should be given.
   - As anti-epileptic medication induces hepatic enzymes, oral vitamin K supplements should be given to mothers in the last week of pregnancy to prevent haemorrhagic disease of the newborn.
   - Folate therapy should be initiated at 5 mg per day to reduce the risk of neural tube defects.
   - If there is a need to stop medication, consider carefully before withdrawing drugs in patients with an epileptic syndrome, structural brain abnormality or a history of prolonged seizures or status epilepticus.
   - Pethidine should be avoided in labour, as it is a potential convulsant.
   - Postpartum monitoring is needed, as levels of anti-epileptic medication may rise to toxic levels.
   - Appropriate contraception should be discussed, as anti-epileptic medication may induce enzymes that metabolize oestrogen-based oral contraceptives.

3. If this patient went into status epilepticus at 29 weeks, I would take the following measures:
   - I would advise urgent management, as status epilepticus carries a 50% risk of fetal death as well as maternal aspiration and mortality.
   - I would call the experts without delay, as this is a medical emergency.

- I would arrange for full resuscitation equipment to be present.
- I would terminate seizures with intravenous diazepam 10–20 mg over 3–5 minutes or intravenous clonazepam 1 mg every 2–3 minutes until the seizures stopped.

The obstetric implications and management of status epilepticus would be the responsibility of the obstetrician.

BUZZ WORDS AND USEFUL TERMINOLOGY

High-risk pregnancy, teratogenic risk, pseudoseizures or non-epileptic seizures, pregnancy planning, status epilepticus.

REFERENCES AND SUGGESTED READING

Barrett C, Richens A 2003 Epilepsy and pregnancy: report of an Epilepsy Research Foundation workshop. Epilepsy Research 52(3):147–187
Crawford P 2002 Epilepsy and pregnancy. Seizure 11(suppl.)A:212–219
Morrow J I, Craig J J 2003 Antiepileptic drugs in pregnancy: current safety and other issues. Expert Opinion on Pharmacology 44(4):445–456
Pschirrer E R 2004 Seizure disorders in pregnancy. Obstetrics and gynecologic clinic of North America 31(2):373–384
Yerby M S 2003 Clinical care of pregnant women with epilepsy: neural tube defects and folic acid supplementation. Epilepsia 44(suppl.)3:33–40
Zhan C A, Morrell M J, Collins S D et al 1998 Management issues for women with epilepsy: a review of the literature. Neurology 51:949–956

A 36-year-old lady, who suffers from a bipolar affective disorder usually of mixed (depressive and hypomanic) presentation, has been stable in the community on 400 mg of lithium for the last 3 years. She has disclosed to you in clinic that she has just discovered she is 6 weeks pregnant. The pregnancy was unplanned but as she is currently engaged to her partner of 8 months they are keen to continue with the pregnancy.

What advice would you give this woman and how would you manage her?

SUGGESTED PROBES

1. What factors would you take into consideration in advising this lady?
2. The patient has suggested trying carbamazepine instead of lithium. What response would you give?
3. In what circumstances could a medico-legal situation arise?

PMP PLAN

TASKS TO DO

The following five areas are relevant to this vignette but are not necessarily all-inclusive. The list is also not exhaustive:

a) Seek evidence of the pregnancy and liaise closely with the patient's partner, midwives and GP.
b) Provide information on the risks involved (deterioration in mental state and teratogenicity), to be balanced against the wishes of the couple. Ensure adequate documentation of all discussions.
c) Demonstrate that the patient will need support and alternative medication if and when she makes the decision to stop medication. Show clear management of this patient on lithium during pregnancy and of other patients who decide to stop lithium.
d) Monitor closely when lithium is stopped, as the patient may suffer from rebound mania.
e) Demonstrate a clear understanding of informed consent, medical negligence and other relevant medico-legal issues.

ISSUES

- Risk of relapse in this lady who has been stable for 3 years, if she stops or alters her medication
- Risk of teratogenicity if she continues lithium in pregnancy
- Medico-legal implications of deciding either way, i.e. to stop or continue lithium in pregnancy.

CLARIFY

- Has the pregnancy been confirmed?
- Has the patient unilaterally stopped medication already?

SEEK MORE INFORMATION

MIDWIVES AND OBSTETRICIAN

- Details of the pregnancy
- Fetal viability at the time of referral
- Plans for future monitoring.

GP

- Opinion on management of the patient to date
- Other medical and relevant psychiatric history.

PSYCHIATRIC SERVICES

- Past presentation, treatment, compliance, relapse and relapse indicators.

PATIENT

- Whether lithium has already been stopped
- What conclusions she and her partner have come to
- Current mental state and risks.

DIFFERENTIAL DIAGNOSIS/DIFFICULTIES

There is no need to elaborate, as the diagnosis has already been given.

APPROACH TO TREATMENT

- Involve partner, GP, midwife and obstetrician.
- Explain the risks, obtain informed consent, and document decisions properly in the notes.
- Inform of problems associated with lithium therapy in pregnancy: respiratory problem in newborn, rhythm disturbances, severe hyperbilirubinaemia, diabetes insipidus, thyroid dysfunction, hypoglycaemia, hypotonia, lethargy and large for gestational age infant.
- Withdraw lithium very slowly and substitute with other medication.

WHAT TREATMENT/ADVICE

- Treatment depends on the decision to withdraw or continue lithium.
- Consider management in the early part of pregnancy— during the time of withdrawal of the medication; the perinatal period—management during late pregnancy and delivery of the baby; and the postnatal period—post-delivery, during breastfeeding, and further follow-up.
- Be clear about the management options whether the patient decides to withdraw the lithium or not, as discussion may generally tend towards one of these options. Generally, most people would advise withdrawal of lithium or reduction of the dose during the embryonic period.

FULL ANSWER

I think the main issue in the case of this 36-year old lady is whether to continue or discontinue lithium now that she is pregnant, given that she has been stable in the community for the last 3 years. The paramount issues on my mind would be the risk of relapse with her mental illness if she stopped the lithium, and also the risk of teratogenicity if she decided to continue on lithium or another mood stabilizer in pregnancy. I would also consider the potential medico-legal implications of my decision.

First of all, I would like to clarify whether this lady is actually pregnant and I would seek evidence from any laboratory investigations, urine and blood pregnancy tests and possibly ultrasound examinations that might have been carried out. I would check straight away that she has not reduced her lithium dose or even stopped completely without the advice of her doctors. I would always keep in mind that, whatever decision this woman takes, it will not be an easy one.

I would seek more information from the patient's GP, midwife and obstetrician, and would look into her medical notes. I would seek information from the local psychiatric services that have been managing her over the years and find out whether she has been pregnant before and, if so, how that was managed. I would ask about her treatment, any relapses and the presentation at that time. It would also be useful to find out about relapse indicators.

I would see her, preferably in the presence of her partner, and would involve the community psychiatric nurse (CPN) who has been following her up. I would find out about her mood at the present time, and examine her main concerns. I would carry out a mental state examination, looking particularly for evidence of elated or depressed mood. I would find out whether she has sought information elsewhere and whether she has made up her own mind about exactly what she wants to do. I would explain why it is necessary to involve her partner in order for her to receive more support, and would find out what kind of support she would have during and after the pregnancy.

In my approach to advising and managing her, I would explain to her the risk of carrying a baby while on lithium or any other mood stabilizer. I would carefully outline the risks if she withdrew the lithium, given that she has been stable in the community for over 3 years. I would explain to her that the risk of a major congenital abnormality during early pregnancy is of the order of 4–12%, compared to about 2%–4% in the untreated population. I would also tell her that using lithium during pregnancy carries a risk of developing major cardiovascular abnormalities such as Ebstein's anomaly, the features of which include redundant valve tissue with downward displacement into the right ventricle, and adherence of portions of the septa and posterior cusp to the right ventricular wall. I would give further advice in conjunction with the obstetrician, who would be able to give her further reassurance. I would state clearly that the risk of developing this abnormality is about 22–140 times higher in people on lithium compared to the general population. I would also inform her about other problems associated with maternal lithium therapy, which include poor respiratory effort and cyanosis in the newborn, rhythm disturbances, severe hyperbilirubinaemia, diabetes insipidus, thyroid dysfunction, hypoglycaemia, hypotonia, lethargy and a large-for-gestational age infant. I would give her the relevant information leaflets to make sure she properly understands the explanations.

I would also explain to her what would happen during the pregnancy, the perinatal period, after she delivers the baby and when she is breastfeeding, if she chooses to continue to use lithium. All this would be necessary in order to enable her to give her informed consent before any steps are actually taken. I would clearly state that the options before her are either taking a drug that may have a teratogenic effect during pregnancy, or suffering the morbidity of discontinuing lithium therapy and risking relapse. I would give her written information and/or leaflets so that she and her partner could look at them and advise them to come back to see me after they have made up their mind. I would say that I would generally favour withdrawing lithium during the pregnancy and treating by alternative means, if that were possible. Ultimately, it is the patient who would make the decision.

The treatment and advice that I would offer would depend on the decision this woman makes as to whether to withdraw from lithium with the risk of relapse in her mental illness or to continue to use lithium or another mood stabilizer. I would recommend stopping lithium unless the patient were adamant or could not tolerate any other medication. If a decision were made to discontinue lithium, we would do this gradually over 10–14 days or a much longer period (15–30 days) to reduce the risk of a recurrence of bipolar manic-depressive illness. The higher the risk to the mother or the pregnancy, the longer would be the period of withdrawal of lithium to avoid adverse withdrawal reaction. I would monitor her mood closely and would continue to see her as an outpatient; if necessary, I would admit her to hospital for lithium withdrawal. If there were any suggestion of a relapse in her mental state, I would consider using haloperidol or a benzodiazepine to treat her symptoms for a short period. (Some doctors have considered reintroducing lithium at a lower divided dose in the second and third trimesters, after which cardiac organogenesis would have taken place.) Since she has already become pregnant while on lithium, I would still suggest she undergoes fetal surveillance as if she were continuing on the drug. In addition to this treatment, I would continue to offer psychological support as necessary.

If this woman decided to continue on lithium, I would suggest that we carry out careful fetal surveillance throughout the pregnancy using a level III anatomic ultrasound and fetal echocardiography up to 20 weeks of gestation. I would give the smallest dose of lithium possible and use smaller divided doses in the last month of pregnancy, monitoring serum lithium levels weekly. As the renal excretion of lithium increases by 30–50% parallel with normal creatinine clearance, the dosage of the maternal lithium (300–1200 mg per day) would be kept to a minimum to achieve levels within a narrow and safe therapeutic window of

0.5–1.2 meq/L. I would suggest monitoring serum lithium levels every 2 days proximal to the date of confinement, and either discontinuing lithium 2–3 days before delivery or decreasing the dose by one-half to one-quarter. This would ensure effective control of symptoms whilst safeguarding against potential toxicity and neonatal withdrawal effects.

I would suggest that the patient's delivery took place in a unit with access to neonatologists and infant resuscitation facilities. After delivery, to reduce the likelihood of an abrupt resurgence of depressive or dysphoric mixed symptoms, I would recommence lithium at an appropriate dose. In line with the American Academy of Pediatrics and other recognized bodies, I would advise against breastfeeding because of the risk of lithium toxicity in the infant with immature kidneys that could not handle lithium excretion. I would continue to give other psychosocial support, as well as support for the partner.

ANSWERS TO SUGGESTED PROBES

1. I would take the following factors into consideration when advising this woman:
   - the importance attached to this baby by the couple, who perhaps may be having their first child
   - the need for prophylaxis, the stage of the pregnancy and the risk of pregnancy loss (cardiogenesis, the formation of the heart in utero, occurs between 3 and 4 weeks of pregnancy, and the risk of this and other malformations continues during pregnancy)
   - the risk of relapse into a severe manic-depressive illness in this patient, who has a severe mental illness that has been largely controlled and stabilized in the community for 3 years
   - the extent of the support that will be available, e.g. medication, partner, midwives, community nurses
   - the need to withdraw lithium as an outpatient or in hospital.
2. If the patient suggested trying carbamazepine, I would inform her that the use of carbamazepine and other mood stabilizers in pregnancy carries a risk of teratogenicity. I would explain that reports have suggested there is an increased incidence of congenital abnormalities such as neural tube and craniofacial defects, finger hypoplasia and developmental delay if mothers take carbamazepine in the first trimester. The fact that she has not also

taken any prophylactic folate (folic acid), as this pregnancy was unplanned, will increase her risk. I would also mention that there is no guarantee that carbamazepine or another mood stabilizer would be able to control her symptoms as well as lithium has done in the last 3 years.

3. A medico-legal situation could arise in the event that:
    *   the patient becomes depressed or manic after lithium withdrawal, and either injures herself or another person or acts in a way that puts herself and others at risk
    *   the lithium is withdrawn and the patient loses the baby
    *   the patient continues on lithium but loses the baby or the baby is deformed
    *   there are other adverse effects, particularly if this patient claims she has not been fully informed of the possible outcomes. Liaison with other professionals and appropriate documentation of discussions will go a long way towards reducing the likelihood of this unpleasant situation.

BUZZ WORDS AND USEFUL TERMINOLOGY

Informed consent, teratogenicity, Ebstein's anomaly, fetal surveillance, medical negligence, medico-legal issues.

REFERENCES AND SUGGESTED READING

Cohen L S, Friedman J, Jefferson J W et al 1994 A re-evaluation of risk of in utero exposure to lithium. Journal of the American Medical Association 271(2):146–150

Suppes T, Baldessarini R J, Faedda G L et al 1991 Risk of recurrence following discontinuation of lithium treatment in bipolar disorder. Archives of General Psychiatry 47:1082–1088

Taylor D, Paton C, Kerwin R 2003 Drug choice in pregnancy. Maudsley Prescribing Guidelines, 7th edn. Martin Dunitz (Taylor & Francis Group) London, pp 204–210

Williams K, Oke S 2000 Lithium and pregnancy. Psychiatric Bulletin 24:229–231

12.4 33-YEAR-OLD WOMAN PRESENTING WITH REPEATED CRYING AND IRRITABILITY 12 WEEKS AFTER CHILDBIRTH

A 33-year-old woman has been referred to you by her GP. Her husband is concerned about her repeated early morning crying and her irritability towards him and their 3-month-old son. She has lost interest in attending to the needs of her baby, and is noticeably losing weight herself.

How would you assess and manage the situation?

SUGGESTED PROBES

1. Would the Edinburgh Postnatal Depression Scale (EPDS) help you in the diagnosis of postnatal depression in this case?
2. What are the risks involved and how would you manage them?
3. What are the alternatives to inpatient management and who else would you involve in this woman's care?

PMP PLAN

TASKS TO DO

The following five areas are relevant to this vignette but are not necessarily all-inclusive. The list is also not exhaustive:

a) Be systematic in your approach.
b) Appreciate the need for multidisciplinary involvement, including health visitors and midwives.
c) Clarify the onset of illness and consider depression and postpartum psychosis as differential diagnoses.
d) Appreciate the need to assess the various risk issues and give consideration to possible predisposing, precipitating and perpetuating factors.
e) Appreciate that this is a potential psychiatric emergency, but at the same time give consideration to both inpatient and outpatient management, depending on the perceived risk and the support system/available services.

ISSUES

- Establishing the cause of the patient's symptoms and distress
- Determining the extent of the risk she poses to herself and her 3-month-old baby
- Deciding on the different management options and settings for such treatment.

CLARIFY

- Who takes care of the baby most of the time and who is taking care of it at the time of referral?
- Has the patient been seen by psychiatric services in the past?
- What does she think about her presentation and the immediate risks and concerns, and is she aware of the referral?
- Are there are any prescribed medications? If so, what are their effects and side-effects, and is the patient compliant?

SEEK MORE INFORMATION

GP

- Past psychiatric history, history of puerperal illness, family history of puerperal and non-puerperal illness.

MIDWIFE/HEALTH VISITOR

- Perspective on presentation
- Arrangements for a joint visit.

PATIENT

- Onset of the problem and progression of the illness
- Evidence of depressive and psychotic symptoms
- Presence of thought disorder and abnormal beliefs about the child
- Suicidal thoughts and thoughts of harming baby or husband.

HUSBAND

- Corroboration of information and views on safety issues/concerns
- Possible predisposing, precipitating and perpetuating factors
- Childcare arrangements if his wife is admitted to hospital.

DIFFERENTIAL DIAGNOSIS/DIFFICULTIES

- *Functional.* Puerperal illness such as postpartum depression, postpartum psychosis; non-puerperal illness such as recurrence of a non-puerperal related depressive illness; psychosocial stressors including adjustment disorder.

APPROACH TO TREATMENT

- Treat as a psychiatric emergency and, as such, give prompt attention.
- Consider immediate, short- and long-term management along biopsychosocial lines.

WHAT TREATMENT/ADVICE

- See Table 12.1.

FULL ANSWER

The main issues that I would like to address in this case are establishing the cause of this lady's symptoms and distress and

Table 12.1 Management plan for postnatal depression

	Biological	Psychological	Social
Immediate	Comprehensive assessment Risk assessment Decide on treatment setting Consider mother and baby unit Psychotropic medication Antipsychotics Antidepressant medication Mood stabilizers Electroconvulsive therapy	Psychoeducation Counselling Nursing observation Cognitive therapy	Assess support network Relationship problems Care of newborn and siblings if mother admitted
Short-term	Treatment optimization Reintroduce safely if previously separated for safety reasons	Continue cognitive therapy Consider family therapy if appropriate Liaison with midwife and health visitor	Community care package Partner support
Long-term	Outpatient follow-up		Support group and CPN input

determining the extent of risk she poses to herself and her baby. I would then outline the different management options and the setting in which such treatment would be carried out. The presentation in this lady raises the possibility of a puerperal illness. As such, I would ensure that the referral was dealt with promptly.

To begin with, I would like to clarify with the GP whether the patient had any major problems when she gave birth, whether the GP has seen the patient or the family recently, and what his or her opinion is on the patient's presentation before referral. I would find out who takes care of the baby most of the time and who is doing so at the time of referral. I would also assess whether there are any immediate risk or safety concerns: for example, if the patient has abnormal beliefs about the baby, or any thoughts of harming herself, the baby or others. I would also like to know whether the GP has prescribed any medication, and if so, what has been the patient's response to medication such as antidepressants. I would find out if the woman and her partner are aware of the referral to mental health services.

In addition, I would seek more information from the GP on the past psychiatric history and history of puerperal illness in both this lady and her family, and also whether there is any history of non-puerperal psychiatric illness. I would also make every effort to talk to both her health visitor and community midwife, if she still has one. I would use the opportunity to get their perspectives on the presentation in this lady and ask if anything similar was suspected or seen before now. If possible, I would arrange a joint visit with her health visitor and community midwife and also with one of the community psychiatric nurses from our team. I would bear in mind that the presence of these different professionals might be overwhelming for the patient. She might feel quite suspicious or fear that the assessment might lead to an admission or separation from her baby. I would therefore ensure that our approach was non-threatening and would carefully explain its purpose.

During the assessment, I would ask her about the onset of the problem and look for evidence of depression (including biological and associated symptoms), psychosis, suicidal thoughts and abnormal beliefs about the baby. I would find out if she has feelings of guilt about not taking care of the baby, and if she has had thoughts of harming herself or the child. I would ask about her personal history of puerperal illness and the treatment she might have received, and whether there is a family history of similar illness. Additionally, I would seek her husband's views on her presentation and try to elicit any possible predisposing, precipitating and perpetuating factors to this illness from him.

I would ask him about the kind of support the woman has been receiving from her family, how he copes himself and whether these developments have had any effect on their relationship. I would enquire whether he has any concerns about his wife's or baby's safety, and how he would cope with the children, should we admit his wife to hospital.

I would include postpartum depression, postpartum psychosis and recurrence of a non-puerperal illness in my differential diagnosis at this point. Given the potential risk in cases like this, my approach would be to treat this as a psychiatric emergency. In order to support a diagnosis of postnatal depression.

Once I was clear that the patient was suffering from a depressive episode, my immediate management plan would be to decide on the type and setting of treatment, guided by the outcome of the various multidisciplinary assessments, risk issues and available resources. I would consider immediate, short- and long-term management, along biopsychosocial lines. As far as possible, the approach would be multidisciplinary, including the patient, GP, midwife, health visitor, CPN and social worker. I would consider inpatient treatment if there were evidence of at least mild to moderate depressive or psychotic illness, a risk to the child or a lack of adequate social support. My preference would be for admission to a mother and baby unit, where the patient could be supported with her child. However, I would bear in mind that this might not be necessary if there were no concerns over the mother's or the baby's safety, and might not be possible if there were no such unit locally. On the other hand, I would consider managing her as an outpatient if there were little or no risk and if she could be supported by family members and community services. In this case I would suggest that one of our CPNs gave the necessary support and monitored the case in the community.

Concerning treatment, I would offer psychoeducation to reassure the woman and her partner and would make sure they had adequate information about the illness and what to expect from treatment. While she might not be able to take in fully all the information, it would still be important to provide it to allay any fears and to prevent or reduce any suspicion or paranoid feelings. Once she was admitted to the hospital, I would start her on appropriate psychotropic medication, taking into consideration whether she was breastfeeding or not. If insomnia were a problem, I would consider prescribing one of the sedative antidepressants. (There is no evidence that any one antidepressant is superior to another in postpartum depression.) These treatments would be coupled with psychosocial support and other psychological approaches. In very rare situations, and after all other options have been adequately explored, electroconvulsive therapy may be given as a last resort. If the patient were admitted to hospital, I would ask nursing staff to give support and observe closely, depending on the degree of risk of self-harm. Nursing staff would also offer reassurance, a listening ear and an opportunity for her to vent her fears and anxieties.

In the short term, the goal would be to optimize any treatment she is already undergoing and give consideration to other psychological (cognitive behaviour and family therapy) and social (community care package) treatments, as appropriate. I would refer her to the team's social worker for social assessment and intervention, which would include, for example, assessing the couple's current support network and care arrangements for the children following the mother's admission to hospital. There would also be a need to give appropriate support to the partner, who might well need treatment in his own right. (A 12-month follow-up of spouses of women with postnatal psychiatric illness by Lovestone and Kumar (1993) showed that the rate of psychiatric illness in these men is higher than in the control group of men whose partners remained well after childbirth and a group of men whose partners were admitted with non-puerperal illness.)

In the long term, I would recommend that this patient be subjected to an enhanced care programme approach (in the UK). This framework of care requires the mental health service to appoint a named key worker, with the responsibility of making sure she has regular follow-up and review, along with an agreed and documented care plan which would detail known relapse indicators and contingency plans. I would suggest joint input from the CPN and the health visitor, at least until there was no further concern about the patient's mental health. I would also give the family information on relevant support groups. In the United Kingdom, there is a group called Newpin for mothers with new babies. Members give each other informal support and some mothers find this beneficial.

ANSWERS TO SUGGESTED PROBES

1. The Edinburgh Postnatal Depression Scale (EPDS) would not help in the diagnosis of postnatal depression in this case. It is a screening tool and not a diagnostic instrument, and is used by non-mental health professionals in large screening programmes of all postnatal women. EPDS would not add anything to a good psychiatric history and mental state examination in making a diagnosis of postnatal depression.

2. The risks in this case are:
   - *Patient.* Suicide: manage by close monitoring, support from staff, risk assessment and treatment of depression.
   - *Baby.* Neonaticide, infanticide and risk of neglect: manage by close monitoring, separation of mother and child if necessary, temporary placements or care by the family, support for the mother, risk assessment and treatment of maternal depression.
   - *Husband.* Stress and/or acute mental illness.
3. Day care would be a useful alternative to inpatient management in this case, with the provision of a full range of interventions including group work, play therapy, motherhood classes, anxiety classes and occupational therapy. As far as possible, the approach should be multidisciplinary and include the patient's GP, midwife, health visitor, CPN and social worker. This is not, however, an alternative to specialist treatment in severe cases, when there are concerns over risk or family support is very limited.

BUZZ WORDS AND USEFUL TERMINOLOGY

Postpartum depression, risk assessment, neonaticide, multidisciplinary assessment, mother and baby unit.

REFERENCES AND SUGGESTED READING

Brockington I 2002 Obstetric and gynaecological conditions associated with psychiatric disorders. In: Gelder M G, López-Ibor Jr J J, Andreasen N C (eds) New Oxford Textbook of Psychiatry, vol. 2. Oxford University Press, Oxford, pp 1202–1207
Lovestone S, Kumar R 1993 Postnatal psychiatric illness: the impact on partners. British Journal of Psychiatry 163:210–216

13

Psychopharmacology, psychotherapy and other treatments

13.1 PATIENT ABOUT TO START TREATMENT WITH CLOZAPINE

A patient with treatment-resistant schizophrenia, whom you have already started working with, is being considered for treatment with clozapine.

What will inform your decision to proceed in this direction and how will you establish this man successfully on the medication?

SUGGESTED PROBES

1. During your discussions with the patient's mother she seems particularly worried about the side-effect profile of clozapine. How would you reassure her?
2. Eight weeks into treatment with clozapine the patient's white blood cell count falls below 2×10^{11} per litre, (coded as 'red' or dangerously low neutropenia). What would you do?
3. Ten weeks after starting clozapine the patient says he is unhappy about continuing on the medication as he has gained 5 kg in weight. What management approach would you take?

PMP PLAN

TASKS TO DO

The following five areas are relevant to this vignette but are not necessarily all-inclusive. The list is also not exhaustive:

a) Discuss the need to establish the diagnosis of treatment-resistant schizophrenia (TRS) and the performance of baseline assessments.

b) Demonstrate the need to give patient and carers clear details about clozapine treatment, its contraindications, side-effects and what to expect.

c) Demonstrate awareness of the protocols involved in establishing a patient on clozapine and of the monitoring arrangements.

d) Show understanding of the measures for assessing improvement, side-effects and associative issues involved in the use of clozapine.

e) Consider other forms of treatment in addition to clozapine in the management of treatment-resistant schizophrenia, i.e. supportive psychotherapy, treatment for addiction and psychosocial treatment.

ISSUES

- Confirming that the diagnosis of treatment-resistant schizophrenia is correct
- Completing all the tasks that need to be done before deciding on clozapine
- Making sure that the patient is suitable for treatment with clozapine and is willing to comply with the mandatory and frequent blood investigations.

CLARIFY

- Is the patient truly treatment-resistant, i.e. has he used at least two antipsychotics from two different classes for a minimum of 6–8 weeks each?

SEEK MORE INFORMATION

MEDICAL NOTES AND STAFF

- Adequacy and duration of the treatment given to date
- Compliance
- Any previous augmentation or combination therapy.

MEDICATION REVIEW

- Past and present drug charts.

PATIENT

- Ask his opinion on the use of clozapine
- Ask whether he would give consent for blood investigations necessary for dispensing and administration of clozapine

- History of allergy and presence of contraindications to the use of clozapine
- Readiness to give blood for therapeutic monitoring
- Expectations in terms of gains and side-effects of treatment
- Use of excessive alcohol and illicit drugs, in particular amphetamine-like drugs, cocaine and cannabis.

DIFFERENTIAL DIAGNOSIS/DIFFICULTIES

Not relevant to this vignette.

APPROACH TO TREATMENT

- Exclude any contraindications to the use of clozapine, such as severe cardiac disorders, active liver disease, severe renal impairment, alcoholic and toxic psychosis, a history of drug-induced neutropenia or agranulocytosis, and bone marrow disorders.
- Exclude organic conditions including brain tumours.
- Obtain informed consent from the patient and seek the cooperation of carers.
- Register him with the Clozaril Patient Monitoring Service (CPMS) and local pharmacy.
- Arrange an initial blood screen, including FBC.
- Obtain an objective baseline assessment using the Brief Psychiatric Rating Scale (BPRS; Overall & Gorman 1962), and carry out and document a mental state examination.

WHAT TREATMENT/ADVICE

- Suggest initial treatment in hospital if it is not possible in the outpatient department.
- Increase the dose of clozapine gradually according to the protocol.
- Monitor side-effects of clozapine treatment: agranulocytosis, other blood dyscrasias, fatigue, sedation, blurred vision, dry mouth, hypersalivation, tremor, weight gain, constipation, paralyticileus, urinary retention/incontinence, seizures in predisposed individuals, and cardiac arrhythmias, postural hypotension and drowsiness.
- Treat embarrassing side-effects, such as hypersalivation.
- Look for evidence of infection.
- Warn the patient not to operate machinery.
- Arrange regular blood testing (including FBC).

- Consider other supportive treatments, such as supportive psychotherapy, cognitive behavioural therapy for psychosis, family therapy, day care and occupational activities. Propose treatment for drug addiction, if concurrent illicit drug use is a problem.
- Consider augmentation of clozapine with combination therapy with other antipsychotics, mood stabilizers or SSRIs.
- Arrange adequate follow-up after discharge.

FULL ANSWER

In attending to this case, I would quickly focus on the basis of the diagnosis of treatment resistance and the need to proceed with clozapine. The main issues that I would like to address would be confirming that the diagnosis of treatment-resistant schizophrenia is correct, ensuring that all the tasks relating to the use of clozapine have been completed, and making sure that the patient is suitable for treatment with clozapine and is willing to comply.

I would reassure myself that the diagnosis of treatment-resistant schizophrenia had been firmly established and that at least two different antipsychotics belonging to different groups had been used for an appropriate duration, i.e. well over 6–8 weeks each. I would also clarify whether appropriate optimal doses had been used and if the patient complied fully with treatment during this period. I would ensure that there had been no compounding issues, such as the use of illicit drugs or the consumption of excessive amounts of alcohol, and that there is no severe affective disorder in this gentleman. I would also ensure that organic conditions, including brain tumour, had been excluded.

Once this had been done, I would seek more information as to whether the patient had yet been informed of the plan to try clozapine and if so, what his response was. I would personally look through the medical notes to assess the adequacy of the treatment given so far, the duration of such treatment and compliance. I would review past and present drug charts to see if there had been any previous augmentation or combination therapy.

I would then assess the patient to find out about his current mental state, the symptoms he is experiencing and how he is coping with them. I would establish whether he has been using excessive alcohol or illicit drugs, in particular amphetamine-like drugs, cocaine and cannabis. I would inform him of the associated benefits from taking clozapine after explaining the side-effects to him. These benefits would include improvement in his mental state and a reduction in distressing symptoms such as voices, less agitation, reduced extrapyramidal side-effects compared to other medication, an improvement in cognitive function, a reduction in aggression and tendency to suicidality, a reduction in the need to readmit frequently and an overall improvement in his quality of life. I would also find out whether he is on any other medication at present, and what psychological and psychosocial support he is receiving. I would elicit his opinion on the need to take clozapine and check that he is happy with the decision and agrees to submit himself for regular blood tests, once a week for the initial 18 weeks of treatment. I would ensure that he has no contraindications to clozapine, such as allergy to the substance itself or any other component of the formulation, a previous history of drug-induced neutropenia, a myeloproliferative disorder, uncontrolled epilepsy, alcoholic and toxic psychosis, drug intoxication, severe cardiac failure, or acute and progressive liver disease.

I would carefully explain the possible side-effects of clozapine, which include agranulocytosis and other blood dyscrasias, fatigue, drowsiness, sedation, blurred vision, dry mouth, hypersalivation, excessive weight gain, marked tremor, constipation, paralytic ileus, urinary retention and incontinence. I would also explain that clozapine has been found to cause some EEG changes and seizures in predisposed people, particularly patients on high doses of medication. I would explain that other side-effects include hyperglycaemia, jaundice and abnormalities on liver function test. (Fulminant hepatic necrosis may rarely occur.) I would reassure him that, even though these side-effects have all been reported, it does not necessarily mean that they will all happen to him. In particular, I would explain the risk of neutropenia leading to agranulocytosis, and tell him that this is an idiosyncratic reaction that has been reported in 1 in 100 patients. I would explain that this is why regular blood testing is necessary. I would find out whether the patient would be prepared to give blood on a weekly basis for the first 18 weeks, then fortnightly for up to 1 year after commencing medication, and then monthly thereafter.

Once I was certain that this man had fully understood this information and he had agreed to commence clozapine, I would start to taper off the conventional antipsychotics very gradually. I would carry out an initial FBC and register the responsible medical officer (usually the consultant) and the patient with the local Clozaril Patient Monitoring Service (CPMS). This would be in compliance with the licensing requirement to monitor the white cell count closely so that clozapine can be promptly withdrawn in patients who are developing severe neutropenia. I would also carry out a baseline mental state examination before starting clozapine, using validated instruments such as the BPRS, GHQ, SAPS and SANS for an objective measurement of psychopathology.

Once these tests had been done, I would consider initiating clozapine treatment in hospital, bearing in mind the need to monitor the patient's physical state, particularly for the risk of postural hypotension. I would give clozapine 12.5 mg once or twice on the first day, to be followed by 25 mg once or twice on the second day, and would continue to increase the dose gradually according to the protocol supplied by the CPMS or as agreed locally. I would continue to use divided doses and would give the larger dose mainly at night. Initially, I would aim for a maintenance dose of about 150–300 mg daily, increasing if necessary to a maximum of 900 mg per day if this case proved very difficult. I would pay particular attention to patient physical status if a very high dose is recommended. If monotherapy with clozapine fails, given that a substantial proportion of patients receiving clozapine will continue to experience disabling symptoms, I will consider augmentation with amisulpiride or other combination therapy, with mood stabilizers or SSRIs.

I would emphasize the need for the patient to be compliant with this medication and would perform the appropriate serum clozapine levels to ensure an adequate level of greater than 0.35 mg per litre was maintained in the blood. I would stress the need to monitor side-effects and also report any evidence of infection, fever, sore throat or pyrexia of unknown origin. As there would be increased sedation and drowsiness, I would initially advise the patient not to drive or operate any heavy machinery that might put him or others at risk of physical injury. I would also consider other forms of treatment, including supportive psychotherapy, family therapy, psychosocial support and help with any concurrent addiction or use of illicit substances.

I would attend to any excessive weight gain by advising on healthy eating, reduction of polysaturated fats, and regular exercise. I would refer to a dietician if the weight gain did not improve despite these measures. I would treat other distressing side-effects such as hypersalivation with hyoscine hydrobromide. Other medication that can be used for excessive oral secretion includes benzatropine, trihexyphenidyl, ipratropium bromide, clonidine, lofexidine and terazosin. I would also consider a reduction in the dose of medication, slow titration and the use of sugarless candy gums in order to combat this embarrassing symptom.

I would hope that, with this approach, the patient would improve on clozapine to the point where he could be safely discharged into the community. In doing so, I would inform the CPMS and make appropriate arrangements in the community for this patient to continue his blood tests and to receive his medication from a named pharmacist. In addition to suggesting that he attend a clozapine clinic attached to the service, I would follow him up in the outpatient clinic.

1. If the patient's mother was worried about the side-effects of clozapine, I would explain that some of these, including neutropenia leading to agranulocytosis (a reduced white blood cell count), have been reported in several people but this does not mean that everyone taking the drug will experience every side-effect. The common ones are fatigue, weight gain, drowsiness, sedation, dizziness, headache, tendency to seizures, dry mouth, blurred vision, hypersalivation, nausea and vomiting, constipation, paralytic ileus, and extrapyramidal side-effects such as tremor and rigidity. I would also inform her that abnormality of liver function tests, jaundice, increased blood sugar, urinary incontinence, urinary retention and priapism have also been reported.

I would also explain that some rare side-effects, including confusion, restlessness, agitation, delirium, neuroleptic malignant syndrome, respiratory depression, circulation collapse and parathyroid gland enlargement, have also been reported. I would, however, reassure her that these have been reported in people from all over the world and would not necessarily all occur in a single individual.

I would emphasize that the effect that gives most concern is neutropenia leading to agranulocytosis, as this can predispose patients to developing infections, but would reassure her that safeguards have been put in place by the manufacturer of clozapine (via the Clozaril Patient Monitoring Service), in the form of regular blood monitoring. This would be carried out weekly for the initial 18 weeks of treatment, then fortnightly for up to 12 months after commencing clozapine, and then monthly after that. This system has been put in place to ensure that clozapine can be immediately withdrawn if there are any signs of agranulocytosis. If these did occur, I would stop the medication and support the patient with an appropriate alternative.

Finally, I would ask her whether she had any other questions, which I would be very happy to answer for her.

2. If, 8 weeks into treatment with clozapine, the white blood cell count fell below 2×10^{11} per litre, I would also check the absolute blood count. If this were less than 1.5×10^{11} per litre I would immediately stop the clozapine and inform the CPMS. If the evidence pointed to a high likelihood of relapse, I would treat with other atypical antipsychotics. I would also monitor for evidence of infection and treat accordingly with antibiotics.

If the white blood cell count fell further and there were a risk of severe infection, I would transfer the patient to a local specialist haematological unit for treatment. The administration of a colony-stimulating factor can usually be carried out at such units. The patient can also be covered with prophylactic antibiotic treatment.

Having stopped clozapine, I would hope that his white cell count would improve to a point where treatment and monitoring could be safely resumed. The next step would be to reintroduce clozapine slowly following the manufacturer's guidelines.

3. If, 10 weeks after starting clozapine, the patient became unhappy about continuing on the medication as he had gained 5 kg, I would inform him that, although I appreciate his concerns, the weight gain caused by clozapine is usually no worse than that caused by other antipsychotics over a long period. I would emphasize that the benefits of using clozapine outweigh the risk of weight gain, and mention that other steps can be usually taken to maintain a healthy weight. I would:

- advise him to eat healthily, particularly large amounts of fruit and vegetables and fewer polysaturated fats
- encourage daily exercise and membership of a weight management group or one of the initiatives available at the local hospital
- refer him to a dietician for appropriate professional advice.

BUZZ WORDS AND USEFUL TERMINOLOGY

Engagement of patient, compliance therapy, augmentation and combination therapy.

REFERENCES AND SUGGESTED READING

Buckley P, Miller A, Olsen J et al 2001 When symptoms persist: clozapine augumentation strategies. Schizophrenia Bulletin 27:615–628

Cree A, Mir S, Fahy T 2001 A review of treatment options for clozapine-induced hypersalivation. Psychiatric Bulletin 25:114–116

Kane J, Honigfeld G, Singer J et al 1988 Clozapine for the treatment of treatment-resistant schizophrenia: a double blind comparison with chlorpromazine. Archives of General Psychiatry 45:789–796

Moncrieff J 2003 Clozapine v. conventional antipsychotic drugs for treatment-resistant schizophrenia: a re-examination. British Journal of Psychiatry 183:161–166

Overall J E, Gorman D R 1962 The brief psychiatric rating scale. Psychological Reports 10:799–812

Tuunainen A ,Wahlbeck K, Gilbody S M 2000 Newer atypical antipsychotic medication in comparison to clozapine: a systematic review of randomized control trials. Schizophrenia Research 56:1–10

13.2 42-YEAR-OLD WOMAN WITH ANXIETY AND DEPRESSION SEEKING SOLELY PSYCHOLOGICAL TREATMENT

A 42-year-old woman, who works as a secretary in the City of London, has been referred to your clinic for psychological treatment for her mild depression and anxiety. She no longer has faith in the medication prescribed for her for the last 3 years.
What treatment would you offer her and why?

SUGGESTED PROBES

1. What information would you seek before embarking on a treatment plan?
2. What are your differential diagnoses?
3. What is the basis of treatment and how would you carry it out?

PMP PLAN

TASKS TO DO

The following five areas are relevant to this vignette but are not necessarily all-inclusive. The list is also not exhaustive:

a) Evaluate previous treatment and response and explore the reasons the patient might have for declining pharmacological treatment.
b) Carry out a comprehensive assessment, including an evaluation of her current symptoms and perpetuating factors.
c) Assess psychological mindedness, readiness to change and suitability for treatment.
d) Demonstrate knowledge of various psychological approaches and discuss one confidently.
e) Assess risk, particularly if the gain of psychological treatment is not realized early.

ISSUES

- Identification of current problems and the psychosocial factors that are perpetuating the patient's illness
- Assessment for suitability, and whether she will engage and benefit from psychological treatment
- Deciding on specific psychological treatment tailored to her specific situation and needs.

CLARIFY

- Is the woman safe and can she engage in psychological treatment?
- How severe is her illness? Is she at risk of self-harm or suicide?

SEEK MORE INFORMATION

GP

- Previous treatment, current symptoms, possible psychosocial maintaining factors and immediate risk issue.

PATIENT

- Past psychiatric history, including details of previous treatment (whether beneficial or not)
- Current anxiety/depressive symptoms and cognitions (negative automatic thoughts both trigger and enhance depressive symptoms)
- Severity of illness and impact on functioning; coping mechanisms (it is important to explore these because the patient could adopt strategies, such as use of alcohol or drugs, that would offer relief in the short term but be unhelpful in the longer term)
- Relevant early life experiences that might have led to the development of current beliefs and assumptions
- Current psychosocial difficulties, including marital or work-related problems
- Reason she gave up on pharmacological treatment
- Previous knowledge and experience of psychological treatment
- Current physical problems (thyroid disease, painful or chronic physical problems) and medications such as beta-blockers and other antihypertensives.

DIFFERENTIAL DIAGNOSIS/DIFFICULTIES

- *Functional.* Axis I diagnoses: mild depression and anxiety, depressive disorder, generalized anxiety, mixed anxiety and depressive disorder, dysthymia. Axis II diagnosis, such as anxious (avoidant) personality disorder
- *Organic.* Organic mood and anxiety disorders secondary to conditions such as thyroid disorders.

Note: whilst it is important to pay attention to the above, they should not affect your decision of whether to offer psychological intervention. This is the patient's choice of treatment and it is for this that she has been referred.

APPROACH TO TREATMENT

- Appraise and reassess the diagnosis prior to embarking on treatment.
- Exclude poor medication compliance due to side-effects, inadequate treatment (doses and duration) with antidepressants, significant physical illness and overwhelming psychosocial difficulties.
- Educate the patient to the effect that her current beliefs may be learned opinion rather than a true reflection of the current state of affairs.
- Suggest cognitive behavioural therapy (CBT) as the first line of psychological treatment, as it has been shown to be consistently effective in depressed patients (Fennell 2002).
- Examine this woman's pre-existing behavioural and cognitive coping skills, acceptance of the cognitive model, willingness to engage in self-help assessment, ease of access to thoughts and feelings, problem specificity, and ability to form a collaborative alliance.

WHAT TREATMENT/ADVICE

Advise cognitive behavioural therapy (CBT), a short-term psychotherapy aimed at changing unhelpful thoughts or behaviours that are causing this woman's problem. It is active, directive, structured and time-limited, typically occupying between 12 and 20 weekly sessions of 1 hour.

CBT would proceed through evaluation of diagnosis, assessment of current situation and problem identification; use of specific cognitive interventions designed to reduce the frequency of negative thoughts; incorporation of behavioural assignments intended to tackle behaviour and reduce any motivational deficits; monitoring and questioning negative automatic thoughts (NATs); relapse prevention.

OBJECTIVES OF THE INITIAL ASSESSMENT INTERVIEW

- Establish a therapeutic alliance.
- Enable case permutation and conceptualization.

- Help the patient to come up with a list of specific problems and corresponding goals, and to select the first problem to tackle.
- Educate her on the cognitive model and explain/illustrate the vicious circle that might possibly be maintaining her illness (see Fig. 13.1 and 'full answer').
- Socialize the CBT model.
- Having identified the patient's problems, demonstrate to her how emotions and behaviour are influenced by negative thinking and relate this to her experience.
- Agree on an assignment to prepare for her next meeting with the therapist. This might involve listening to an audiotape of the session that has taken place or a reading and self-monitoring assignment.
- Teach her behavioural interventions such as distraction techniques, activities monitoring and planning.
- Maximize engagement in activities that provide a sense of pleasure and mastery through early behavioural intervention to reduce the negative thoughts and the depression.

SECOND STAGE OF TREATMENT

This is composed of symptom-focused cognitive and behavioural reattribution through cognitive and behavioural techniques. There is an overlap between these two.

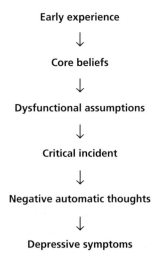

Fig. 13.1 The cognitive behavioural model.

Examples of cognitive techniques include:

- identifying and labelling thinking errors
- addressing the validity of her NATs through questioning of the evidence and reviewing the counter-evidence. The dysfunctional thought record is a useful tool for this purpose
- addressing the usefulness of the NATs
- using the dysfunctional thought record to identify and record unpleasant emotions, situations in which emotion is involved, and NATs associated with emotion
- teaching the patient how to question her NATs and how to develop the ability to generate alternative views to her thoughts
- problem-solving.

Examples of behavioural techniques include:

- activity monitoring and scheduling
- exposure
- experiments.

CLOSING STAGES OF TREATMENT

- Focus on re-evaluating and addressing any dysfunction assumption using the principle of Socratic questioning. This is an essential tool during the assessment and engagement phase of CBT. Essentially, it involves helping the client to develop alternative explanations for their experience. For example, patients can be helped to draw on their own doubts and experiences in order to realize that there are other ways of making sense of their experience. It does not involve any attempt to persuade patients that they are wrong in their beliefs.
- Consolidate what has been learnt and prepare for setbacks.

OTHER TREATMENT MODALITIES

- Psychodynamic psychotherapy.
- Brief focal psychotherapy.
- Interpersonal psychotherapy.

FULL ANSWER

The history in this 42-year-old woman is very suggestive of someone who has not benefited from pharmacological treatment for her anxiety and depression and who is now seeking psychological treatment. The important issue in this presentation is the need to identify and understand her current problems and the psychosocial factors that are perpetuating her illness. I would also focus on assessment of her suitability to engage with and benefit from various psychological treatments. I would then decide on a specific treatment that would be tailored to her specific situation and needs. However, in order to clarify the exact nature of the problem and what the patient really wants, I would first need to clarify with her GP what her current symptoms are, details of previous treatments, and possible psychosocial maintaining factors of her illness. I would also make enquiries about any immediate risk issues, whether the woman is currently stable, and if the GP thinks she is ready for treatment.

I would arrange to see the patient at the outpatient clinic to seek more information on her current anxiety and depressive symptoms, the treatment she has received so far, and why she has lost faith in pharmacological treatment. I would ask her what she thinks triggers and maintains her depressive illness and if she currently has overwhelming psychosocial problems related to her work, relationship or family. I would use the opportunity to examine for the presence of a distorted way of thinking, including negative automatic thoughts (NATs). In addition, I would enquire about relevant early life experiences, such as loss of her mother or parental separation at an early age, which might have predisposed her to depression and developing dysfunctional assumptions or beliefs. This information might be used to educate her that any negative or dysfunctional assumption she holds about herself is a learnt opinion and not a reflection of the truth. I would ask about her past psychiatric history, details of previous treatment, current physical health problems such as thyroid disease or other painful or chronic disorders. I would ask if she is on any prescribed or non-prescribed substances such as beta-blockers or other medication that might be depressogenic. I would assess the severity of her illness and ask her what impact it has on her daily functioning. I would like to know exactly how she has been coping since the illness began, in order to exclude the use of strategies that would offer relief in the short term but would be unhelpful in the long term: for example, the use of alcohol or drugs. I would ask her why she has given up on using medication, if she has any specific psychological treatment in mind, and what she already knows about the treatments available.

Before proceeding to offer another type of treatment, I would reassure myself that the patient had been rightly diagnosed, and that other possible differential diagnoses, including organic mood and anxiety disorders secondary to thyroid disorders, had been excluded. I would also exclude compounding physical and overwhelming psychosocial problems. Unless a new and significant finding emerged, I would proceed to psychological intervention, as this is the patient's choice of treatment and the main reason that she has been referred.

In planning for psychological treatment, I would assess whether this patient is psychologically minded, and suitable and ready for treatment. My approach would be to discuss the various options, provide the patient with written information on the various types of treatment and give her time to think about them. The main options would be cognitive behavioural therapy (CBT), interpersonal psychotherapy and psychodynamic psychotherapy. In this case, I would suggest the patient considered CBT, which, as well as being a tried and popular technique, has consistently been shown to be effective in patients with depression and anxiety. Should she accept this argument, I would examine her pre-existing behavioural and cognitive coping skills, acceptance of the cognitive model, willingness to engage in self-help assessment, ease of access to thoughts and feelings, problem specificity, and ability to form a collaborative alliance. I would then offer her CBT.

Unless I had a special interest, skill or experience in this form of therapy, I would refer her to a psychotherapist. Nevertheless, I would educate her that CBT is an individual, short-term psychotherapy in which she would have to collaborate with the therapist in order to achieve alteration of the unhelpful thoughts or behaviours that are causing or perpetuating her depression and anxiety. I would inform her that CBT usually lasts between 12 and 20 weeks. The hour-long weekly sessions normally proceed through diagnosis, assessment and problem identification. The therapist would use specific cognitive interventions to reduce the frequency of negative thoughts; use behavioural assignments to tackle behavioural and motivational deficits; monitor and question NATs; and engage in relapse prevention. The main objective of the initial session would be to establish a therapeutic relationship, to attempt a case permutation and conceptualization, to help the patient come up with a list of specific problems and corresponding goals, and to select the first problem to tackle. I would socialize her on the CBT model, and explain or illustrate to her the vicious circle that might possibly be maintaining her illness. I would explain the link between early experiences, core beliefs, dysfunctional assumptions, a critical incident, NATs and depressive symptoms. I would use her identified problems to show how negative thinking influences emotions and behaviours, and how this relates to her own experience. We would agree on an assignment for her to work on in preparation for the next meeting and this might include listening to an audiotape, reading or a self-monitoring assignment.

During the second phase of treatment, the therapist would attempt a symptom-focused cognitive and behavioural reattribution through cognitive and behavioural techniques. There is an overlap between these two. I or the therapist would focus on helping her to learn how to identify and label thinking errors, and also challenge NATs with the aim of reducing her distress and allowing her to find constructive solutions to her problems. I would address the validity of her NATs through questioning of the evidence and reviewing the counter-evidence. I would suggest that she use a dysfunctional thought record to identify and record unpleasant emotions, the situations in which emotions occur, and the NATs associated with the emotions. Once she was able to challenge and question her NATs, I would encourage her to generate alternative views to her negative thoughts and also attempt problem-solving. During the closing stages of treatment the focus would be on re-evaluating and addressing any dysfunctional assumption using the principle of Socratic questioning, consolidating what has already been learnt and preparing for setbacks. Essentially, Socratic questioning involves helping the patient to develop alternative explanations for their experience. For example, patients can be helped to draw on their own doubts and experiences in order to realize that there are other ways of making sense of their experience. It does not involve any attempt to persuade patients that they are wrong in their beliefs.

I would also teach the patient behavioural interventions like distraction techniques, activity monitoring scheduling and planning. Exposure techniques and other experiments could also be carried out. The overall goal of this early behavioural intervention would be to maximize engagement in activities, which provide a sense of pleasure and mastery. These hopefully would help reduce the negative thoughts and depression.

Note: do not waste too much time asking whether this lady has had full courses of antidepressants or anxiolytics at different doses. There would be a problem too, if you jumped to the conclusion that she had agoraphobia or a panic disorder without that information being given in the vignette, just because you had rehearsed those topics.

ANSWERS TO SUGGESTED PROBES

1. The information I would need before embarking on a treatment plan is covered in the full answer.

2. My differential diagnoses are covered in the full answer.
3. The basis of treatment would be cognitive behavioural therapy, which has been shown to be consistently effective in depressed patients. The full answer explains how I would carry it out.

BUZZ WORDS AND USEFUL TERMINOLOGY

Case permutation and conceptualization, engagement, diaries, homework, dysfunctional schema, poor coping skills, negative automatic thought patterns, fundamental assumptions, reattribution, hypothesis generation and testing, activities scheduling, self-monitoring, feedbacks and triggers.

REFERENCES AND SUGGESTED READING

Fava G A 2002 Cognitive behavior approach to loss of clinical effect during long-term antidepressant treatment: a pilot study. American Journal of Psychiatry 159:2094–2095
Fennell M J 2002 Cognitive–behaviour therapy for depressive disorders. In: Gelder M G, López-Ibor Jr J J, Andreasen N C (eds) New Oxford Textbook of Psychiatry, vol. 2. Oxford University Press, Oxford, pp 1394–1405

13.3 43-YEAR-OLD WHO IS ANXIOUS AND UNABLE TO LEAVE HER HOME

A 43-year-old woman who has been finding it increasingly difficult to leave her home unaccompanied has been referred to you for further advice and management. She suffered a minor fall at work 9 months ago and has not returned to work since then. Her GP, who has tried several antidepressants, can no longer cope with her repeated demand for benzodiazepines and is certain that she needs psychological treatment.

What would be your approach to management and what treatment would you give?

SUGGESTED PROBES

1. What are your differential diagnoses?
2. Other than psychological treatment, what else would help in the management of this patient?
3. What other issue would you pay attention to in the assessment and management of this patient?

PMP PLAN

TASKS TO DO

The following five areas are relevant to this vignette but are not necessarily all-inclusive. The list is also not exhaustive:

a) Discuss the possibility of comorbid depression and the issue of risk (self-neglect, self-harm or suicide).
b) Discuss possible predisposing, precipitating and perpetuating factors to the illness.
c) Carry out a systematic and comprehensive assessment, to include agoraphobia as a differential diagnosis, and also consider other anxiety disorders (including post-traumatic stress disorder (PTSD), obsessive-compulsive disorder (OCD)) and substance misuse (benzodiazepine dependence) as comorbid conditions.
d) Include a broad range of biopsychosocial interventions in your management plan.
e) Discuss a preferred psychological treatment for agoraphobia.

ISSUES

- Identification of the current problems and determination of the roles of anxiety (agoraphobia), past trauma and benzodiazepine use in this lady's presentation
- Assessment of whether the patient would engage with and benefit from psychological treatment
- Deciding on a psychological treatment tailored to her specific situation and needs.

CLARIFY

- When was the onset of her current difficulties and how long have they lasted?
- How soon does the GP want her to be seen?
- Are there any immediate risks or safety concerns?

SEEK MORE INFORMATION

GP

- Past psychiatric and medical history; previous treatment and response
- Current medication: duration of benzodiazepine treatment, dependency on benzodiazepines, other non-prescribed drugs or substances such as alcohol
- Home situation, i.e. partner and children, financial and other possible psychosocial difficulties.

PATIENT/FAMILY

- Comprehensive psychiatric assessment, with the emphasis on the onset and duration of her anxiety about leaving home. What happened when she last attempted this, where she was going, what psychological and physical symptoms she suffered, and her response. Site- or situation-specific anxiety, i.e. which occurs only when going to a particular place (as opposed to it happening in other situations). Factors that make it worse or better. Autonomic symptoms of anxiety, such as headache, breathing difficulty, palpitations, excessive sweating and 'butterflies in the stomach'. Panic attacks and their duration; fear of dying during these attacks
- Possible predisposing (family history), precipitating (recent fall at work or other work- or family-related difficulties) and perpetuating factors (avoidance of going out alone, safety

behaviours, attentional deficits, i.e. focusing on physical accompaniments of her anxiety, faulty beliefs, attitude and beliefs of significant others in her life and abuse of prescribed and non-prescribed medication—for example, tranquillizers which cause sleep disturbance, or painkillers which cause derealization)

- Use of alcohol as a coping mechanism prior to going out
- Presence of comorbid PTSD, OCD or depressive disorders
- Understanding of what the threat of going out means to the patient, and development of a cognitive behavioural formulation of the presentation to form the blueprint to help organize and develop a programme of cognitive behavioural therapy (CBT).

DIFFERENTIAL DIAGNOSIS/DIFFICULTIES

- *Functional.* Phobic anxiety disorder (agoraphobia, panic disorder, social phobia), depressive illness and substance misuse disorder
- *Organic.* Although not likely, hyperthyroidism, hypothyroidism or an early menopause.

APPROACH TO TREATMENT

- Exclude risk issues.
- Look out for and treat any mental illness and substance misuse.
- Identify the patient's negative beliefs and evidence for them.

WHAT TREATMENT/ADVICE

PSYCHOLOGICAL

- Organize CBT (the principles of this are described in vignette 13.2, p. 455), relaxation therapy/anxiety management.
- Give education on anxiety disorder, preferably linking it with the patient's irrational fears; also cover the cognitive model of anxiety, how the triggers for her anxiety lead to the production of negative automatic thoughts relating to the feared outcome, and how these are maintained by her decision not to go out.
- Carry out cognitive restructuring, either by imagery or by identifying observations that contradict her negative beliefs.

- Build up a systematic exposure to going out alone, initially by imagery and then in real life, while engaging her in more relaxing activities.
- Propose family therapy, if appropriate.

MEDICAL

- Give antidepressants, preferably sedative.
- Arrange benzodiazepine or alcohol detoxification.

SOCIAL

- Advise the patient to contact the Citizens Advice Bureau (in the UK): for example, for help with money management if she has financial difficulties.

FULL ANSWER

A history of difficulty going out unaccompanied and possible dependence on benzodiazepines in this 43-year-old lady arouses the suspicion of a possible phobic anxiety disorder such as agoraphobia. The main issues in this vignette are identification of the current problems, and determination of the roles that anxiety (agoraphobia), past trauma and benzodiazepine use play in this presentation. The other issue is the assessment of the patient's suitability to engage in and benefit from psychological treatment, and deciding on a psychological treatment tailored to her specific situation and needs.

I would first like to clarify with the GP how bad the situation is and whether the patient is considered to be at risk of self-neglect, neglect of others, medical and physical complications from benzodiazepine misuse, self-harm or suicide. I would ask about the onset and duration of the current difficulties and how soon she needs to be seen. Once I was satisfied that there were no immediate risk or safety concerns, I would arrange to see her as soon as possible.

In order to have a good understanding of her illness and offer advice on diagnosis and management, I would seek more information from her GP on her past psychiatric and medical history, previous treatment and response, and also on her current medication and present home situation. I would ask why the GP is reluctant to prescribe further benzodiazepines and if he or she considers that the woman has been on benzodiazepines for too long or is becoming dependent on them. Following this, I would arrange to see her in the outpatient clinic, advising her to come with a close friend or family member if at all possible. It might be necessary to see her at home with one of my colleagues (preferably female if I was a male doctor), if the patient found it very difficult to make the journey to the clinic.

On seeing her, I would ask about the onset, duration, frequency and progression of her inability to go out alone. I would ask her what happened when she last attempted to leave the house unaccompanied and if she suffered any psychological and/or physical symptoms. I would ask specifically whether she suffered any panic attacks, how long they lasted, and whether she experienced autonomic symptoms of anxiety such as headache, breathing difficulty, palpitations, excessive sweating and butterflies in the stomach. I would ask her what was going through her mind at the time, if she felt she was going to die with each panic attack, what were the aggravating and the relieving factors, and what she did to reduce her anxiety. I would also find out if her symptoms only occur when she is going to a particular place or in particular situations. I would examine whether she has faulty beliefs and attitudes or abnormal beliefs about significant others in her life. I would pay attention to possible predisposing factors, such as family history, precipitating factors, such as a recent fall at work or other work- or family-related difficulties, and perpetuating factors, such as avoidance of going out alone, undue engagement in safety behaviours, and undue focusing on physical accompaniments of her anxiety. I would also consider adverse psychosocial circumstances such as an unhealthy relationship with her partner, distress from taking care of young children or financial difficulties. I would assess for the presence of comorbid anxiety, depressive disorders, and substance misuse, including excessive use of either prescribed or non-prescribed medication. For example, tranquillizers can cause sleep disturbance, whilst painkillers can cause derealization, and both would only serve to maintain her anxiety. I would also ask if she has been using alcohol to cope prior to going out. I would hope through this assessment to develop a cognitive behavioural formulation of her presentation to form a blueprint to help organize and develop a programme of cognitive behavioural therapy (CBT).

I would consider phobic anxiety disorder high on the list of differential diagnoses, with agoraphobia being the main problem in this lady. Other possibilities would include social phobia, panic disorders or generalized anxiety disorder. I would also consider a comorbid depression with anxiety disorder, depending on my findings on history and mental state examination. There would also be the possibility of comorbid post-traumatic stress disorder, and misuse of or dependence on drugs such as benzodiazepines or alcohol. Although not likely in this case, I would exclude possible underlying organic problems such as hyperthyroidism, hypothyroidism or even an early menopause which may be contributing to her anxiety state.

In managing this patient, my approach would be to address any attendant risk issues and to exclude the differential diagnoses and comorbid illnesses that I have listed. If she were dependent on alcohol or benzodiazepines, there might be a need to detoxify her first before embarking on psychological treatment. I would also consider the use of antidepressants, such as the selective serotonin re-uptake inhibitors (SSRIs) paroxetine or fluoxetine. I would consider using a more sedative SSRI like venlafaxine if there were problems with sleeping. Buspirone, a $5HT_{1A}$ agonist with no addictive potential, might be given as a substitute to the benzodiazepine.

As far as psychological treatment is concerned, I would offer CBT with the aim of identifying this woman's negative beliefs and her evidence for such beliefs. I would educate her about anxiety disorders, preferably linking this with her fears. I would also introduce her to the cognitive model of anxiety and how the triggers for her anxiety lead to the production of negative automatic thoughts relating to the feared outcome and are maintained by her decision not to go out on her own. Cognitive restructuring, either by imagery or by identifying observations that contradict her negative beliefs, would also be used. She might also be offered systematic desensitization, which would involve her initially going out accompanied, preferably by a therapist, and then going out on her own, with the distance from her home gradually increasing.

There might also be a need for social interventions, by way of dealing with any marital or other psychosocial and work-related problems. If there were financial difficulties, I would refer her to the local debt settlement advice agency (Citizens Advice Bureau in the UK) for assistance.

ANSWERS TO SUGGESTED PROBES

1. Differential diagnoses are discussed in the full answer.
2. Other than psychological treatment, antidepressants and psychosocial intervention as appropriate would help in the management of this patient.
3. In the assessment and management of this patient I would pay attention to comorbid substance misuse, which might need treatment in its own right.

BUZZ WORDS AND USEFUL TERMINOLOGY

Comprehensive assessment of presentation in terms of antecedent, behaviour and consequence, cognitive behavioural formulation, biopsychosocial intervention.

REFERENCES AND SUGGESTED READING

Beck A T, Emery G, Greenberg R L 1985 Anxiety Disorders and Phobias: a Cognitive Perspective. Basic Books, New York
Clark D M 2002 Cognitive behaviour therapy for anxiety disorders. In: Gelder M G, López-Ibor Jr J J, Andreasen N C (eds) New Oxford Textbook of Psychiatry, vol. 2. Oxford University Press, Oxford, pp 1373–1386
Marks I M 1975 Behavioural treatment of phobic and obsessive-compulsive disorders. In: Hersen M, Fisher R M, Miller P M (eds) Progress in Behaviour Modification. Academic, New York, pp 66–158

13.4 MAN WHO IS SELF-HARMING AFTER SEPARATION FROM HIS WIFE

A 35-year-old man has been referred to your community mental health team by his GP for consideration for psychotherapy. He has a long history of deliberate self-harm and attempted suicide, usually in response to psychosocial stressors. He has been through a divorce recently and has started self-harming again, but he is adamant that he has no plans to end his life.

How would you assess and manage this man?

SUGGESTED PROBES

1. What are your differential diagnoses and how would you assess his risks?
2. How would you assess this man for suitability for psychotherapy?
3. What psychotherapy options would you consider?

PMP PLAN

TASKS TO DO

The following five areas are relevant to this vignette but are not necessarily all-inclusive. The list is also not exhaustive:

a) Show an ability to pose relevant questions to get to the root of the underlying problems.
b) Demonstrate an understanding of the psychodynamic factors influencing this man's presentation.
c) Demonstrate an understanding of the procedures for assessment of the patient's potential to engage in and benefit from different treatments.
d) Show knowledge of psychotherapeutic treatment options in dealing with life-long problems of deliberate self-harm.
e) Draw up a risk assessment and management plan if this man continues to self-harm despite offers of psychological treatment.

ISSUES

- Diagnosis and establishing what might be responsible for this man's behaviour
- The risk he poses and how to manage it
- Identification of suitable and safe psychological treatment.

CLARIFY

- Is there any life-threatening condition?
- Are there immediate life stressors that need to be dealt with straight away?

SEEK MORE INFORMATION

GP

- Why the referral is occurring now and the level of deliberate self-harm (DSH) (increased risk?)
- Repeated presentation at the GP's surgery; malignant alienation from the practice.

PATIENT

- Presenting complaint and previous history
- History of and factual information about the previous level of self-harm and its context
- Changes (or lack of them) in the patient or the context since any self-harm or suicide attempt
- Mental state examination – evidence of mental disorder and of hopelessness (as hopelessness is the cognitive feature most consistently related to suicidal ideation), extent of planning for DSH, and intent. Present intent and willingness to seek help, evidence of risk to others. (A review of classification studies revealed three types of suicide attempters: mild, severe and mixed. Severe: harder methods followed by serious physical consequences, older (> 40 years in age), many precautions to avoid discovery, high-level suicidal preoccupation, high suicidal intent, self-directed motivation, previous attempted suicides, depression, drug dependence, high degree of overall dysfunction, poor physical health, previous psychiatric treatment. The risk of repetition is higher in the severe type.)

COLLATERAL INFORMATION

- Interviewing people who have known the patient for some time (it is important to obtain the patient's consent before seeking information elsewhere).

SUITABILITY FOR PSYCHOTHERAPY

- Assessment of whether the patient is suitably stable to enter a course of psychotherapy or whether a period of stabilization

at the community health team level is required. Negative aspects include severe thoughts of self-harm or of violence to others, moderate to severe psychoactive substance use or problems, active psychosis, severe depression or mania
- CBT: specific area on which the work can be focused, suitability of a more pragmatic, problem-focused approach for this patient, clear gains from developing practical skills
- Psychodynamic therapy: wish for self-understanding in the context of relationships with others, willingness to forego the prospect of immediate symptomatic relief, willingness to tolerate uncertainty, willingness to consider another point of view, ability to accept some responsibility, signs of success or achievement (even if limited) in some area of life (study, work, relationships) and some degree of proper self-esteem in relation to this.

DIFFERENTIAL DIAGNOSIS/DIFFICULTIES

- *Functional.* Mood disorder, personality disorder—emotionally unstable, borderline; substance use disorder, adjustment disorder.

APPROACH TO TREATMENT

- Even if the patient does not meet the criteria for severe suicide attempt, treat seriously. Between 10–15% DSH attempters eventually die of suicide. There is a continuing risk, even after many years of DSH, and an increased risk in older people.

WHAT TREATMENT/ADVICE

PSYCHOTHERAPEUTIC

- Give consideration to specific therapies such as dialectical behavioural therapy (DBT), cognitive behavioural therapy (CBT), psychodynamic psychotherapy and cognitive analytical therapy (CAT). The strongest evidence base exists for DBT and psychodynamically informed therapy in the treatment of DSH and patients with borderline personality disorder.

DIALECTICAL BEHAVIOURAL THERAPY

DBT has its roots in principles of behaviour, cognitive treatment and Zen practice. Zen is characterized by the humanistic assumption that all individuals have an inherent capacity for enlightenment and truth. This is referred to in DBT as 'wise mind'. Principles of Zen practice have been introduced into DBT, largely due to the need for patients to develop an attitude of greater acceptance towards a reality that is often painful. Some of the most vital Zen principles and practice relevant to DBT are the importance of being mindful of the present moment, accepting reality without judgment, and finding a middle way. DBT focuses on problem-solving, skills training, contingency management and cognitive modification. A randomized control trial has shown the superiority of DBT in reducing the incidence and severity of parasuicide, dropout from therapy, and the number of inpatient psychiatric days.

PSYCHODYNAMIC THERAPY

This therapy can be carried out as a day hospital or outpatient programme for borderline personality disorder. It consists of a psychoanalytically based exploration of the patient's internal object relational system within the transference and countertransference relationship. The treatment can be given individually or within a group setting. It is known to reduce the frequency of suicide attempts, acts of self-harm, self-report measures of depression, anxiety and general distress, and to improve interpersonal functioning and social adjustment. In their paper Bateman & Fonagy (2001) describe this as a 'partial hospitalization' programme, which helps to maintain the gains of treatment.

COGNITIVE BEHAVIOURAL THERAPY

This is a time-limited, problem-focused approach, which relies on collaborative empiricism to treat concrete target problems. Dysfunctional thoughts and their accompanying feelings and behaviours are conceptualized and treated through a wide range of cognitive and behavioural techniques. Five sessions of CBT have been shown to reduce DSH.

COGNITIVE ANALYTICAL THERAPY (CAT)

This is an approach drawn from an integration of psychodynamic and cognitive ideas. CAT is time-limited (approximately 16 sessions), and places the emphasis on developing a non-collusive relationship with the patient, and on the reformulation, recognition and revision of problem procedures/patterns in thinking, feeling and acting. The patient's state shifts and the reciprocal roles (e.g. contemptuous versus contemptible) that the patient elicits are the focus of therapy.

OTHER TREATMENTS

- Vocational therapy.
- Day hospital attendance.

FULL ANSWER

In dealing with the main issues in this case, I would like to consider the diagnosis and what might be responsible for this man's behaviour. I would also look at the risk he poses and how to manage it. I would then proceed to the identification of suitable and safe psychological treatments to reduce this pattern of behaviour.

In the first instance I would clarify that there is no life-threatening condition secondary to his repeated self-harm. I would also assess whether there were immediate life stressors that needed to be dealt with straight away. Once I was reassured about this, I would make arrangements to see him in the clinic or at home with another colleague, preferably our team psychologist or social worker, particularly if the patient had evidence of disturbing psychosocial stressors that might need practical attention.

Before seeing the patient, I would seek more information from the referring GP as to why the man was referred at this particular time, and the nature and level of his deliberate self-harm (DSH). It is possible that the referral is being made now because there is an increased risk or because the patient has been presenting repeatedly at the surgery. It is also possible that there is a form of a malignant alienation from the practice due to the patient's behaviour. I would find out what has changed in the patient or the context since the recent self-harm attempts. I would elicit the presenting complaint and examine his previous history and current mental state for evidence of a mental disorder. I would assess for evidence of hopelessness, as this is the cognitive feature most consistently related to suicidal ideation, intent and completion. I would again assess his present intentions and his willingness to seek help. I would examine for evidence of risk to others. After seeing the patient and obtaining consent, I would seek further collateral information from people who have known him over a period of time.

I would obtain his history of the previous level of self-harm to assist me in determining what kind of suicide attempts he has made, and whether they were mild, severe or mixed. I would consider him severe due to his numerous attempted suicides, particularly if he used harder methods followed by serious physical consequences, if he took precautions to avoid discovery, if he has a high level of suicidal preoccupation and if he has expressed high suicidal intent. This man would also be considered as severe if there were evidence of depression, drug dependence, a high degree of overall dysfunction, poor physical health and previous psychiatric treatment. This is important, as the risk of repetition is higher in the severe type. Even if he did not meet the criteria for a severe suicide attempter, I would still take him seriously, as between 10 and 15% of DSH attempters eventually die of suicide. Given the limitations of actuarial and clinical data in assessing risk, I would take into account his past behaviour and the context in which it occurred during the risk assessment and while planning for treatment.

My approach would be to assess his suitability for psychotherapeutic intervention before offering any form of treatment. While this is the stated reason for the referral, I would establish whether the patient is sufficiently stable to enter a course of psychotherapy at the present time, or whether a period of stabilization with the community mental health team is required. Aspects that might indicate that the patient is not at a stage to use psychotherapy include severe thoughts of self-harm or of violence to others, moderate to severe psychoactive substance use, active psychosis, severe depression or mania. I would give consideration to specific therapy and to cognitive behavioural therapy (CBT), for which I would assess whether there seem to be specific areas on which work would be focused and also if the patient wants a more pragmatic, problem-focused approach. I would also find out if there seem to be clear gains to be made from developing practical skills. For psychodynamic therapy, I would assess whether the patient has a wish for self-understanding in the context of relationships with others and the willingness to forego the prospect of immediate symptomatic relief and to tolerate uncertainty. It is important for the patient to be willing to consider another point of view and accept some responsibility. I would also look for signs of success or achievement, even if limited, in some area of life (study, work, relationships) and some degree of proper self-esteem in relation to this.

Concerning psychotherapeutic treatments, the strongest evidence base exists for dialectical behavioural therapy (DBT) and psychodynamically informed therapy in the treatment of DSH and patients with borderline personality disorder. DBT has its roots in principles of behaviour, cognitive treatment and Zen practice. The dialectic consists of the need for both acceptance and change. DBT focuses on problem-solving, skills training, contingency management and cognitive modification. A randomized controlled trial of DBT has shown its superiority in reducing the incidence and severity of parasuicide, dropout from therapy, and number of inpatient psychiatric days. The treatment usually consists of weekly (or sometimes twice weekly) visits to the therapist and can continue for as long as 24 months.

The alternative is psychodynamic therapy and this treatment, which can be offered as a day patient or outpatient programme for borderline personality disorder, has been well described. It consists of psychoanalytically based exploration of the patient's internal object relational system within the transference and countertransference relationship. It can be carried out individually or within a group setting, and it might help reduce the frequency of suicide attempts, acts of self-harm, depression, anxiety and general distress in this man. The treatment would also help to improve his interpersonal functioning and social adjustment, thereby making him less preoccupied with his self-harm behaviour. The partial hospitalization programme, described by Bateman & Fonagy (2001), might be useful for maintaining the gains of treatment.

Treatment for this man might also take the form of CBT, which is a time-limited, problem-focused approach relying on collaborative empiricism to treat concrete target problems. Dysfunctional thoughts and their accompanying feelings and behaviours are conceptualized and treated through a wide range of cognitive and behavioural techniques. Five sessions of CBT have been shown to reduce deliberate self-harm, but in this gentleman allowance should be made for up to 12 sessions.

Last but not the least, there is also the option of cognitive analytical therapy (CAT), which is an approach drawn from the integration of psychodynamic and cognitive ideas. CAT is time-limited (approximately 20 sessions), with an emphasis on developing a non-collusive relationship with the patient (by not accepting the reason for his self-harm behaviour as valid), and on the reformulation, recognition and revision of problems and patterns of thinking, feeling and acting.

The other thing to consider in this gentleman are non-medical and non-psychological options focused on engaging him in a way that puts regular structure into his life rather than allowing him to be preoccupied with responding to psychological pain by self-harming. It is possible that, despite these approaches, the patient would continue to behave in this way. Effort would then have to be directed towards harm minimization strategies and health education about the risks of physical harm, infection and accidental death, given that he has engaged in this self-harm behaviour over a period of time without actually wanting to end his life.

ANSWERS TO SUGGESTED PROBES

1. The differential diagnosis includes the functional disorders of mood disorder, borderline personality disorder (emotionally unstable type), substance use disorder and adjustment disorder.

   The main risk is that of further self-harm or suicide. The risk can be assessed by considering historical, static and dynamic factors:

   Historical: History of previous self-harm/attempted suicide, severity of episodes. History of poor engagement with services (including psychological approaches). Previous use of dangerous item or weapon. History of previous careful planning, suicide notes. History of suicide in family.
   Static: Male gender, young age.
   Dynamic: Presence of depression or other mental illness. Current use of alcohol and drugs increases risk. Poor impulse control. Further failed relationships. Failure in other domains of life. Isolation, homelessness, other psychosocial adversities, e.g. court cases, debt problems, child custody and maintenance problems, unemployment, bereavement.

2. The assessment of this man's suitability for psychotherapy has been covered in the full answer.

3. Psychotherapy options are described in the full answer.

BUZZ WORDS AND USEFUL TERMINOLOGY

Dialectical behaviour therapy, vocational therapy, partial hospitalization.

REFERENCES AND SUGGESTED READING

Bateman A W 1997 Borderline personality disorder and psychotherapeutic psychiatry: an integrative approach. British Journal of Psychotherapy 13(4):489–498

Bateman A, Fonagy P 2001 Treatment of borderline personality disorder with psychoanalytically orientated partial hospitalization: an 18-month follow-up. American Journal of Psychiatry 158:36–42

Linehan M M, Armstrong H E, Suarez A et al 1991 Cognitive behavioural treatment of chronically parasuicidal borderline patients. Archives of General Psychiatry 48:1060–1064

Maris R W 1992 The relationship of non-fatal suicide attempts to completed suicide. In: Maris R W, Berman A L, Maltsberger J T et al (eds) Assessment and Prediction of Suicide. Guilford Press, New York, pp 362–380

Salkosvskis P M, Atha C, Storer D 1990 Cognitive behavioural problem solving in the treatment of patients who repeatedly attempt suicide: a controlled trial. British Journal of Psychiatry 157:871–876

14

Professional practice and relations

You are deputizing for your consultant, who is currently away on leave. One of the CPNs involved in the management of an elderly lady with dementia asks you to join in a meeting with the patient's family. They complain they were not 'kept informed' about her diagnosis, treatment and eventual transfer to residential care. They feel 'disgusted' at having to pay for her residential care, while other patients have their nursing care paid for.

How would you deal with this situation?

SUGGESTED PROBES

1. Would you involve the patient's GP? If so, why?
2. What are the possible reasons behind this presentation?
3. Is there a need to involve the rest of the team?
   If so, why?

PMP PLAN

TASKS TO DO

The following five areas are relevant to this vignette but are not necessarily all-inclusive. The list is also not exhaustive:

a) Appreciate the need to be empathic and involve the multidisciplinary team in your approach.
b) Appreciate the need to familiarize yourself with the local complaints procedure and gather as much information as possible before seeing the family. Advise the complaints manager.
c) Need to gather clear systematic information on the process of arriving at the decision which is the subject of the complaint.

d) Show your familiarity with government guidelines on the funding of residential and nursing care, and understanding of the financial implications of residential rather than nursing care for the family.

e) Appreciate the need to look into the issue of carer stress and support, and also consider the possibility of the family's difficulty in coping with the recent transfer of their relative to a nursing home.

ISSUES

- Understanding the reasons behind this family's dissatisfaction
- Provision of an opportunity to hear and respond to the views of the family
- Addressing any concerns about or shortcomings in the information supplied or the care provided.

CLARIFY

- Why are you being involved?
- What are the family's main concerns?
- Which family members are attending the meeting?
- What is your role and who should lead the meeting?
- Are any other team members involved?

SEEK MORE INFORMATION

CPN

- Basis of the decision to transfer to a nursing home rather than a residential home
- Family involvement in the past
- Any suggestion of stress in the carer or the rest of the family. If so, counselling offered.

MEDICAL NOTES

- Details of previous medical, nursing, nursing needs and psychological assessments
- Results of previous investigations, diagnosis and management
- Documentation of the team's involvement with the family and what has been discussed and agreed in the past.

GP

- Any knowledge of the complaint
- Whether the patient's family has ever approached the GP on the issues of diagnosis and treatment
- Recent contact with the patient's husband or other supporting family members
- Any suggestion that the relatives are not coping
- Any family members who are receiving help from the GP or other psychiatric services
- Attendance at the meeting.

MULTIDISCIPLINARY TEAM

- Encouragement for the CPN to organize a multidisciplinary team meeting, preferably with the team manager in attendance, if the meeting cannot wait for the consultant to return from leave
- Views of team members who have been involved in the patient's care.

DIFFERENTIAL DIAGNOSIS/DIFFICULTIES

Not relevant in this vignette.

APPROACH TO TREATMENT

- Gather all the information first, find a witness for the meeting and agree to attend.
- Adopt a no-blame approach and be non-judgmental.
- Encourage the family to choose a spokesperson and to write down exactly what they are dissatisfied with.
- Allow the family to express their views with limited interruptions, but keep control of the meeting.
- Once the family have expressed their concerns, take time to advise them accordingly.
- Invite the social worker along to explain the intricacies of welfare policies as they relate to the funding of residential placement and nursing homes.

WHAT TREATMENT/ADVICE

- Give a full explanation to the family: demonstrate empathy, while explaining their relative's presentation, the basis of the diagnosis, the treatment she has received so far and how the team arrived at the main decisions they took.

PROFESSIONAL PRACTICE AND RELATIONS

- Give the carer support: pay attention to any evidence of stress in the carer and be awake to the possibility that the whole family, in particular the partner, may be going through a process of adjustment following the transfer of this lady to a residential home.
- Give family education and counselling: educate about government policy on the funding of residential care and nursing placement, which unfortunately most families know little about until they become directly involved.
- Carry out a financial assessment and provide advice: the decision to transfer the patient to a residential home might have financial implications for the partner. Therefore, the issue of finances should be clarified and dealt with appropriately, preferably with the help of a social worker.
- If the relatives are unhappy with the outcome of the meeting, give them the opportunity for a second meeting with the deputizing consultant or the responsible medical officer (the patient's own consultant) when he or she is back from leave. Encourage the family to make a formal complaint if they are still not satisfied.
- Give the family contact details for relevant carer support associations or advocacy groups.
- Write a follow-up letter (very important).

FULL ANSWER

The main issues involved in this scenario are the need to understand the reasons behind this family's dissatisfaction, and the provision of an opportunity for them to air their views and grievances. The other issue is how the service should respond to their views and complaints in order to address any concerns about or shortcomings in the information supplied or the care provided as a whole. The nurse's request might suggest either that she expects difficulties in dealing with this family's needs on her own, or that there is a requirement for a medical or team perspective on the various issues raised by the family.

I would clarify with the CPN why she wants me to be involved and what the main concerns are. I would ask what my role would be and who would chair the meeting. I would also ask if any other team members were involved and in what capacity. I would also clarify which of the family members were attending and what role they would have. As far as possible I would suggest that family members who have been closely involved in the care of this lady attend. I would suggest that the relatives write down the main points causing dissatisfaction and that they limit attendance to a maximum of four family members, which might mean that they would need to choose a spokesperson.

I would review the care this woman has received and familiarize myself with the case so that I could make a positive contribution. I would seek more information in her medical and nursing notes, and review the results of psychological and occupational therapy assessments. In addition, I would look at the results of previous investigations, including the dementia screen and CT scan, medical diagnosis, treatment and agreed management plan. I would contact the GP to ask whether he or she is aware of the family's complaints, has discussed the issue of diagnosis and treatment with the family before, and has any concerns about stress in the carer or other family members. I would invite the GP to the meeting. I would ask the CPN to organize a multidisciplinary team meeting, preferably with the team manager in attendance, if the meeting could wait for the consultant to return from leave. I would seek the views of team members who have been involved in the patient's care and information on the role of the key players.

Whilst I am aware that the UK government does not currently fund residential placements, I would familiarize myself with how the decision was made to transfer this patient to a residential home and would examine whether that decision was based on the woman's nursing needs assessment. I would invite the responsible social worker for a discussion on how the issue of funding was decided, so that I could pass the information on to the family when we met. I would find out whether the patient's relatives' concerns about not being kept adequately informed on her diagnosis and illness are justified. I would find out when the diagnosis was made, what the main symptoms were on presentation, and what her final agreed diagnosis was. I would also find out how involved the family has been in her care, who the main carer is and if the CPN has noticed anything to suggest stress in the carer or family as a whole. I would ask if a carer's assessment of need was carried out, as this would be very good practice, quite apart from being mandatory under the National Service Framework in England and Wales. If there had been stressors, I would also look at the specific help the family received in terms of practical support and counselling. Having taken the above steps, I would hope to familiarize myself properly with the care this patient received, even though I might have had little or no involvement with the patient myself.

Once I had agreed to attend, I would ask the CPN to arrange a meeting with the family at a mutually convenient time. I would encourage the family to choose a spokesperson and write down the main points causing dissatisfaction. I would bring along a witness to document the minutes of the meeting and the points raised. As far as possible I would adopt a 'no-blame', non-judgmental approach and I would use the opportunity to try to understand what might have gone wrong in the overall care of and communication with this family. I would apologize for the distress they have experienced regarding their relative's care. I would bear in mind the need to be empathic, given that the recent transfer of this lady to a residential home might have come as a shock to them. I would allow the family to express their views with limited interruptions and give them adequate time to express what they are unhappy about, but at the same time keep control of the meeting. I would ask for their views on the patient's illness and diagnosis and explain how we arrived at our various decisions. I would also listen to any alternative suggestions they might have and what role they would be playing in the future. This approach would also give me the opportunity to assess their knowledge of dementia as a whole, its treatment and the issue of funding. This would guide me on how much education I would need to provide for this family.

Once the patient's family had expressed their concerns, I would then explain how the team arrived at the various decisions and the steps taken to communicate these to the relatives. I would advise that, under current policies, the government would not fund residential placement for those considered to have adequate resources because the 'residence' is the patient's place of domicile and as such attracts no funding from the state. I would also explain that, under existing policies, the state would only pay for those patients subject to compulsory aftercare arrangements (under Section 117 of the Mental Health Act 1983 in the UK) or those in need of nursing care. I would explain that the word 'nursing' means that these people are in need of treatment and so they would not pay for that treatment, just like any other UK citizen. I would mention that this is the case with their mother, who was recommended for residential placement rather than a nursing home, following detailed multidisciplinary assessment lasting several weeks. I would pay attention to anything that might suggest stress in the carers or other family members, as I might need to advise them to contact their GP for help. This would also be in line with the government National Service Framework for Older Adults (NSF, 1999) for mental health. If there were financial concerns or worries on the part of the family, I would ask our social worker to look into any benefits entitlement.

If we were able to satisfy the family on how and why we took the decisions we did, I would aim for closure in this case and would inform the hospital's complaints office. I would document carefully what we discussed, the family's satisfaction and responses, other issues emanating from the meeting and what action the two parties agreed to take. I would send the minutes of the meeting to the family to ensure that the record was a true reflection of what we discussed and agreed. This would prevent unnecessary revisits to this issue in the future. It is possible that, despite efforts to inform the family as to how we arrived at our decisions, the family might remain unhappy with the outcome of this meeting. I would ask them to arrange to meet the deputizing consultant, who would be more experienced and better able to reassure them. The alternative would be for us to meet again after we had gathered more information to reassure the family, or they might decide to see the responsible consultant on his or her return from leave. If they were still not satisfied, I would encourage them to speak to staff at the advocacy, complaints and patient affairs department, with a view to making a formal complaint so that the issues could be dealt with properly. The patient's family would also have the opportunity to raise their complaints with the local community health organization or the government ombudsman responsible for mental health and long-term care. In line with this support, I would inform them of the local carers' association and the Patient Advocacy Liaison Services (PALS), who might be able to provide more information and support.

Finally, I would follow up with a letter detailing what was discussed, what further points remain to be pursued, and who is responsible for each task. This would ensure that what is documented is indeed what everyone agreed to during the meeting, and would hopefully reduce the risk of future complaints.

Note: this vignette is aimed at testing how candidates would handle complaints from relatives, rather than assessing their knowledge of long-term care arrangements for older adults. These arrangements differ between jurisdictions, counties and countries, and sadly do not exist in most of the less developed countries.

ANSWERS TO SUGGESTED PROBES

1. I would involve the GP, who probably had a hand in the discharge planning process. The GP would be likely to know the family better than we do and thus might be able to give more information on their background. He or she might also have picked up on family or carer stress as a result of this woman's illness. More details are given in the full answer.

2. The possible reasons behind this presentation are:
   - family or carer stress
   - the prospect of loss of inheritance, if the patient has to move from her house and dispose of most of her assets to fund residential placement
   - the financial burden for the family of having to pay for residential care, if the patient does not have sufficient means of paying for long-term residential placement herself.

3. It would be important to seek the views of other members of the team who might have been involved in the care of this patient. They might also have had similar difficulties in the past and thus be able to share their experience on how previous cases were dealt with.

BUZZ WORDS AND USEFUL TERMINOLOGY

Carer's view, carer's stress and support, carer's assessment, multidisciplinary liaison and management advocacy, formal complaint, complaints manager, closure.

REFERENCES AND SUGGESTED READING

Mayberry M K 2002 The NHS complaint system. Postgraduate Medical Journal 78(925):651–653

Seelos L, Adamson C 1994 Redefining NHS complaint handling – the real challenge. International Journal of Healthcare Quality Assurance 7(6):26–31

Thornicroft G 2000 National Service Framework for Mental Health. Psychiatric Bulletin 24:203–206

Wood D 1996 Acting on complaints about mental health services. Implication of power imbalances. Journal of Management and Medicine 10(3):31–38

You are sitting in the doctor's mess with a female colleague early one morning before you start work. She approaches you and confides that she has been drinking excessively and has to steady her nerves in the morning. She injects ketamine very occasionally. She is worried she will draw attention to herself when on duty for ECT next week and fears being sacked.

She has asked for your help and advice. What would you do?

SUGGESTED PROBES

1. What are the sensitive issues in this scenario and what problems would you envisage in obtaining help for this colleague?
2. What psychosocial stressors would you consider in this case?
3. You advise her to seek treatment and she is off sick for a week. The following week, she starts avoiding you after you hint that you think she is still drinking. What would you do?

PMP PLAN

TASKS TO DO

The following five areas are relevant to this vignette but are not necessarily all-inclusive. The list is also not exhaustive:

a) Appreciate the sensitivity of dealing with another colleague (especially one of the opposite gender) who has private and personal problems that might affect her clinical practice and career. Discuss issues of confidentiality and stigma.
b) Discuss concerns about risk (to patients, to the doctor's career and the legal risk to the hospital and health authority if there is an adverse incident) and the actions to be taken to forestall these problems.
c) Discuss the treatment options available to this addicted professional practitioner, including ongoing support.
d) Discuss medical registration council guidelines (from the General Medical Council (GMC) in the UK) on reporting medical practitioners considered unfit to practise. This would obviously be different from one area (or country) of practice to another.
e) Discuss treatments available, reintegration at work, monitoring and ongoing support.

ISSUES

- Giving appropriate advice to a colleague whose activities and habits may seriously affect her clinical practice
- Maintaining confidentiality with regard to a professional colleague and balancing this against one's professional duty to put the interests of the patient first at all times
- Legal responsibility to disclose activities that may be injurious to patients' welfare.

CLARIFY

- How long has your colleague had these problems?
- Have there been any major incidents or near misses in the past, to which she feels her habits might have contributed? Does she foresee any in the future?
- Has she received any help or treatment in the past?
- Has she sought help from her supervisor, consultant or occupational health department?

SEEK MORE INFORMATION

COLLEAGUE

- History of drug use and addiction, source of substances, particularly ketamine, access to drugs, use of drugs at work and use of drugs to continue to function
- Assessment of whether her difficulties meet the usual criteria for substance dependence
- Psychosocial stressors and bullying at work
- Problems with career progression, including examinations
- Relationship and family difficulties, financial problems
- Depressive disorder or other mental health needs.

DIFFERENTIAL DIAGNOSIS/DIFFICULTIES

- Alcohol and other polysubstance misuse disorder
- Anxiety and depressive disorder, adjustment depressive disorder with substance misuse.

APPROACH TO TREATMENT

- Be as sensitive about issues concerning a colleague as you would be with patients.
- Remember patients' interests are paramount, but also appreciate the need to help your colleague to seek more

appropriate advice in order to protect both patients and her own career.

- Advise her to take sick leave for safety reasons.
- Involve others (with her consent) to give support and ensure confidentiality.
- Seek assistance from the local occupational health department.

WHAT TREATMENT/ADVICE

MEDICAL

- Suggest treatment for addicted professionals, including detoxification and antidepressants.
- Refer to the Sick Doctors' Trust.
- Supervise and monitor post-treatment.

PSYCHOLOGICAL

- Provide counselling, practical problem-solving and cognitive behavioural therapy (CBT).

PSYCHOSOCIAL

- Deal with situations such as livelihood and family responsibilities.
- Revisit occupational health for clearance.
- Return to work under supervision.

ENVIRONMENTAL

- Consider redeployment.
- Try flexible working.
- Take a part-time shift or job initially.

FULL ANSWER

I think this must be a difficult situation for a professional to find herself in. The main issues in this vignette are to ensure that appropriate advice is given to this colleague, whose activities and habits might seriously affect her clinical practice, and also the need to balance confidentiality against one's professional duty to put the interests of the patient first at all times. There is also the issue of the legal responsibility to disclose activities that might be injurious to patients' welfare.

I would thank my colleague for letting me know about this serious issue in her private life that might have strong implications for her professional practice and career. While I would reassure her with regard to confidentiality, I would encourage her to be open and honest, if I am to give any reasonable assistance. I would be mindful that she is in fact a colleague and not my patient, and would handle this situation with great sensitivity and care. I would clarify when these problems first started, and encourage her to be honest about any major risks or incidents to which she feels her habit might have contributed. I would enquire about any previous help or treatment she has received, and whether she has sought help from her supervisor or consultant.

I would seek more information and take a brief history of her drug use and addiction, trying to discover the source of the substances, in particular ketamine. I would find out whether she uses drugs while at work, and if she needs drugs to function effectively in her job. I would examine whether her difficulties meet the usual criteria for substance dependence, in terms of compulsion to use substances, primacy, tolerance, salience, withdrawal reaction when substances are not used, and reinstatement after a period of abstinence. I would ask why she continues to use these drugs despite knowing the potential consequences of her behaviour for her career and on patients' care and safety. I would also like to know if there are relevant psychosocial stressors such as perceived bullying at work, excessive workload, problems with particular staff or patient(s), and problems with career progression, including examinations. I would enquire about worries and concerns with regard to physical illness, such as alcoholic liver diseases, hepatitis and other infections such as AIDS. I would find out if there are any relationship and family difficulties or financial problems that can be addressed. Finally, I would enquire about any symptoms of a depressive disorder and also ask whether this doctor has ever contemplated taking her life.

Given her self-disclosure, the diagnosis is likely to be alcohol and other polysubstance misuse disorder or dependence, but I would consider other problems in my differential diagnosis, such as anxiety and depressive disorders, adjustment depressive disorder with substance misuse and psychosocial difficulties as I have detailed.

In my approach to advising her, I would be very sensitive, bearing in mind that she is a professional colleague and not a patient. I would consider patients' interests and safety to be paramount and balance this against the need for this colleague to protect herself and her career. I would encourage her to seek the help of others, particularly her own consultant who usually would be her direct line manager, especially if she had to take long-term sick leave. I would also suggest seeking help from the hospital or trust occupational health department, who would usually be able to summon appropriate help in this kind of situation. If an untoward adverse event such as a medication error had been committed, I would encourage her to disclose this to her consultant so that the necessary risk management could be carried out, before someone was put in serious danger by her practice. I would encourage her to seek the necessary support aimed at rectifying the errors, in a way that does not lay emphasis on apportioning blame to the doctor. I would advise her to see her own GP for referral for treatment and to take sick leave for safety reasons. I would encourage her to seek assistance from the local sick/addicted doctors' treatment programme, which would be able to arrange appropriate specialist treatment and monitor her in an honest and confidential manner. I would encourage her not to hurry back to work but to make sure she has received all the help she needs to deal with the addiction and contributing psychosocial difficulties.

As part of the treatment, I would suggest that this colleague seeks more appropriate help, involving detoxification from alcohol and any illicit substances, preferably in an area remote from her area of practice. If there were any evidence of a mental illness such as mild depression, I would suggest medical treatment with the use of an antidepressant. I would also suggest psychological treatment aimed at helping her cope with her current life situation and stressors. A cognitive behavioural therapy (CBT) approach would also be useful in dealing with any mild to moderate depression. It would be important to deal with some of those factors that might have contributed to the problem, such as pressure of work, access to drugs or a difficult psychosocial situation. I would consider reintegration to work as a crucial part of the treatment process. In an ideal situation, it would be useful if this doctor could start in another unit, where she could be given proactive and practical help. This would be carefully chosen to ensure that she did not have direct access to drugs that could be abused or misused. I hope that, by receiving appropriate help, my colleague would put an end to this difficult situation and her life could return to normal.

It is possible that, despite this approach, the doctor would not seek or receive appropriate help and she might continue to practise dangerously. I would explain kindly to her that, if she does not seek help, the situation might arise when I would have to breach confidentiality, as I would have to consider the overall interests and safety of patients, as well as the interests of the establishment we work for. If things got this far, I would inform my own supervising consultant and possibly the clinical manager of the service, who I would expect to involve other decision-makers and to offer this doctor assistance before any untoward incident occurred. I would also seek the advice of my medical defence union without disclosing the identity of the doctor involved. Before doing this, I would inform the doctor of my intention to inform the authority if she continues to practise in a way that might be dangerous to patients and other colleagues. I would say to her that I would do this as a matter of necessity, pointing out my professional duty under the General Medical Council (GMC) guidelines (in the UK). I would explain to her that I would be liable if I did not report a totally preventable occurrence before it happened. I would emphasize that, rather than breach her confidence, I would rather support her in disclosing her own difficulties to the authorities and her employer, but I might not have any other option if she did not choose to do so herself.

Once I had reported the situation to the relevant authority, I would expect immediate action to be taken to address the situation. Equally, I would expect managers and service directors to act at this stage, if necessary suspending her from practising in the hospital and reporting her to the local medical licensing body. In the rare case of nothing proactive being done by the managers, and if I considered that this doctor was still practising in a way that might be inimical to the health and safety of patients and others, I would have the obligation to report the situation directly to the medical director myself. I would report her to the medical licensing authority, the GMC in the UK and the Irish Medical Council in Ireland. These bodies have the legal and statutory obligation of withdrawing the licence to practise from any practitioner found unfit. This might eventually be necessary to encourage this colleague to seek treatment through the occupational therapy department and her GP.

Apart from dealing with the acute problem with detoxification, treatment would also involve active psychological and professional support. This might be through the Addicted Doctors Scheme or another arrangement. The GMC in the UK might stipulate conditions for returning to practice, including medical supervision under specialists endorsed by the GMC. These specialists would be in a position to give a confidential report to the licensing body on the compliance of the doctor and the progress being made. The GMC or the local medical licensing body would then have to decide at a later date if this doctor was fit to practise again. The doctor would need continuous support from her supervisors and the hospital's occupational health department while settling back into work.

14

PROFESSIONAL PRACTICE AND RELATIONS

ANSWERS TO SUGGESTED PROBES

1. The following sensitive issues might arise in this scenario:
   - The colleague might deny the problem and isolate herself or even leave work.
   - There might be difficulties in accessing help due to stigma-related problems, fear of breach of confidence, fear of jeopardy to her reputation, professional accreditation and employment.
   - The colleague might find it difficult to accept the role of patient.
   - She might run the risk of being treated as a colleague rather than a patient by others, who might therefore have higher expectations for her recovery.
   - It could be difficult to find a suitable environment for treatment and rehabilitation.
   - Unfortunately, though this is rare, the colleague might maliciously accuse you of improper conduct (including sexual harassment, particularly if you are male).

2. I would consider the following psychosocial stressors:
   - perceived bullying at work
   - excessive workload
   - problems with particular staff or patients
   - problems with career progression, including examinations
   - problems with family and relationships.

3. If my colleague started avoiding me, I would express my concern that I think she is still abusing alcohol and possibly still injecting ketamine. If she did not voluntarily seek help, I would have no choice but to breach her confidence. The processes discussed in the full answer might then follow.

BUZZ WORDS AND USEFUL TERMINOLOGY

Addicted doctor, confidentiality, relapse prevention, fitness to practise, duty of care.

REFERENCES AND SUGGESTED READING

General Medical Council 2002 Referring a Doctor to the GMC: A Guide for Health Professionals. GMC, London

Joiner I 2000 The Sick Doctors Trust Addicted Physicians Programme. In: Ghodse H, Mann S, Johnson P (eds) Doctors and Their Health. Centre for Addiction Studies, St George's Medical School, London

Strang J, Wilks M, Wells B et al 1998 Missed problems and missed opportunities for addicted doctors: we need a special service for doctors addicted to drugs and alcohol. British Medical Journal 316(7129):405–406

Working Group on the Misuse of Alcohol and other Drugs by Doctors 1998 The Misuse of Alcohol and other Drugs by Doctors. British Medical Association, London

15

Additional practice questions – not indexed

15.1 34-YEAR-OLD MAN WITH BORDERLINE PERSONALITY DISORDER

A 34-year-old male with borderline personality disorder (emotionally unstable type) has presented himself to the medical ward requesting that he be admitted. He smells noticeably of alcohol and has multiple old scars on his body. He has a history of self-harm. You have been asked to advise on further management, including whether he should stay on the medical ward or be transferred to a psychiatric unit.

What advice would you give and what would be your strategy for management?

15.2 16-YEAR-OLD BOY WITH REPEATED HAND-WASHING

A 16-year-old boy living with his parents has been playing the piano a lot in the last 5 weeks. His parents have noticed that, after playing the piano, he cleans his hands repeatedly. He bullies his parents, who have tried to discuss this with him, and will not listen to them.

What are the differential diagnoses, and how would you assess and manage this boy?

15.3 25-YEAR-OLD DRUG USER WHO THINKS SHE IS BEING PERSECUTED

The registrar at the local accident and emergency department has asked you to see a 25-year-old female who was brought in by the police. She thinks there is a plot against her and has been running away from her perceived persecutors in busy traffic. She uses cannabis and amphetamines regularly.

What are your differentials and your strategy for assessment and management?

15.4 63-YEAR-OLD EX-BOXER WITH IRRITABILITY, LOSS OF TEMPER AND FORGETFULNESS

A 63-year-old former professional boxer has been referred to you after his wife expressed concerns about his irritability, loss of temper and forgetfulness in the last 6 months.

How would you go about further management and assessment?

15.5 27-YEAR-OLD WOMAN WHO IS UNABLE TO LEAVE HER HOME

A 27-year-old lady was referred to you after she lost three members of her immediate family in a road traffic accident 18 months ago. She has not returned to work since then and said she has nothing to live for. Her GP was of the opinion that she needs psychological help as antidepressants have not helped.

How would you approach this case and what treatment would you give?

15.6 77-YEAR-OLD MAN WITH LOW MOOD AND SOCIAL WITHDRAWAL

A 77-year-old man presents with low mood and social withdrawal. He has been known to neglect himself and has become slow. His neighbour, who is not aware of any relatives, is finding the daily task of checking up on him stressful.

Discuss your differential diagnosis. What features would you look for in your assessment to aid further management?

15.7 22-YEAR-OLD MAN SEEKING DIAMORPHINE

You have been asked to see a 22-year-old male by the casualty officer. He is well known to the department, having presented on numerous occasions demanding to be given diamorphine and threatening to kill himself on each occasion if his demand is not met.

How would you manage this situation?

15.8 MIDDLE-AGED HOMELESS MAN SEEKING HELP IN GIVING UP ALCOHOL

A middle-aged man is brought to your clinic by a support worker from a homeless persons hostel, with a request for help in giving up alcohol.

How would you manage the situation?

15.9 43-YEAR-OLD LADY IN A ROAD TRAFFIC ACCIDENT

A 43-year-old lady was involved in a road traffic accident in which she suffered a whip-lash injury to her neck. She returned to work 6 weeks after but subsequently developed weakness and loss of function in her right limbs 5 months after her accident. Neurological investigations and other tests have not revealed any organic pathology.

How would you assess and manage this lady? What recommendations would you give?

15.10 YOUNG BOY EXPOSING HIMSELF AT SCHOOL

You have received a telephone call from the head teacher of a nearby primary school. A boy known to have a learning difficulty has dropped his trousers in front of other pupils on two occasions, and has been having tantrums since an attempt was made to prevent further episodes of similar behaviour.

How would you go about further assessment and management?

15.11 35-YEAR-OLD DOWN'S SYNDROME PATIENT WITH ANXIETY AND AGITATION

A 35-year-old Down's syndrome patient who lives with his elderly parents is referred to you by his GP following concern over his increased anxiety and agitation.

What are the possible reasons for this development and how would you manage?

15.12 26-YEAR-OLD MAN WITH LEARNING DISABILITIES, WHO HAS SEXUALLY ATTACKED A 14-YEAR-OLD GIRL

You have been asked to write a court report on a 26-year-old patient with learning disabilities, who recently attacked a 14-year-old secondary schoolgirl sexually in a public car park. He has been arrested in the past for two other minor sexual offences.

How would you deal with this request? What factors would inform your advice on the best way to manage this patient safely and on the setting of such treatment?

15.13 19-YEAR-OLD BOY WITH LEARNING DISABILITIES EXPOSING HIMSELF

The attention of the police has been drawn to a 19-year-old boy with learning disabilities, who has been exposing his lower parts through the window of the community home where he lives.

How would you assess and manage?

15.14 35-YEAR-OLD WOMAN WITH CONSTANT DOUBTS ABOUT HER HUSBAND'S FIDELITY

A 35-year-old female has been referred to your clinic by her GP. Her husband is worried that her constant doubts about his fidelity are about to break up their 18-month-old marriage. She has had three other relationships in the past but none of them lasted more than 12 months. Her mother died when she was 4 years old and her father later remarried. She resents her father, who she claims deserted her for his new family.

What are the possible explanations for this woman's experience in psychodynamic terms?

15.15   15-YEAR-OLD BALLET STUDENT WITH WEIGHT LOSS AND VOMITING

A 15-year-old ballet student has been brought to the accident and emergency department by her mother, who is concerned about her recent weight loss. She now frequently eats on her own, and when she does eat with the rest of the family, she is sick shortly afterwards.

What are the possible diagnoses, and how would you assess and manage her care?

15.16   24-YEAR-OLD WOMAN WITH A BMI OF 11.8

A 24-year-old patient with an eating disorder was admitted to your unit 5 days ago. She has not eaten any solids for several weeks and has been surviving on juice. She has had several admissions in the past and has always rapidly regained her weight. On examination, she seems very distractible, with a BMI of 11.8.

How would you manage and what physical complications would you pay attention to?

15.17   25-YEAR-OLD MAN WITH DISRUPTIVE AND THREATENING BEHAVIOUR

A 25-year-old patient has been referred to your team by his GP, who has been having difficulty managing his behaviour. He has presented to the surgery repeatedly in the recent past, making various 'unreasonable demands' and threatening to set the surgery alight if he was not referred to the psychiatric service. He believes this will help his application for rehousing, having been ejected from his council flat recently for disruptive behaviour and threats to kill.

What are the diagnostic possibilities and how would you manage this situation?

15.18 29-YEAR-OLD WOMAN WITH BORDERLINE PERSONALITY DISORDER AND A RECENT INCREASE IN SELF-MUTILATION

A 29-year-old female with a well-established diagnosis of borderline personality disorder has once more been referred to your community mental health team by her GP, who is rather worried about the recent increase in frequency of her self-mutilation.

How would you assess and manage this patient?

15.19 DEPRESSED AND SUICIDAL 40-YEAR-OLD WHO HAS BEEN ABUSING HIS DAUGHTER

A 40-year-old man self-presents to the psychiatric emergency clinic, complaining of feeling depressed and suicidal. He reports feeling very guilty about abusing his 14-year-old daughter, who has been living with him since he and his wife divorced 10 years ago. He sees killing himself as the only way of getting himself out of this 'misery'.

How would you manage?

15.20 45-YEAR-OLD MARRIED MAN WHO IS FREQUENTLY MASTURBATING

A local GP has referred to you a 45-year-old man who has recently been behaving out of character. He was caught by his wife masturbating in front of the mirror. She has threatened to divorce him unless he seeks help, after she found three female dolls in their bedroom.

What are the differential diagnoses and how would you manage?

15.21 PATIENT WITH A LEARNING DISABILITY REFUSING CONSENT FOR SURGERY

You have been asked by a consultant surgeon to sign consent for laparotomy for one of your patients who has a learning disability. He has refused to consent on numerous occasions and the surgeon now doubts the patient's ability to understand the nature of the procedure.

What would be your response, what advice would you give, and how would you manage the situation?

15.22 34-YEAR-OLD MAN EXPOSING HIMSELF AND CLAIMING TO HAVE BEEN SENT BY GOD

As duty psychiatrist in a busy inner city hospital, you have been asked to assess a 34-year-old male who has been exposing himself in the middle of the street. He claims to have been sent by God to cleanse the world of evil people.

How would you assess and manage him?

15.23 32-YEAR-OLD WOMAN ALLEGING THAT SHE WAS RAPED IN HOSPITAL

You have been asked to see a 32-year-old woman on the general adult psychiatric ward. She is alleging that she was raped during the night but is unsure of the perpetrator. She has never made allegations like this before and nurses are worried because of the implications of her complaint.

How would you assess and manage this situation?

15.24 24-YEAR-OLD WOMAN WHO FEELS PEOPLE ARE ACCUSING HER

A 24-year-old woman is terrified of going back to her library job, as she feels people are accusing her of stealing the books. Her family says that she has been keeping to herself at home recently and occasionally mumbles to herself.

What are your differential diagnoses and how would you manage her?

15.25 42-YEAR-OLD BARRISTER WHO IS GRANDIOSE

You have been asked to assess a 42-year-old barrister who was admitted to the emergency clinic last night after taking an overdose of 40 tablets of paracetamol. He is due in court for fraudulent activities after spending excessively on his credit card. He reports that he has no need to sleep, as he is busy preparing for taking up the post of chief executive of his employer's multinational company.

How would you proceed with assessment and management?

15.26 ANGRY PARENTS ACCUSING YOUR DEPARTMENT OF NOT MONITORING A PATIENT WHO ALLEGEDLY INTERFERED WITH (OR SEXUALLY ABUSED) A CHILD

You have been asked by an approved social worker to see a man who is already one of your patients, as he has been accused of interfering with (sexually abusing) a child who lives nearby. The child's parents are furious that the mental health services have let them down and they have threatened to take action against the hospital if something is not done quickly.

How would you deal with this situation?

15.27   53-YEAR-OLD WIDOWER WHO IS SUICIDAL AFTER BEING MADE REDUNDANT

You have been called to the accident and emergency department to see a 53-year-old widower. He took an overdose of co-dydramol after being told that he is to be made redundant from his highly paid job. This is his third overdose in the space of 3 weeks.

How would you proceed with further assessment and management?

15.28   76-YEAR-OLD WOMAN WITH MODERATE DEMENTIA AND AN UNHELPFUL SON

A GP has phoned you to say that he is worried about a 76-year-old lady who is currently living with her son. She was assessed 18 months ago and was diagnosed as having moderate dementia. She has been seen wandering and was picked up by the police 4 days ago. The last time the GP saw her, her son had been drinking heavily and was quite uncooperative.

How would you proceed?

15.29   71-YEAR-OLD WOMAN WORRIED THAT SHE IS DEVELOPING ALZHEIMER'S DEMENTIA

A 71-year-old woman has been referred to you because she feels that her memory has deteriorated. Her mother suffered from Alzheimer's dementia and the daughter is very fearful that she too will develop the disease. Her health is failing and she has high blood pressure.

How would you assess and manage?

15.30   27-YEAR-OLD MAN COUNTING JACKETS IN A CLOTHES SHOP

A 27-year-old man who works in a clothes shop has been found counting jackets in the shop over and over again. This habit has been disrupting his work. His wife thinks he behaves in a similar manner at home and she is getting fed up with his preoccupation with arranging everything in order.

How would you assess with a view to arriving at a diagnosis and managing appropriately?

15.31   72-YEAR-OLD WOMAN WITH DEPRESSION REFUSING TO EAT OR DRINK

A 72-year-old woman with depression is refusing to eat or drink and is now preventing home helps and carers from coming into her house. She has no known relative.

How would you assess and manage this situation?

15.32   32-YEAR-OLD WOMAN WITH WORSENING DEPRESSION

A 32-year-old woman has been referred to you, who lost her father 4 years ago and her grandfather 6 months ago. She has been on antidepressant treatment for over a year, but despite treatment her symptoms have recently got worse.

How would you assess and manage?

15.33 73-YEAR-OLD LADY HAVING HALLUCINATIONS AFTER SURGERY

You have been asked to see a 73-year-old lady who had surgery for a ruptured appendix 4 days ago. She has become increasingly agitated and has pulled out her intravenous line. She later talks about giants coming on to the ward and was screaming obscenities.

What would be your advice on how to manage the situation?

15.34 59-YEAR-OLD MAN WHO HAS OVERDOSED FOLLOWING ACCUSATIONS OF CHILD ABUSE

A 59-year-old man presents to the accident and emergency department after taking an overdose of sleeping tablets. He has been accused of abusing his 15-year-old daughter until she reached the age of 14. It appeared his wife had 'turned a blind eye' at the time but now regrets not acting sooner.

How would you proceed with assessment and management?

15.35 17-YEAR-OLD MALE WITH LEARNING DISABILITIES ACCUSED OF TOUCHING HIS HOUSEMATES

A 17-year-old male who has mild to moderate learning disabilities has been referred to you because he has been touching the female residents in his hostel on the breast and buttocks. He currently attends a carpentry course at the local college.

How would you assess and manage?

15.36 32-YEAR-OLD WORRIED THAT HER CURRENT PREGNANCY WILL BE AS DIFFICULT AS THE LAST ONE

A 32-year-old woman who is 28 weeks pregnant has become increasingly depressed and anxious. She is continuously worried about having a stillborn or a malformed baby. Her previous pregnancy ended in a complicated delivery and premature birth. Her GP has asked for your advice on her management.

How would you proceed?

15.37 23-YEAR-OLD MOTHER WITH ABNORMAL BELIEFS ABOUT HER NEW BABY

A 23-year-old woman was delivered of a baby boy 7 weeks ago. Her mother-in-law has reported to the GP that the new mother has been attempting to put cotton wool in the baby's nostrils, believing that the child is breathing out 'toxic gases from heaven'.

How would you plan further assessment and management?

15.38 ELDERLY WOMAN WITH CONFUSION, BRUISING AND BLISTERS

You have been asked to see a confused elderly lady who has been attempting to leave the day hospital. She has significant bruising on her body and blisters on her feet.

What are the diagnostic possibilities and how would you manage?

15.39 73-YEAR-OLD WOMAN WITH ABNORMAL BELIEFS AND IDEAS

A GP has asked you to make a domiciliary visit to a 73-year-old lady who is currently living alone. Her doctor has noticed that the house smells of rotten food and reports that there is also a large collection of rubbish in the front room, which the lady says she plans to use to invent a device to attack UFOs and 'aliens'.

How would you assess and manage this lady?

15.40 27-YEAR-OLD MOTHER CHARGED WITH KILLING HER 9-MONTH-OLD BABY

A 27-year-old mother of two has been arrested and charged with killing her 9-month-old child. You have been asked to assess her, with a view to providing a report for the court. The woman has a history of bipolar affective disorder but was thought to be free of symptoms at the time of the incident.

What would be the basis of your report, and what recommendation would you make?

Index